THE
ABSITE
REVIEW 7th EDITION

THE
ABSITE
REVIEW 7th EDITION

Steven M. Fiser, MD

Cardiac Surgery Specialists
Bon Secours Heart and Vascular Institute
Richmond, Virginia

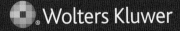 Wolters Kluwer

Philadelphia · Baltimore · New York · London
Buenos Aires · Hong Kong · Sydney · Tokyo

Acquisitions Editor: Keith Donnellan
Development Editor: Lindsay Ries
Editorial Coordinator: Remington Fernando
Senior Production Project Manager: Sadie Buckallew
Marketing Manager: Kirsten Watrud
Design Coordinator: Stephen Druding
Manufacturing Coordinator: Beth Welsh
Prepress Vendor: Absolute Service, Inc.

Seventh Edition

10 9 8 7 6 5 4 3 2

Printed in Mexico

Library of Congress Cataloging-in-Publication Data

Names: Fiser, Steven M., 1971- author.
Title: The ABSITE review / Steven M. Fiser.
Description: Seventh edition. | Philadelphia : Wolters Kluwer, [2022] |
  Includes bibliographical references and index.
Identifiers: LCCN 2021053855 (print) | LCCN 2021053856 (ebook) | ISBN
  9781975190293 | ISBN 9781975190323 (epub)
Subjects: MESH: Surgical Procedures, Operative | Clinical Medicine |
  Outline
Classification: LCC RD37.2 (print) | LCC RD37.2 (ebook) | NLM WO 18.2 |
  DDC 617.0076--dc23/eng/20211124
LC record available at https://lccn.loc.gov/2021053855
LC ebook record available at https://lccn.loc.gov/2021053856

shop.lww.com

QUADM0923

Dedicated to Garrett, Elle, and the rest of my wonderful family

CONTENTS

CREDITS

Figure on the page number listed below is reprinted with permission from: Rosdahl CB, Kowalski MT. Textbook of Basic Nursing. Philadelphia, PA: Wolters Kluwer Health; 2012.

160

Figure on the page number listed below is adapted with permission from: Dimick JB, Upchurch GR, Alam HB, Pawlik TM, Hawn MT, Sosa JA. Mulholland & Greenfield's Surgery: Scientific Principles & Practice, 7th ed. Philadelphia, PA: Lippincott Williams & Wilkins; 2021.

Abbas AK, Lichtman AH, and Pillali S. Cellular and Molecular Immunology, 9th ed. Philadelphia, PA: Elsevier, Inc; 2018.

57

Figure on the page number listed below is adapted with permission from:

Block GE, Michelassi F, Tanaka M, et al. Crohn's disease. *Curr Probl Surg.* 1993;30:173–265.

Greenfield's Surgery: Scientific Principles & Practice, 4th ed. Mulholland MW, Lillemoe KD, Doherty GM, Maier RV, Upchurch GR, eds. Philadelphia, PA: Lippincott Williams & Wilkins; 2006.

250

Figure on the page number listed below is adapted with permission from:

Haggitt RC, Glotzbach RE, Soffen EE, et al. Prognostic factors in colorectal carcinomas arising in adenomas: implications for lesions removed by endoscopic polypectomy. *Gastroenterology* 1985;89:328.

Mulholland MW, Lillemoe KD, Doherty GM, Upchurch GR, Alam HB, Pawlik TM. Greenfield's Surgery: Scientific Principles & Practice, 6th ed. Mulholland MW, Lillemoe KD, Doherty GM, Upchurch GR, Alam HB, Pawlik TM, eds. Philadelphia, PA: Lippincott Williams & Wilkins; 2016.

258

TABLE CREDITS

Tables on the page numbers listed below are reprinted and/or modified with permission from: Mulholland MW, Lillemoe KD, Doherty GM, Maier RV, Simeone DM, Upchurch GR. Greenfield's Surgery: Scientific Principles & Practice, 5th ed. Philadelphia, PA: Lippincott Williams & Wilkins; 2011.

60, 66, 95, 107, 138, 143, 144, 206, 243, 264

Tables on the page numbers listed below are reprinted and/or modified with permission from: Dimick JB, Upchurch GR, Alam HB, Pawlik TM, Hawn MT, Sosa JA. Mulholland & Greenfield's Surgery: Scientific Principles & Practice, 7th ed. Philadelphia, PA: Lippincott Williams & Wilkins; 2021.

33, 34, 38, 89, 214, 245, 319

Tables on the page numbers listed below are reprinted and/or modified with permission from: Fischer JE, Bland KI, et al. Mastery of Surgery. 5th ed. Philadelphia, PA: Lippincott Williams & Wilkins; 2007, with permission.

96, 135, 171, 265

Table on the page number listed below is adapted from:

Bernard GR, Artigas A, Brigham KL, et al. The American-European Consensus Conference on ARDS. Definitions, mechanisms, relevant outcomes, and clinical trial coordination. *Am J Respir Crit Care Med* 1994;149:818–824.

Mulholland MW, Lillemoe KD, Doherty GM, Maier RV, Simeone DM, Upchurch GR. Greenfield's Surgery: Scientific Principles & Practice, 5th ed. Philadelphia, PA: Lippincott Williams & Wilkins; 2011.

94

Table on the page number listed below is modified from: O'Connell C, Dickey VL. Blueprints: Hematology and Oncology. Philadelphia, PA: Lippincott Williams & Wilkins; 2005, with permission.

47

Table on the page number listed below is reprinted and/or modified with permission from: Shah SS, Hu KK, Crane HM, eds. Blueprints Infectious Diseases. Philadelphia, PA: Lippincott Williams & Wilkins; 2006.

159

Table on the page number listed below is reprinted and/or modified with permission from: Sleisenger MH, Fordtran JS. Gastrointestinal Disease. 5th ed. Philadelphia, PA: WB Saunders; 1993:898.

248

Table on the page number listed below is reprinted from Neuroblastoma Treatment (PDQ®) – Health Professional Version, originally published by the National Cancer Institute.

309 (top)

Tables and boxes on the page numbers listed below are reprinted and/or modified with permission of the American College of Surgeons, Chicago, Illinois. The original source for this information is the AJCC Cancer Staging System (2020).

147, 154, 261, 289, 290 (top), 290 (bottom)

PREFACE TO THE FIRST EDITION

Each year, thousands of general surgery residents across the country express anxiety over preparation for the American Board of Surgery In-Training Examination (ABSITE), an exam designed to test residents on their knowledge of the many topics related to general surgery.

This exam is important to the future career of general surgery residents for several reasons. Academic centers and private practices searching for new general surgeons use ABSITE scores as part of the evaluation process. Fellowships in fields such as surgical oncology, trauma, and cardiothoracic surgery use these scores when evaluating potential fellows. Residents with high ABSITE results are looked upon favorably by general surgery program directors, as high scorers enhance program reputation, helping garner applications from the best medical students interested in surgery.

General surgery programs also use the ABSITE scores, with consideration of feedback on clinical performance, when evaluating residents for promotion through residency. Clearly, this examination is important to general surgery residents.

Much of the anxiety over the ABSITE stems from the issue that there are no dedicated outline-format review manuals available to assist in preparation. *The ABSITE Review* was developed to serve as a quick and thorough study guide for the ABSITE, such that it could be used independently of other material and would cover nearly all topics found on the exam. The outline format makes it easy to hit the essential points on each topic quickly and succinctly, without having to wade through the extraneous material found in most textbooks. As opposed to question-and-answer reviews, the format also promotes rapid memorization.

Although specifically designed for general surgery residents taking the ABSITE, the information contained in *The ABSITE Review* is also especially useful for certain other groups:

- General surgery residents preparing for their written American Board of Surgery certification examination
- Surgical residents going into another specialty who want a broad perspective of general surgery and surgical subspecialties (and who may also be required to take the ABSITE)
- Practicing surgeons preparing for their American Board of Surgery recertification examination

PREFACE TO THE SEVENTH EDITION

The seventh edition of *The ABSITE Review* dives deeper in found in the ABSITE with new information on surgical oncology, trauma, vascular, critical care, nutrition, and a number of other topics. Like previous editions, *The ABSITE Review* provides a quick, easy review of important surgical topics while still providing sufficient explanation, so readers do not feel lost.

Again, I thank all of the residents who gave me feedback on the books or who I met at surgical meetings saying, "I used your books in residency and they were great." I am glad I could help out.

Thank you again and good luck on the ABSITE.

1 Cell Biology

CELL MEMBRANE

- A **lipid bilayer** that contains protein channels, enzymes, and receptors
- **Cholesterol** increases membrane fluidity.
- Cells are negative inside compared to outside; based on Na/K ATPase (3 Na$^+$ out/2 K$^+$ in)
- The **Na$^+$ gradient** that is created is used for **co-transport** of glucose, proteins, and other molecules.

Electrolyte Concentrations of Intracellular and Extracellular Fluid Compartments

	Extracellular Fluid (mEq/L)	Intracellular Fluid (mEq/L)
CATIONS		
Na$^+$	140	12
K$^+$	4	150
Ca^{2+}	5	10^{-4}
Mg^{2+}	2	7
ANIONS		
Cl$^-$	103	3
HCO$_3^-$	24	10
SO$_4^{2-}$	1	—
HPO$_4^{3-}$	2	116
Protein	16	40
Organic anions	5	—

- **Desmosomes/hemidesmosomes** – adhesion molecules (cell–cell and cell–extracellular matrix, respectively), which anchor cells
- **Tight junctions** – cell–cell occluding junctions; form an impermeable barrier (eg epithelium)
- **Gap junctions** – allow communication between cells (connexin subunits)
- **G proteins** (are GTPases) – intramembrane proteins; transduce signal from receptor to response enzyme
- **Ligand-triggered protein kinase** – receptor and response enzyme are a single transmembrane protein (eg receptor tyrosine kinase)

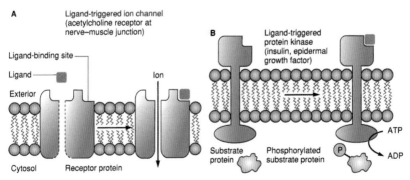

Types of cell surface receptors. (A) Ligand-activated ion channel; binding results in a conformational change, opening or activating the channel. **(B)** Ligand-activated protein kinase; binding activates the kinase domain, which phosphorylates substrate proteins. *(continued)*

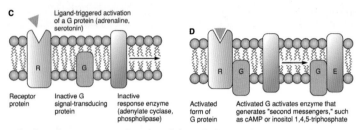

C Ligand-triggered activation of a G protein (adrenaline, serotonin)

Receptor protein	Inactive G signal-transducing protein	Inactive response enzyme (adenylate cyclase, phospholipase)

D

Activated form of G protein	Activated G activates enzyme that generates "second messengers," such as cAMP or inositol 1,4,5-triphosphate

Types of cell surface receptors. *(continued)* **(C and D)** Ligand activation of a G protein, which then activates an enzyme that generates second, or intracellular, messengers.

- **ABO blood-type antigens** – glycolipids on cell membrane
- **HLA-type antigens** – glycoproteins (Gp) on cell membrane
- **Osmotic equilibrium** – water will move from an area of low solute concentration to an area of high solute concentration and approach osmotic equilibrium

CELL CYCLE

- **G1, S** (protein synthesis, chromosomal duplication), **G2, M** (mitosis, nucleus divides)
- G1 most variable, determines <u>cell cycle length</u>
- **Growth factors** affect cell during G1.
- Cells can also go to G0 (quiescent) from G1.
- **Mitosis**
  - **Prophase** – centromere attachment, centriole and spindle formation, nucleus disappears
  - **Metaphase** – chromosome alignment
  - **Anaphase** – chromosomes pulled apart
  - **Telophase** – separate nucleus reforms around each set of chromosomes

NUCLEUS, TRANSCRIPTION, AND TRANSLATION

- **Nucleus** – double membrane, outer membrane continuous with rough endoplasmic reticulum
- **Nucleolus** – inside the nucleus, no membrane, **ribosomes** are made here
- **Transcription** – DNA strand is used as a template by **RNA polymerase** for synthesis of an mRNA strand

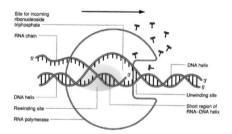

Transcription of DNA. RNA polymerase acts to unwind the DNA helix, catalyzes the formation of a transient RNA–DNA helix, and then releases the RNA as a single-strand copy while the DNA rewinds. In the process, the polymerase moves along the DNA from a start sequence to a stop sequence.

- **Transcription factors** – bind DNA and help the transcription of genes
  - **Steroid hormone** – binds receptor in cytoplasm, then enters nucleus and acts as transcription factor
  - **Thyroid hormone** – binds receptor in nucleus, then acts as a transcription factor
  - Other transcription factors – AP-1, NF-κB, STAT, NFAT
- **Initiation factors** – bind RNA polymerase and initiate transcription
- **DNA polymerase chain reaction** – uses oligonucleotides to amplify specific DNA sequences
- **Purines** – guanine, adenine
- **Pyrimidines** – cytosine, thymidine (only in DNA), uracil (only in RNA)
  - Guanine forms 3 hydrogen bonds with cytosine.
  - Adenine forms 2 hydrogen bonds with either thymidine or uracil.
- **Translation** – mRNA used as a template by **ribosomes** for the synthesis of **protein**

Ribosomes – have small and large subunits that read mRNA, then bind appropriate tRNAs that have amino acids, and eventually make proteins

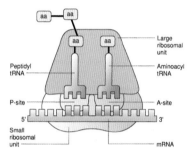

Schematic view of the elongation phase of protein synthesis on a ribosome. As the ribosome moves along the mRNA, incoming aminoacyl–tRNA complexes bind to the A-site on the ribosome, after which a new peptide bond is formed with the nascent polypeptide chain previously attached to the peptide tRNA. The ribosome then moves, ejecting the now-empty tRNA and opening the A-site for the next aminoacyl–tRNA complex.

CELLULAR METABOLISM

- **Glycolysis** – 1 glucose molecule generates 2 ATP and 2 pyruvate molecules
- **Mitochondria** – 2 membranes, Krebs cycle on inner matrix, NADH/FADH$_2$ created
  - **Krebs cycle** (citric acid cycle) – the 2 pyruvate molecules (from the breakdown of 1 glucose) create NADH and FADH$_2$
  - NADH and FADH$_2$ enter the electron transport chain, leading to formation of a H$^+$ gradient and creation of ATP by ATP synthase.
  - Overall, 1 molecule of glucose produces 36 ATP.
  - Amino acids, ketones, and short-chain fatty acids can also enter the Krebs cycle to produce ATP.
- **Gluconeogenesis** – mechanism by which **lactic acid** (Cori cycle) and **amino acids** (#1 alanine) are converted to glucose
  - Used in times of starvation or stress (basically the glycolysis pathway in reverse)
  - **Fat and lipids** are not available for gluconeogenesis because acetyl CoA (breakdown product of fat metabolism) cannot be converted back to pyruvate.
- **Cori cycle** – mechanism in which the **liver** converts **muscle lactate** into new **glucose**; pyruvate plays a key role in this process

OTHER CELL ORGANELLES, ENZYMES, AND STRUCTURAL COMPONENTS

- **White blood cells** – contain nuclear material
- **Red blood cells** and **platelets** – do <u>not</u> contain nuclear material
- **Rough endoplasmic reticulum** – synthesizes proteins that are exported (increased in pancreatic acinar cells)
- **Smooth endoplasmic reticulum** – lipid/steroid synthesis, detoxifies drugs (increased in liver and adrenal cortex)
- **Golgi apparatus** – modifies proteins with **carbohydrates**; proteins are then transported to the cellular membrane, secreted, or targeted to lysosomes
- **Lysosomes** – have digestive enzymes that degrade engulfed particles and worn-out organelles
- **Phagosomes** – engulfed large particles; these fuse with lysosomes
- **Endosomes** – engulfed small particles; these fuse with lysosomes
- **Major signaling pathways** – phospholipase C, protein kinase A, and MAPK/ERK pathway
  - Utilize second messengers for signal transduction
- **Phospholipase C** – cleaves phospholipid phosphatidylinositol 4,5-bisphosphonate (PIP_2) into diacylglycerol (DAG) and inositol 1,4,5-triphosphate (IP_3)
  - IP_3 causes release of calcium from the smooth endoplasmic reticulum.

Protein kinase C – activated by **calcium** and **diacylglycerol** (DAG); phosphorylates other enzymes and proteins
Protein kinase A – activated by **cAMP**; phosphorylates other enzymes and proteins

- **MAPK/ERK** – very complex pathway
- **Myosin** – thick filaments, uses ATP to slide along actin to cause **muscle contraction**
- **Actin** – thin filaments, interact with myosin above
- **Intermediate filaments** – keratin (hair/nails), desmin (muscle), vimentin (fibroblasts)
- **Microtubules** – form specialized cellular structures such as cilia, neuronal axons, and mitotic spindles; also involved in the transport of organelles in the cell (form a latticework inside the cell)
  - **Centriole** – a specialized microtubule involved in cell division (forms spindle fibers, which pull chromosome apart)

INTRODUCTION

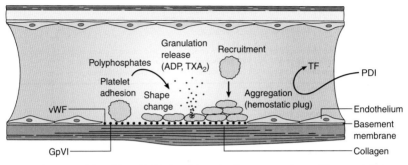

Primary hemostasis is achieved initially with a platelet aggregation as illustrated. Note that platelet adhesion, shape change, granule release followed by recruitment, and the hemostatic plug at the area of subendothelial collagen and collagen exposure are the initial events for thrombus formation.

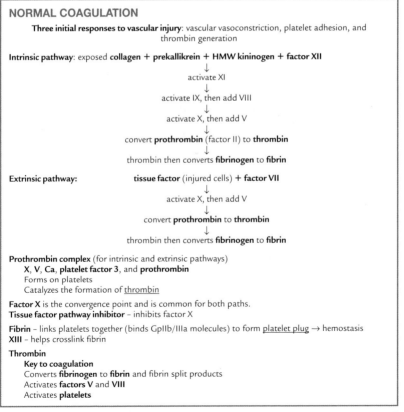

NORMAL COAGULATION

Three initial responses to vascular injury: vascular vasoconstriction, platelet adhesion, and thrombin generation

Intrinsic pathway: exposed **collagen + prekallikrein + HMW kininogen + factor XII**
↓
activate XI
↓
activate IX, then add VIII
↓
activate X, then add V
↓
convert **prothrombin** (factor II) to **thrombin**
↓
thrombin then converts **fibrinogen** to **fibrin**

Extrinsic pathway: **tissue factor** (injured cells) **+ factor VII**
↓
activate X, then add V
↓
convert **prothrombin** to **thrombin**
↓
thrombin then converts **fibrinogen** to **fibrin**

Prothrombin complex (for intrinsic and extrinsic pathways)
X, V, Ca, platelet factor 3, and **prothrombin**
Forms on platelets
Catalyzes the formation of <u>thrombin</u>

Factor X is the convergence point and is common for both paths.
Tissue factor pathway inhibitor – inhibits factor X

Fibrin – links platelets together (binds GpIIb/IIIa molecules) to form <u>platelet plug</u> → hemostasis
XIII – helps crosslink fibrin

Thrombin
Key to coagulation
Converts **fibrinogen** to **fibrin** and fibrin split products
Activates **factors V** and **VIII**
Activates **platelets**

NORMAL ANTICOAGULATION

Antithrombin III (AT-III)
    Key to anticoagulation
    Binds and inhibits **thrombin**
    Inhibits **factors IX, X, and XI**
    Heparin activates **AT-III** (up to 1000× normal activity).
Protein C – vitamin K–dependent; degrades **factors V** and **VIII**; degrades **fibrinogen**
Protein S – vitamin K–dependent, <u>protein C cofactor</u>
Fibrinolysis
    Tissue plasminogen activator – released from endothelium and converts plasminogen to plasmin
    Plasmin – degrades **factors V** and **VIII**, **fibrinogen**, and **fibrin** → lose platelet plug
    Alpha-2 antiplasmin – natural inhibitor of plasmin, released from endothelium

---

- **Factor VII** – shortest half-life
- **Factors V** and **VIII** – labile factors, activity lost in stored blood, <u>activity not lost in FFP</u>
- **Factor VIII** – only factor *not* synthesized in liver (synthesized in **endothelium** along with von Willebrand's Factor [vWF])
- **Factor II** – prothrombin
- **Vitamin K–dependent factors** – II, VII, IX, and X; proteins C and S
- **Vitamin K** – IV form takes <u>12 hours</u> to start effect and **24 hours** for full effect
- **FFP** – effect is <u>immediate</u> after infusion (takes **2 hours** to thaw and complete infusion)
- **PCC** (prothrombin complex concentrate; eg Kcentra) – effect is <u>immediate</u> after infusion (which takes **30 minutes**)
- **Normal half-life** – <u>RBCs</u>: 120 days; <u>platelets</u>: 7 days; <u>PMNs</u>: 1–2 days
- **Prostacyclin** (PGI$_2$)
  - From **endothelium**
  - <u>Decreases platelet aggregation</u> and promotes <u>vasodilation</u> (antagonistic to TXA$_2$)
  - <u>Increases cAMP in platelets</u>
- **Thromboxane** (TXA$_2$)
  - From **platelets**
  - <u>Increases platelet aggregation</u> and promotes <u>vasoconstriction</u>
  - Triggers release of **calcium** in platelets → exposes **GpIIb/IIIa receptor** and causes platelet-to-platelet binding; platelet-to-collagen binding also occurs (**GpIb receptor**)

COAGULATION FACTORS

- **Cryoprecipitate** – contains highest concentrations of **vWF** and **factor VIII**; used in von Willebrand's disease and hemophilia A (factor VIII deficiency), also high levels of **fibrinogen**
- **FFP** (fresh frozen plasma) – has high levels of all coagulation factors, protein C, protein S, and AT-III
- **DDAVP** and **conjugated estrogens** – cause release of **VIII** and **vWF** from endothelium

COAGULATION MEASUREMENTS

- **PT/INR** (prothrombin time; extrinsic pathway) – measures II, V, VII, and X; fibrinogen; best for **liver synthetic function**
  - Measures **warfarin** anticoagulation (want **INR 2–3** for routine anticoagulation)
- **PTT** (partial thromboplastin time; intrinsic pathway) – measures most factors *except VII and XIII (thus does <u>not</u> pick up factor VII deficiency)*; also measures fibrinogen
  - Measures **heparin** anticoagulation (want **PTT 60–90 sec** for routine anticoagulation)

- **ACT** = activated clotting time
  - Want **ACT 150–200 sec** for routine anticoagulation, > **400 sec** for cardiopulmonary bypass
- INR > 1.5 – relative contraindication to performing surgical procedures
- INR > 1.3 – relative contraindication to central line placement, percutaneous needle biopsies, and eye surgery
- **Bleeding time** – tests platelet function
- **TEG** (Thromboelastography)
  - **Elevated R** (reaction time) Tx: **FFP**
  - **Elevated K** (K time) Tx: **cryoprecipitate**
  - **Low angle** (clot kinetics) Tx: **cryoprecipitate**
  - **Low MA** (maximum altitude) Tx: **platelets/DDAVP**
  - **High LY30** (lysis 30 minutes after MA) Tx: **aminocaproic acid** or **tranxemic acid**

BLEEDING DISORDERS

- **Incomplete hemostasis** – most common cause of surgical bleeding
- **von Willebrand's disease**
  - *Most common congenital bleeding disorder*
  - MC Sx – epistaxis
  - Types I and II are autosomal dominant; type III is autosomal recessive.
  - **vWF** links **GpIb receptor** on **platelets** to **collagen**.
  - PT normal; PTT can be normal or abnormal.
  - Have long **bleeding time** (ristocetin test)
  - **Type I** is **most common** (70% of cases) and often has only mild symptoms.
  - **Type III** causes the **most severe bleeding**.
  - **Type I** – reduced quantity of vWF
    - Tx: recombinant VIII:vWF, **DDAVP**, cryoprecipitate
  - **Type II** – defect in vWF molecule itself, vWF does not work well
    - Tx: recombinant VIII:vWF, **cryoprecipitate, DDAVP**
  - **Type III** – complete vWF deficiency (rare)
    - Tx: recombinant VIII:vWF; **cryoprecipitate** (highest concentration of vWF:VIII)
      - *DDAVP will not work for type III.*
- **Hemophilia A** (VIII deficiency)
  - Sex-linked recessive
  - MC Sx – hemarthrosis
  - Need levels 100% preop; keep at 80%–100% for 10–14 days after surgery.
  - **Prolonged PTT** and normal PT (follow PTT Q 8 hours after surgery)
  - **Factor VIII** crosses **placenta** → newborns may not bleed at circumcision
  - Hemophiliac **joint bleeding** – *do not aspirate*
    - Tx: ice, keep joint mobile with range of motion exercises, **factor VIII** concentrate or **cryoprecipitate**
  - Hemophiliac **epistaxis, intracerebral hemorrhage**, or **hematuria**
    - Tx: **recombinant factor VIII** or **cryoprecipitate**
- **Hemophilia B** (IX deficiency) – Christmas disease
  - Sex-linked recessive
  - Need level 100% preop; keep at 30%–40% for 2–3 days after surgery
  - **Prolonged PTT** and normal PT
  - Tx: **recombinant factor IX** or **FFP**
- **Factor VII deficiency** – **prolonged PT** and normal PTT, bleeding tendency.
  Tx: **recombinant factor VII** concentrate or **FFP**
- **Platelet disorders** – cause bruising, epistaxis, petechiae, purpura
  - **Acquired thrombocytopenia** – can be caused by H_2 blockers, heparin

- **Glanzmann's thrombocytopenia** – GpIIb/IIIa receptor deficiency on platelets (cannot bind to each other)
  - Fibrin normally links the GpIIb/IIIa receptors together.
  - Tx: **platelets**
- **Bernard Soulier** – GpIb receptor deficiency on platelets (cannot bind to collagen)
  - vWF normally links GpIb to collagen.
  - Tx: **platelets**
- **Uremia** (BUN > 60-80) – inhibits platelet function, mainly by inhibiting release of vWF
  - Tx: **hemodialysis** (1st-line Tx), DDAVP (for acute reversal), cryoprecipitate (for moderate to severe bleeding)
- **Heparin-induced thrombocytopenia** (HIT)
  - Thrombocytopenia due to **anti-heparin antibodies** (IgG heparin-PF4 antibody) results in platelet destruction.
  - Can also cause platelet aggregation and **thrombosis** (HITT; **T** = thrombosis)
  - Clinical signs: platelets < 100, a drop in platelets > 50% admission levels, or thrombosis while on heparin
  - Forms a **white clot**
  - Can occur with low doses of heparin
  - Dx: ELISA for heparin Ab's (initial screen); serotonin release assay (confirmation)
  - Tx: ***Stop heparin***; start **argatroban** (direct thrombin inhibitor) to anticoagulate.
  - *Avoid giving platelets (risk of thrombosis).*
- **Disseminated intravascular coagulation** (DIC)
  - **Decreased platelets, low fibrinogen, high fibrin split products** (high D-dimer)
  - Prolonged PT and prolonged PTT
  - Often initiated by **tissue factor**
  - Tx: need to treat the underlying cause (eg sepsis)
- **ASA** – stop 7 days before surgery; patients will have prolonged bleeding time
  - **Inhibits cyclooxygenase** in platelets and **decreases TXA$_2$**
  - Platelets lack DNA, so they cannot resynthesize cyclooxygenase.
- **Clopidogrel** (Plavix) – stop 7 days before surgery; ADP receptor antagonist
  - Tx for **bleeding**: platelets
  - Coronary stent and need to stop Plavix for elective surgery – Tx: bridge with Integrilin (eptifibatide [GpIIb/IIIa inhibitor])
- **Coumadin** – stop 7 days before surgery, consider starting heparin while Coumadin wears off
  - Tx for **bleeding**: **PCC** (fastest) or **FFP**; Vit K if you have time
- **Platelets** – want them > 50,000 before surgery, > 20,000 after surgery
- **Prostate surgery** – can release **urokinase**, activates plasminogen → thrombolysis
- Tx: **ε-aminocaproic acid** (Amicar; inhibits fibrinolysis)
- **H and P** – best way to predict bleeding risk
- **Normal circumcision** – does not rule out bleeding disorders; can still have clotting factors from mother
- **Abnormal bleeding with tooth extraction or tonsillectomy** – picks up 99% patients with bleeding disorder
- **Epistaxis** – common with vWF deficiency and platelet disorders
- **Menorrhagia** – common with bleeding disorders

HYPERCOAGULABILITY DISORDERS

- Present as venous or arterial thrombosis/emboli (eg DVT, PE, stroke)
- **Factor V Leiden mutation** – 30% of spontaneous venous thromboses
  - ***Most common congenital hypercoagulability disorder***
  - Causes **resistance to activated protein C**; the defect is on **factor V**.
  - Tx: heparin, warfarin

- ⊕ **Hyperhomocysteinemia** – Tx: **folic acid** and **B$_{12}$**
- ⊕ **Prothrombin gene defect G20210 A** – Tx: heparin, warfarin
- ⊕ **Protein C or S deficiency** – Tx: heparin, warfarin
- ⊕ **Antithrombin III deficiency**
  - *Heparin does <u>not</u> work in these patients.*
  - Can develop after previous heparin exposure
  - Tx: recombinant AT-III concentrate or FFP (highest concentration of AT-III) followed by heparin, then warfarin
- ⊕ **Dysfibrinogenemia, dysplasminogenemia** – Tx: heparin, warfarin
- ⊕ **Polycythemia vera** – from bone marrow overproduction; can get **thrombosis**
  - Keep Hct < 48 and platelets < 400 before surgery.
  - Tx: phlebotomy, ASA, hydroxyurea
- ⊕ **Anti-phospholipid antibody syndrome**
  - Sx's: DVT/PE; loss of pregnancy; may have symptoms of lupus
  - Not all of these patients have SLE.
  - **Procoagulant** (get prolonged PTT but are **hypercoagulable**)
  - Caused by **antibodies** to phospholipids including **cardiolipin** (mitochondria) and **lupus anticoagulant** (cell membrane)
  - Dx: **prolonged PTT** (not corrected with FFP), positive Russell viper venom time, false-positive RPR test for syphilis
  - Tx: heparin, warfarin
- ⊕ **Acquired hypercoagulability** – **tobacco** (most common factor causing acquired hypercoagulability), malignancy, inflammatory states, inflammatory bowel disease, infections, oral contraceptives, pregnancy, rheumatoid arthritis, postop patients, myeloproliferative disorders
- ⊕ **Cardiopulmonary bypass** – factor XII (Hageman factor) activated; results in consumptive coagulopathy
  - Tx: heparin to prevent
- ⊕ **Warfarin-induced skin necrosis**
  - Occurs when placed on Coumadin without being heparinized first
  - Due to short half-life of proteins C and S, which are first to decrease in levels compared with the procoagulation factors; results in relative hyperthrombotic state
  - *Patients with relative **protein C deficiency** are especially susceptible.*
  - Tx: heparin if it occurs; prevent by placing patient on heparin before starting warfarin
- ⊕ **Key elements in the development of venous thromboses** (Virchow's triad) – stasis, endothelial injury, and hypercoagulability
- ⊕ **Key element in the development of arterial thrombosis** – endothelial injury

DEEP VENOUS THROMBOSIS (DVT)

- ⊕ Stasis, venous injury, and hypercoagulability (Virchow's triad) are risk factors.
- ⊕ The majority of adult surgery inpatients should receive DVT prophylaxis.
- ⊕ **Duration of anticoagulation for DVT/PE:**
  - **3 months** for – 1st time calf DVT <u>or</u> a provoked DVT or PE (eg postop patient)
  - **Lifetime** for – 2nd time calf DVT, unprovoked proximal DVT or PE, cancer (until cured), or a hypercoagulable state
- ⊕ **IVC filters** (some are removable) – indicated for patients with either:
  1. Contraindications to anticoagulation
  2. PE while on anticoagulation
  3. Free-floating IVC, ilio-femoral, or deep femoral DVT (controversial)
  4. Recent pulmonary embolectomy
     - Place IVC <u>below</u> the renal veins (caudad to renal veins).
     - PE with filter in place – likely arise from SVC (upper extremities), IVC above filter, or gonadal veins

PULMONARY EMBOLISM (PE)

- If clinical suspicion is high, do <u>not</u> wait on CT scan results, just **give heparin bolus** unless there is a contraindication.
- If the patient is in shock despite massive inotropes and pressors, go to OR for open removal or angiography for suction catheter Tx; otherwise, give heparin (thrombolytics have not shown an improvement in survival) or suction catheter–based intervention.
- Most commonly from the **ilio-femoral** region

HEMATOLOGIC DRUGS

- **Procoagulant agents** (anti-fibrinolytics)
  - **ε-Aminocaproic acid** (Amicar)
    - Inhibits fibrinolysis by inhibiting **plasmin**
  - Used in DIC, persistent bleeding following cardiopulmonary bypass, *thrombolytic overdoses*
- Anticoagulation agents
  - **Warfarin** – inhibits VKORC (inhibition <u>prevents decarboxylation of glutamic residues</u> on vitamin K–dependent factors); need to follow INR level
    - Half-life – **40 hours**
    - *Contraindicated* in pregnancy
  - Dabigatran (**Pradaxa**), apixaban (**Eliquis**), and rivaroxaban (**Xarelto**) – novel oral anticoagulants (NOACs) that do not use INR levels; used for patients **with atrial fibrillation** not due to a heart valve problem and in patients with **DVT** or **PE**
    - Pradaxa is a **direct thrombin inhibitors**
    - **Half-life** and **reversal agents**:
      - <u>Pradaxa</u> (half-life **12 hours**) – **Praxbind** (idarucizumab; monoclonal Ab that binds drug), dialysis
      - <u>Eliquis</u> (half-life **12 hours**) and <u>Xarelto</u> (half-life **6 hours**) – **Andexxa** (andexanet alfa; decoy receptor for Eliquis/Xarelto)
      - PCC can give partial reversal.
  - **Sequential compression devices** – improve venous return but also induce fibrinolysis with compression (release of tPA [tissue plasminogen activator] from endothelium)
  - **Heparin**
    - Binds and activates **anti-thrombin III** (1000× more activity); increases neutralization of factors IIa (prothrombin) and Xa
    - Reversed with **protamine** (binds heparin)
    - Half-life of heparin is **60–90 minutes** (want PTT 60–90 <u>seconds</u>).
    - Is cleared by the **reticuloendothelial system** (spleen; macrophages)
    - **Long-term heparin** – osteoporosis, alopecia
    - Heparin does <u>not</u> cross placental barrier (can be used in pregnancy) → warfarin does cross the placental barrier (not used in pregnancy)
      - **Protamine** – cross-reacts with NPH insulin or previous protamine exposure; 1% get protamine reaction (hypotension, bradycardia, and decreased heart function)
  - **Low molecular weight heparin** (eg enoxaparin) – lower risk of HIT compared to unfractionated heparin; binds and activates antithrombin III but inhibits just factor **Xa**
    - *Weakly* reversed with protamine
    - Can check **anti-Factor Xa levels** (LMWH assay) to determine effectiveness
    - Half-life – **6 hours**
  - **Argatroban** – direct thrombin inhibitor; metabolized in the **liver**, half-life is 50 minutes, often used in patients w/ **HITT**
  - **Bivalirudin** (Angiomax) – direct thrombin inhibitor, metabolized by **proteinase enzymes** in the blood; half-life is 25 minutes; can be used in patients w/ **HITT**

- **Hirudin** (Hirulog; from leeches) – direct thrombin inhibitor; metabolized by **kidneys**; half-life is 40 minutes; is the <u>most potent</u> direct inhibitor of thrombin; high risk for bleeding complications
- **Thrombolytics** – usually used for thrombosis; given with heparin
  - **tPA** (MC; tissue plasminogen activator) and **streptokinase** (has high antigenicity)
  - Both activate **plasminogen** which breaks down **fibrinogen**.
  - Need to follow **fibrinogen levels** – fibrinogen < 100 associated with increased risk and severity of bleeding
  - *Tx for thrombolytic overdose – **ɛ-aminocaproic acid** (Amicar)*

Contraindications to Thrombolytic Use (Urokinase, Streptokinase, tPA)	
Degree	**Contraindications**
Absolute	Active internal bleeding; recent CVA or neurosurgery (<3 mo); intracranial pathology, recent GI bleeding
Major	Recent (<10 d) surgery, organ biopsy, or obstetric delivery; left heart thrombus; active peptic ulcer; recent major trauma; uncontrolled hypertension, recent eye surgery
Minor	Minor surgery; recent CPR; atrial fibrillation with mitral valve disease; bacterial endocarditis; hemostatic defects (ie renal or liver disease); diabetic hemorrhagic retinopathy; pregnancy

3 Blood Products

INTRODUCTION

All blood products carry the risk of HIV and hepatitis except **albumin** and **serum globulins** (these are heat treated).

Donated blood is screened for HIV, HepB, HepC, HTLV, syphilis, and West Nile virus.

CMV-negative blood – use in low-birth-weight infants, bone marrow transplant patients, and other transplant patients

Type O blood – universal donor, contains no antigens

Type AB blood – contains both A and B antigens

Females of childbearing age should receive Rh-negative blood.

Stored blood is low in 2,3-DPG → causes left shift (increased affinity for oxygen)

Type and crossmatch – determines ABO compatibility

Type and screen – determines ABO compatibility and looks for preformed Ab's to minor antigens

One unit of **pRBCs** should raise the Hgb by 1 (Hct 3–5).

One six-pack of **platelets** should raise platelet count by 50,000.

HEMOLYSIS REACTIONS

- **Acute hemolysis** – from **ABO incompatibility**; antibody mediated (type II hypersensitivity)
  - Back pain, chills, tachycardia, fever, hemoglobinuria
  - Can lead to ATN, DIC, shock
  - **Haptoglobin < 50** mg/dL (binds Hgb, then gets degraded), **free hemoglobin > 5** g/dL, increase in **unconjugated bilirubin**
  - Tx: fluids, diuretics, HCO_3^-, pressors
  - In anesthetized patients, transfusion reactions may present as **diffuse bleeding**.
- **Delayed hemolysis** (mild jaundice) – antibody-mediated against minor antigens from donor
  - Tx: Observe if stable.
- **Nonimmune hemolysis** – from squeezed blood
  - Tx: fluids and diuretics

OTHER REACTIONS

- **Febrile nonhemolytic transfusion reaction** – *most common transfusion reaction*
  - Usually **recipient antibody** reaction against **donor WBCs** (cytokine release)
  - Tx: Discontinue transfusion if patient had previous transfusions or if it occurs soon after transfusion has begun.
  - Use WBC filters for subsequent transfusions.
- **Urticaria** (rash) – usually nonhemolytic
  - Usually **recipient antibodies** against **donor plasma proteins** (eg peanuts) or **IgA** in an IgA-deficient patient
  - Tx: histamine blockers (Benadryl), supportive
- **Anaphylaxis** – bronchospasm, hypotension, angioedema, urticaria
  - Usually **recipient antibodies** against **donor IgA** in an IgA-deficient recipient
  - Can be an **airway emergency**
  - Tx: **epinephrine**, fluids, pressors, steroids, histamine blockers (Benadryl)
- **Transfusion-related acute lung injury** (TRALI) – rare
  - Caused by **donor** antibodies to **recipient's** WBCs, clot in pulmonary capillaries
  - Leads to noncardiogenic pulmonary edema in < 6 hours (ARDS)
  - *MCC of death from transfusion reaction*

OTHER TRANSFUSION PROBLEMS

- **Cold – poor clotting** can be caused by cold products or cold body temperature (coagulopathy due to slowing of enzyme reactions); patient needs to be warm to clot correctly
- Dilutional **thrombocytopenia** and dilution of **coagulation factors** occur with massive transfusion.
- **Hypocalcemia** – can cause poor clotting; occurs with massive transfusion; Ca is required for the clotting cascade; hypocalcemia can also cause hypotension
- **Citrate** used in stored blood binds Ca after transfusion and causes hypocalcemia.
- Most common bacterial contaminate – **GNRs** (usually *E. coli*)
- Most common blood product source of contamination – **platelets** (not refrigerated)
- **Chagas' disease** – can be transmitted with blood transfusion

4 Immunology

T CELLS (THYMUS) – CELL-MEDIATED IMMUNITY

- **Helper T cells** (CD4)
  - Release **IL-2**, which mainly causes maturation of **cytotoxic T cells**
  - Release **IL-4**, which mainly causes **B-cell** maturation into **plasma cells**
  - Release **interferon-gamma** which activates **macrophages**
  - Involved in **delayed-type hypersensitivity** (type IV; brings in inflammatory cells by chemokine secretion)
- **Suppressor T cells** (CD8) – regulate CD4 and CD8 cells
- **Cytotoxic T cells** (CD8) – recognize and attack non–self-antigens attached to **MHC class I receptors** (eg viral gene products); responsible for the majority of liver injury due to HepB
- Cell-mediated immunity does <u>not</u> require Ab's.
- Effector cells in cell-mediated immunity – macrophages, cytotoxic T cells, natural killer cells
- **Intradermal skin test** (ie TB skin test) – used to test cell-mediated immunity; takes 2–3 days
- *Infections associated with defects in cell-mediated immunity – intracellular pathogens (TB, viruses)*

B CELLS (BONE) – ANTIBODY-MEDIATED IMMUNITY (HUMORAL)

- IL-4 from helper T cells stimulates B cells to become plasma cells (antibody secreting).
- 10% become memory B cells which can be reactivated.
- IgG (as opposed to IgM) is secreted with reinfection.

MHC CLASSES

- **MHC class I** (A, B, and C)
  - **CD8** cell activation
  - Present on **all nucleated cells**
  - Single chain with 5 domains
  - *Target for cytotoxic T cells (bind T-cell receptor)*
- **MHC class II** (DR, DP, and DQ)
  - **CD4** cell activation
  - Present on **antigen-presenting cells** (APCs; eg dendrites [most important], monocytes)
  - 2 chains with 4 domains each
  - *APCs activate helper T cells (bind T-cell receptor) when passing through lymph nodes.*
  - *Stimulates antibody formation after interaction with B cells*

Viral infection – endogenous viral proteins produced, are bound to class I MHC, go to cell surface, and are recognized by CD8 cytotoxic T cells

Bacterial infection – endocytosis, proteins get bound to class II MHC molecules, go to cell surface, recognized by CD4 helper T cells → B cells which have already bound to the antigen are then activated by the CD4 helper T cells; they then produce the antibody to that antigen and are transformed to plasma cells and memory B cells

NATURAL KILLER CELLS

- Not restricted by MHC, do not require previous exposure, do not require antigen presentation
- Not considered T or B cells
- *Recognize cells that **lack self-MHC***
- Part of the body's natural immunosurveillance for cancer
- Also attack cells with bound Ab (have Fc receptor)

14

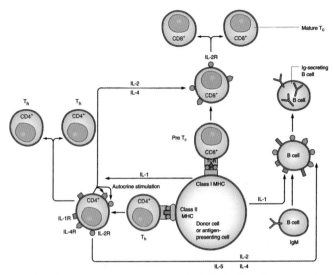

T-cell and B-cell activation. Two signals are required. First, alloantigen binds to anti-gen-specific receptors—the TCR (T cells) or surface IgM (B cells). The second, or costimulatory, signal is provided by IL-1 released by the antigen-presenting cell. CD4 helper T cells (T_h) release IL-2 and IL-4, which provide help for CD8 T cells (T_c) and for B-cell activation.

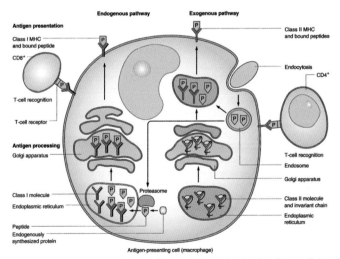

Antigen processing and presentation. Endogenously synthesized or intracellular proteins are degraded into peptides that are transported to the ER. These peptides bind to **class I MHC** molecules and are transported to the surface of the antigen-presenting cell. CD8$^+$ cells recognize the foreign peptide bound to class I MHC by way of the TCR complex. Exogenous antigen is endocytosed and broken down into peptide fragments in endosomes. **Class II MHC** molecules are transported to the endosome, bind the peptide, and are delivered to the surface of the antigen-presenting cell, where they are recognized by CD4$^+$ cells.

ANTIBODIES

- **IgM** – initial antibody secreted after exposure to antigen (**primary** immune response). It is the largest antibody, having 5 domains (10 binding sites); MC Ab in the spleen
- **IgG** – most abundant antibody in body. Responsible for **secondary** immune response. Can cross the placenta and provides protection in newborn period. MC Ab overall
- **IgA** – found in secretions, in Peyer's patches in gut, and in breast milk (additional source of immunity in newborn); helps prevent microbial adherence and invasion in gut
- **IgD** – membrane-bound receptor on B cells (serves as an antigen receptor)
- **IgE** – allergic reactions, parasite infections (type I hypersensitivity reactions, see below)
- **IgM** and **IgG** are **opsonins**.
- **IgM** and **IgG** fix **complement** (requires 2 IgGs or 1 IgM).
- All Ab's have **2 antigen-binding sites** except **IgM** (which has 10 antigen-binding sites).
- **Variable region** – antigen recognition
- **Constant region** – recognized by PMNs, macrophages, and natural killer cells
  - Fc fragment does <u>not</u> carry variable region.
- **Polyclonal antibodies** have multiple binding sites to the antigen at multiple epitopes.
- **Monoclonal antibodies** have only 1 binding site to the antigen at 1 epitope.
- **Basophils** – major source of histamine in blood
- **Mast cells** – major source of histamine in tissue; main cell type for type I hypersensitivity
- **Primary lymphoid organs** – liver, bone, thymus
- **Secondary lymphoid organs** – spleen and lymph nodes
- **Immunologic chimera** – 2 different cell lines in one individual (eg bone marrow transplant patients)

Hypersensitivity Reactions

Type	Description	Examples
I	**Immediate hypersensitivity reaction** (allergic reaction; anaphylaxis) – **IgE** receptors on **mast cells** and **basophils** react with the antigen and cause release of **histamine**, serotonin, and bradykinin	Bee stings, peanuts, hay fever, Lymphazurin blue dye; Sx's – urticaria, hypotension, bronchoconstriction, angioedema; Tx: epinephrine, airway management
II	**IgG or IgM reacts with cell-bound antigen.**	ABO blood incompatibility, hyperacute rejection, myasthenia gravis
III	**Immune complex deposition**	Serum sickness, SLE
IV	**Delayed-type hypersensitivity** – APCs present antigen to helper T cells, which then activate macrophages to destroy the antigen; only hypersensitivity reaction not to involve Ab's (cell-mediated immunity)	TB skin test (PPD), contact dermatitis Generally takes 2–3 days

IL-2

- Converts lymphocytes to **lymphokine-activated killer** (LAK) cells by enhancing their immune response to tumor
- Also converts lymphocytes into **tumor-infiltrating lymphocytes** (TILs)
- Has shown some success for melanoma

TETANUS

- **Non–tetanus-prone wounds** – give **tetanus toxoid** only if patient has received < 3 doses or tetanus status is unknown, or > 10 years since booster
- **Tetanus-prone wounds** (> 6 hours old; obvious contamination and devitalized tissue; crush, burn, frostbite, or missile injuries) – always give **tetanus toxoid** unless patient has had ≥ 3 doses and it has been < 5 years since last booster
- **Tetanus immune globulin** (given intramuscular near wound site) – give only with tetanus-prone wounds in patients who have not been immunized or if immunization status is unknown

5 Infection

INTRODUCTION
Malnutrition – most common immune deficiency; leads to infection

MICROFLORA
- Stomach – virtually sterile; some GPCs, some yeast
- Proximal small bowel – 10^5 bacteria, mostly GPCs
- Distal small bowel – 10^7 bacteria, GPCs, GPRs, GNRs
- Colon – 10^{11} bacteria, almost all anaerobes, some GNRs, GPCs
- **Anaerobes** (anaerobic bacteria)
  - Most common organisms in the GI tract
  - More common than aerobic bacteria in the colon (1,000:1)
  - Need low-oxygen environment (lack superoxide dismutase and catalase, making them vulnerable to oxygen radicals)
  - *Bacteroides fragilis* – most common anaerobe in the colon
- *Escherichia coli* – most common aerobic bacteria in the colon

FEVER
- MC fever source **within 48 hours**   **Atelectasis**
- MC fever source **48 hours – 5 days**   **Urinary tract infection**
- MC fever source **after 5 days**   **Wound infection**
- **Fever sources** (sequentially over time) – atelectasis, urinary tract infection, pneumonia, DVT, wound infection, intra-abdominal abscess

GRAM-NEGATIVE SEPSIS
- *E. coli* most common
- **Endotoxin** (lipopolysaccharide **lipid A**) is released.
- Endotoxin triggers the release of **TNF-α** (most potent stimulus; released from macrophages, triggers inflammation), activates complement, and activates coagulation cascade.
- Early gram-negative sepsis – ↓ insulin, ↑ glucose (impaired utilization)
- Late gram-negative sepsis – ↑ insulin, ↑ glucose secondary to insulin resistance
- **Hyperglycemia** – often occurs just before the patient becomes clinically septic
- **Optimal glucose level in a septic patient**: < 180 mg/dL

CLOSTRIDIUM DIFFICILE COLITIS (PSEUDOMEMBRANOUS COLITIS)
- Sx's: foul-smelling diarrhea; nursing home or ICU patients
- Dx: ELISA for **toxin A**; elevated WBCs (often in 30–40's)
- Tx: **oral** – vancomycin or Flagyl; **IV** – Flagyl; lactobacillus can also help
- Pregnancy – oral vancomycin (no systemic absorption)
- Fluid resuscitation; stop other antibiotics or change them.
- Fulminant (eg severe sepsis, perforation) pseudomembranous colitis – Tx: total abdominal colectomy with ileostomy

ABSCESSES
- 90% of abdominal abscesses have anaerobes.
- 80% of abdominal abscesses have both anaerobic and aerobic bacteria.
- Abscesses are treated by **drainage** (usually percutaneous).
- Usually occur **7–10 days** after operation

- Antibiotics for an abscess are needed in patients with diabetes, cellulitis, clinical signs of sepsis, fever, or who have bioprosthetic hardware (eg mechanical valves, hip replacements).

WOUND INFECTION (SURGICAL SITE INFECTION)
- **Clean** (hernia): 2%
- **Clean contaminated** (elective colon resection with prepped bowel): 3%–5%
- **Contaminated** (gunshot wound to colon with repair): 5%–10%
- **Gross contamination** (abscess): 30%
- **Prophylactic antibiotics** are given to **prevent surgical site infections**.
  - Give antibiotics **within 1 hour** of incision.
  - Stop **within 24 hours** of end operation time, except cardiac, which is stopped within 48 hours of end operation time.
- *Staphylococcus aureus* – <u>coagulase-positive</u>
  - **Most common organism overall** in surgical site infections
- *Staphylococcus epidermidis* – <u>coagulase-negative</u>
- **Exoslime** released by staph species is an **exopolysaccharide matrix**.
- *E. coli* – most common **GNR** in surgical wound infections
- *B. fragilis* – most common **anaerobe** in surgical wound infections
  - Recovery from tissue indicates necrosis or abscess (only grows in low redox state).
  - Also implies translocation from the gut
- $\geq 10^5$ bacteria needed for wound infection; less bacteria is needed if foreign body present
- **Risk factors for wound infection**: long operations, hematoma or seroma formation, advanced age, chronic disease (eg COPD, renal failure, liver failure, diabetes mellitus), malnutrition, immunosuppressive drugs
- **Tx wound infection** (erythema, warmth, tenderness) – antibiotics, may need to open wound if wound abscess is present (get U/S if not sure)
- **Surgical infections within 48 hours of procedure**
  - **Injury to bowel** with leak
  - **Invasive soft tissue infection** – *Clostridium perfringens* and beta-hemolytic strep can present within hours postoperatively (produce exotoxins)
- Most common infection in surgery patients – **urinary tract infection**
  - Biggest risk factor – **urinary catheters**; most commonly *E. coli (GNRs)*
  - Tx: remove urinary catheter, abx's
- Leading cause of infectious death after surgery – **nosocomial pneumonia**
  - Related to the length of ventilation; aspiration from duodenum thought to have a role
  - Most common organisms in ICU pneumonia – **#1 *S. aureus*, #2 *Pseudomonas*, #3 *E. coli***
  - GNRs #1 class of organisms in ICU pneumonia

LINE INFECTIONS
- **#1 *S. epidermidis*, #2 *S. aureus*, #3 yeast**
- **Femoral lines** at higher risk for infection compared to subclavian and intrajugular lines; subclavian lines have the lowest risk
- 50% line salvage rate with antibiotics (important for patients requiring long-term central access; 2 weeks of antibiotics); much less likely with yeast line infections
- **Suspected line infection** (temporary line) → move to new site or pull out the central line and place peripheral IVs if central line not needed

NECROTIZING SOFT TISSUE INFECTIONS
- Beta-hemolytic *Streptococcus* (group A), *C. perfringens*, or mixed organisms
- Usually occur in patients who are immunocompromised (eg diabetes mellitus, AIDS) or who have poor blood supply
- Can present very quickly after injury or surgical procedures (within hours)

- Pain out of proportion to skin findings (infection starts deep to the skin), mental status changes, WBCs > 20, thin gray drainage that is foul-smelling, can have skin blistering/necrosis, induration and edema, crepitus or soft tissue gas on x-ray, can be septic
- **Necrotizing fasciitis** – usually **beta-hemolytic group A strep** or **MRSA**
  - Overlying skin can look normal in the early stages (spreads along fascial planes).
  - Overlying skin progresses from pale red to purple with blister or bullae development.
  - Thin, gray, foul-smelling drainage; crepitus
  - GPCs without PMNs
  - Beta-hemolytic group A strep and MRSA have **exotoxin**.
  - Tx: **early debridement**, high-dose penicillin; may want broad spectrum if thought to be poly-organismal
- **C. perfringens** infections
  - **Necrotic tissue** decreases oxidation-redux potential, setting up environment for C. perfringens.
  - C. perfringens has **alpha toxin** (major source of morbidity).
  - Pain out of proportion to exam; may not show skin cellulitis (is a deep infection)
  - Gram stain shows GPRs without WBCs.
  - **Myonecrosis** and **gas gangrene** – common presentations
  - Can occur with farming injuries (dirty wounds)
  - Tx: **early debridement**, high-dose penicillin
- **Fournier's gangrene**
  - Severe infection in perineal and scrotal region
  - Risk factors – diabetes mellitus and immunocompromised state
  - Caused by mixed organisms (GPCs, GNRs, anaerobes)
  - Tx: **early debridement**; try to preserve testicles if possible; antibiotics

FUNGAL INFECTION

- Need fungal coverage for positive blood cultures, 2 sites other than blood, 1 site with severe symptoms, endophthalmitis, or patients on prolonged bacterial antibiotics with failure to improve
- **Actinomyces** (not a true fungus) – pulmonary symptoms most common; can cause tortuous abscesses in cervical, thoracic, and abdominal areas; characteristic yellow sulfur granules on Gram stain
  - Tx: **drainage** and **penicillin G**
- **Nocardia** (not a true fungus) – pulmonary and CNS symptoms most common
  - Tx: **drainage** and **sulfonamides** (Bactrim)
- **Candida** – common inhabitant of the respiratory tract; MCC of fungemia
  - Tx: **fluconazole** (some *Candida* resistant), **anidulafungin** for severe infections
  - Candiduria – Tx: remove urinary catheter only (anti-fungal not necessary)
- **Aspergillosis**
  - Tx: **voriconazole** for severe infections
- **Histoplasmosis** – pulmonary symptoms usual; Mississippi and Ohio River valleys
  - Tx: **liposomal amphotericin** for severe infections
- **Cryptococcus** – CNS symptoms most common; usually in AIDS patients
  - Tx: **liposomal amphotericin** for severe infections
- **Coccidioidomycosis** – pulmonary symptoms; Southwest
  - Tx: **liposomal amphotericin** for severe infections
- **Mucormycosis** – extensive burns or widespread trauma patients at risk; area turns black
  - Tx: debridement; **liposomal amphotericin**

SPONTANEOUS BACTERIAL PERITONITIS (SBP; PRIMARY)

- Sx's: mental status changes, fever, abdominal pain in a cirrhotic patient
- **Low protein** (< 1 g/dL) in peritoneal fluid – risk factor
- **Monobacterial** (50% **E. coli**, 30% *Streptococcus*, 10% *Klebsiella*)

- Secondary to decreased host defenses (intrahepatic shunting, impaired bactericidal activity in ascites); not due to transmucosal migration
- Fluid cultures are negative in many cases.
- **Peritoneal fluid with PMNs > 250 or positive cultures are** diagnostic.
- Tx: **ceftriaxone** or other 3rd-generation cephalosporin
- Need to rule out intra-abdominal source (eg bowel perforation) if not getting better on antibiotics or if cultures are polymicrobial
- Liver transplantation not an option with active infection
- Weekly **fluoroquinolones** good for **SBP prophylaxis** (norfloxacin; indicated **for ascites** total protein < 1 g/dL or a previous history of SBP)
- Cirrhotic patients with **active UGI bleeds** should be placed on Abx's (eg norfloxacin) for a **7 day** course

SECONDARY BACTERIAL PERITONITIS

- Intra-abdominal source (implies perforated viscus)
- Polymicrobial – *B. fragilis, E. coli, Enterococcus* most common organisms
- Tx: usually need laparotomy to find source

HIV

- AIDS – loss of cell mediated immunity (decreased CD4 cells) leading to opportunistic infections
- RNA virus with reverse transcriptase
- **Exposure risk**
  - HIV blood transfusion 70%
  - Infant from positive mother 30%
  - Needle stick from positive patient 0.3%
  - Mucous membrane exposure 0.1%
  - Seroconversion occurs in 6–12 weeks.
  - **AZT** (zidovudine, reverse transcriptase inhibitor) and **ritonavir** (protease inhibitor) can help decrease seroconversion after exposure.
  - Antivirals should be given within 1–2 hours of exposure.
- **Opportunistic infections** – most common indication for laparotomy in HIV patients (CMV infection most common)
  - Neoplastic disease – 2nd most common reason for laparotomy (lymphoma most common)
- **CMV colitis** – most common intestinal manifestation of AIDS (can present with pain, bleeding, or perforation)
- **Kaposi's sarcoma** – MC neoplasm in AIDS patients (although surgery rarely needed)
- **Lymphoma in HIV patients** – stomach most common followed by rectum
  - MC malignancy requiring laparotomy
  - Mostly non-Hodgkin's (B cell)
  - Tx: chemotherapy usual; may need surgery with significant bleeding or perforation
- **GI bleeds – lower GI bleeds** are more common than upper GI bleeds in HIV patients
  - **Upper GI bleeds** – Kaposi's sarcoma, lymphoma
  - **Lower GI bleeds** – CMV, bacterial, HSV
- **CD4 counts**: 800–1,200 normal; 300–400 symptomatic disease; < 200 opportunistic infections

HEPATITIS C

- Now rarely transmitted with blood transfusion (0.0001%/unit)
- 1%–2% of population infected
- Fulminant hepatic failure rare
- Chronic infection in 60%; cirrhosis in 15%; hepatocellular carcinoma in 1%–5%
- MC indication for liver TXP
- Now curable with Sovaldi (sofosbuvir) in combination with ribavirin

CMV INFECTION

- Transmitted via **leukocytes**
- MC infection in TXP patients
- MC manifestation – **febrile mononucleosis** (sore throat, adenopathy)
- Most deadly form – **CMV pneumonitis**
- Dx: biopsy – shows characteristic **cellular inclusion bodies**; CMV serology
- Tx: **ganciclovir**; **CMV immune globulin** (Cytogam) indicated for severe infections or a CMV-negative patient receiving a CMV-positive organ

OTHER INFECTIONS

- **Aspiration pneumonia** – MC in the superior segment of the right lower lobe
  - Strep pneumonia MC organism; also need to cover anaerobes
- Highest sensitivity test for **osteomyelitis** – MRI (avoid bone Bx)
- **Brown recluse spider bites** – Tx: oral **dapsone** initially; avoid early surgery; may need resection of area and skin graft for large ulcers later
- **Acute septic arthritis** – *Gonococcus*, staph, *H. influenzae*, strep
  - Tx: **drainage**, 3rd-generation cephalosporin and vancomycin until cultures show organism
- **Diabetic foot infections** – mixed staph, strep, GNRs, and anaerobes
  - Tx: broad-spectrum antibiotics (Unasyn, Zosyn)
- **Cat/dog/human bites** – polymicrobial infection usual (MC – *Strep pyogenes*)
  - *Eikenella* found only in human bites; can cause permanent joint injury
  - *Pasteurella multocida* found in cat and dog bites
  - Tx: broad-spectrum antibiotics (Augmentin)
- **Impetigo**, **erysipelas**, **cellulitis**, and **folliculitis** – staph (most common) and strep
- **Furuncle** – boil; usually *S. epidermidis* or *S. aureus*. Tx: drainage ± antibiotics
- **Carbuncle** – a multiloculated furuncle
- **Peritoneal dialysis catheter infections**
  - Sx's: cloudy fluid, abdominal pain, fever; usually monobacterial
  - *S. epidermidis* (#1), *S. aureus*, and *Pseudomonas* most common organisms
  - Fungal infections hard to treat
  - Tx: intraperitoneal vancomycin and gentamicin; increased dwell time and intraperitoneal heparin may help; IV antibiotics not as effective as intraperitoneal
  - Removal of catheter for peritonitis that lasts for 4–5 days
  - Fecal peritonitis requires laparotomy to find perforation.
  - Some say need removal of peritoneal dialysis catheter for all fungal, tuberculous, and *Pseudomonas* infections.
- **Sinusitis**
  - **Risk factors** – nasoenteric tubes, intubation, patients with severe facial fractures
  - Usually polymicrobial
  - CT head shows air–fluid levels in the sinus.
  - Tx: broad-spectrum antibiotics; rare to have to tap sinus percutaneously for systemic illness
- **Prevention of nosocomial infections** (hospital-acquired infections)
  - Hand washing – best prevention strategy
  - Highest risk patients – burn patients
  - If patient is on isolation, leave gloves and gown in the room.
- **Prevention of surgical site infections**
  - Use **clippers** preoperatively instead of razors.
  - Keep glucose 80–120.
  - Keep PO_2 elevated (give 100% oxygen).
  - Keep patient warm (keep OR 70°F; warm air conduction [Bair Hugger] best for warming patients).
  - Chlorhexidine prep with iodine-impregnated drapes

6 Antibiotics

INTRODUCTION
- **Antiseptic** – kills and inhibits organisms on body
- **Disinfectant** – kills and inhibits organisms on inanimate objects
- **Sterilization** – all organisms killed
- **Common antiseptics in surgery**
  - **Iodophors** (Betadine) – good for GPCs and GNRs; poor for fungi
  - **Chlorhexidine gluconate** (Hibiclens) – good for GPCs, GNRs, and fungi

ANTIBIOTIC MECHANISM OF ACTION
- **Inhibitors** of **cell wall synthesis** – penicillins, cephalosporins, carbapenems, monobactams, vancomycin
- **Inhibitors** of the **30s ribosome and protein synthesis** – tetracycline, aminoglycosides (tobramycin, gentamicin)
- **Inhibitors** of the **50s ribosome and protein synthesis** – erythromycin, clindamycin, Synercid, linezolid
- **Inhibitor** of **DNA helicase** (DNA gyrase) – quinolones
- **Inhibitor** of **RNA polymerase** – rifampin
- **Produces oxygen radicals** that **breakup DNA** – metronidazole (Flagyl)
- **Sulfonamides** – PABA analogue, inhibits purine synthesis
- **Trimethoprim** – inhibits dihydrofolate reductase, which inhibits purine synthesis
- **Bacteriostatic antibiotics** – tetracycline, clindamycin, erythromycin (all have reversible ribosomal binding), Bactrim
- **Aminoglycosides** – have irreversible binding to ribosome and are considered **bactericidal**

MECHANISM OF ANTIBIOTIC RESISTANCE
- **PCN resistance** – due to plasmids for beta-lactamase (eg *Staphylococcus aureus*)
- **Transfer of plasmids** – most common method of antibiotic resistance
- **Methicillin-resistant *S. aureus*** (MRSA) – resistance caused by a **mutation of cell wall–binding protein**
- **Vancomycin-resistant *Enterococcus*** (VRE) – resistance caused by a **mutation in cell wall–binding protein**
- **Gentamicin resistance** – resistance due to modifying enzymes leading to a **decrease in active transport of gentamicin** into the bacteria

APPROPRIATE DRUG LEVELS
- **Vancomycin** – peak 20–40 μg/mL; trough 5–10 μg/mL
- **Gentamicin** – peak 6–10 μg/mL; trough < 1 μg/mL
- **Peak too high** → decrease amount of each dose
- **Trough too high** → decrease frequency of doses (increase time interval between doses)

SPECIFIC ANTIBIOTICS
- **Penicillin**
  - **GPCs** – streptococci, syphilis, *Neisseria meningitides* (GPR), *Clostridium perfringens* (GPR), beta-hemolytic *Streptococcus*, anthrax
  - Not effective against *Staphylococcus* or *Enterococcus*
- **Oxacillin**, **methicillin**, and **nafcillin**
  - **Anti-staph** penicillins (staph only)

- **Ampicillin** and **amoxicillin**
  - Same as penicillin but also picks up <u>enterococci</u>
- **Unasyn** (ampicillin/sulbactam) and **Augmentin** (amoxicillin/clavulanic acid)
  - Broad spectrum – pick up **GPCs** (staph and strep), **GNRs**, ± anaerobic coverage
  - Effective for enterococci; <u>not</u> effective for *Pseudomonas, Acinetobacter*, or *Serratia*
  - **Sulbactam** and **clavulanic acid** are beta-lactamase inhibitors.
- **Ticarcillin** and **piperacillin** (antipseudomonal penicillins)
  - **GNRs** – enterics, *Pseudomonas, Acinetobacter*, and *Serratia*
  - Side effects: **inhibits platelets**; high salt load
- **Timentin** (ticarcillin/clavulanic acid) and **Zosyn** (piperacillin/tazobactam)
  - Broad spectrum – pick up **GPCs** (staph and strep), **GNRs**, and **anaerobes**
  - Effective for enterococci; effective for *Pseudomonas, Acinetobacter*, and *Serratia*
  - Side effects: **inhibits platelets**; high salt load
  - **Zosyn** has **QID dosing**.
- **First-generation cephalosporins** (cefazolin, cephalexin)
  - **GPCs** – staph and strep
  - <u>Not</u> effective for *Enterococcus*; does not penetrate CNS
  - Ancef (cefazolin) has the longest half-life → best for prophylaxis
- **Second-generation cephalosporins** (cefoxitin, cefotetan)
  - **GPCs, GNRs**, ± anaerobic coverage; lose some staph activity
  - <u>Not</u> effective for *Enterococcus, Pseudomonas, Acinetobacter*, or *Serratia*
  - Effective only for community-acquired GNRs
  - Cefotetan has longest half-life → best for prophylaxis
- **Third-generation cephalosporins** (ceftriaxone, cefepime)
  - **GNRs** mostly, ± anaerobic coverage
  - <u>Not</u> effective for *Enterococcus*; effective for *Pseudomonas, Acinetobacter*, and *Serratia*
  - Side effects: **cholestatic jaundice**, sludging in gallbladder (ceftriaxone)
- **Monobactam** (aztreonam)
  - **GNRs**; picks up *Pseudomonas, Acinetobacter*, and *Serratia*
- **Carbapenems** (meropenem, imipenem) – is given with cilastatin
  - Broad spectrum – **GPCs, GNRs**, and **anaerobes**
  - <u>Not</u> effective for **MEP**: MRSA, *Enterococcus*, and *Proteus*
  - **Cilastatin** – prevents renal hydrolysis of the drug and increases half-life
  - Side effects: **seizures**
- **Bactrim** (trimethoprim/sulfamethoxazole)
  - **GNRs**, ± GPCs
  - <u>Not</u> effective for *Enterococcus, Pseudomonas, Acinetobacter*, and *Serratia*
  - Side effects (numerous): teratogenic, allergic reactions, renal damage, Stevens–Johnson syndrome (erythema multiforme), hemolysis in G6PD-deficient patients
- **Quinolones** (ciprofloxacin, levofloxacin, norfloxacin)
  - Some **GPCs**, mostly **GNRs**
  - <u>Not</u> effective for *Enterococcus*; picks up *Pseudomonas, Acinetobacter*, and *Serratia*
  - 40% of MRSA sensitive; same efficacy PO and IV
  - **Ciprofloxacin** has **BID dosing**; **levofloxacin** has **QD dosing**.
  - Side effects: **tendon ruptures**
- **Aminoglycosides** (gentamicin, tobramycin)
  - **GNRs**
  - Good for *Pseudomonas, Acinetobacter*, and *Serratia*; not effective for anaerobes (need O_2)
  - Resistance due to **modifying enzymes** leading to **decreased active transport**
  - Synergistic with ampicillin for *Enterococcus*
  - Beta-lactams (ampicillin, amoxicillin) facilitate aminoglycoside penetration.
  - Side effects: reversible **nephrotoxicity**, irreversible **ototoxicity**

- **Erythromycin** (macrolides)
  - **GPCs**; best for community-acquired pneumonia and atypical pneumonias
  - Side effects: **nausea** (PO), **cholestasis** (IV)
  - Also binds motilin receptor and is **prokinetic** for bowel
- **Vancomycin** (glycopeptides)
  - **GPCs**, *Enterococcus*, *Clostridium difficile* (with PO intake), MRSA
  - Binds cell wall proteins
  - Resistance develops from a **change in cell wall–binding protein**.
  - Side effects: HTN, **Redman syndrome** (histamine release), nephrotoxicity, ototoxicity
- **Synercid** (streptogramin – quinupristin-dalfopristin)
  - **GPCs**; includes MRSA, VRE
- **Linezolid** (oxazolidinones)
  - **GPCs**; includes MRSA, VRE
- **Tetracycline**
  - **GPCs, GNRs, syphilis**
  - Side effects: tooth discoloration in children
- **Clindamycin**
  - **Anaerobes**, some GPCs
  - Good for aspiration pneumonia
  - Can be used to treat *C. perfringens*
  - Side effects: pseudomembranous colitis
- **Metronidazole** (Flagyl)
  - **Anaerobes**
  - Side effects: disulfiram-like reaction, **peripheral neuropathy** (long-term use)
- **Antifungal drugs**
  - **Amphotericin** – binds **ergosterols** in wall and alters membrane permeability
    - Side effects: **nephrotoxic**, fever, hypokalemia, hypotension, anemia
    - Liposomal type has fewer side effects.
  - **Voriconazole** – inhibits ergosterol synthesis (needed for cell wall)
  - **Anidulafungin** (Eraxis), micafungin, caspofungin – inhibit synthesis of **cell wall glucan**
  - **Prolonged broad-spectrum antibiotics** ± fever → **anidulafungin** (or other fungin drug)
  - **Invasive aspergillosis** → **voriconazole**
  - **Candidemia** → **anidulafungin** (or other fungin drug)
  - **Fungal sepsis** other than candida and aspergillus → **liposomal amphotericin**
- **Antituberculosis drugs**
  - **Isoniazid** – inhibits mycolic acids (give with pyridoxine)
    - Side effects: hepatotoxicity, **B_6 deficiency**
  - **Rifampin** – inhibits RNA polymerase
    - Side effects: hepatotoxicity; GI symptoms; high rate of resistance
  - **Pyrazinamide**
    - Side effect: hepatotoxicity
  - **Ethambutol**
    - Side effect: **retrobulbar neuritis**
- **Antiviral drugs**
  - **Acyclovir** – inhibits viral DNA polymerase; used for **HSV** infections, EBV
  - **Ganciclovir** – inhibits viral DNA polymerase; used for **CMV** infections
    - Side effects: decreased bone marrow, CNS toxicity
- Broad-spectrum antibiotics can lead to **superinfection**.
- **Effective for *Enterococcus*** – ampicillin/amoxicillin, vancomycin, Timentin/Zosyn
  - *Enterococcus is resistant to all cephalosporins.*
- **Effective for VRE** (vancomycin-resistant *Enterococcus*) – Synercid, linezolid

- **Effective for *Pseudomonas*, *Acinetobacter*, and *Serratia*** – ticarcillin/piperacillin, Timentin/Zosyn, third-generation cephalosporins, aminoglycosides (gentamicin and tobramycin), meropenem/imipenem, or fluoroquinolones
- **Effective for MRSA** – vancomycin, Synercid, linezolid
- **Double cover *Pseudomonas***
  - Has an alginate mucoid biolayer; can colonize tubes and lines

7 Medicines and Pharmacology

INTRODUCTION

- **Sublingual** and **rectal drugs** – do not pass through liver first (no first-pass metabolism); have higher bioavailability compared to oral drugs
- **Skin absorption** – based on lipid solubility through the epidermis
- **CSF absorption** – restricted to nonionized, lipid-soluble drugs
- **Albumin** – largely responsible for binding drugs (PCNs and warfarin 90% bound)
- **Sulfonamides** – will displace unconjugated bilirubin from albumin in newborns (avoid in newborns; can cause kernicterus [damages brain])
- **Tetracycline** and **heavy metals** – stored in bone
- **0 order kinetics** – constant amount of drug is eliminated regardless of dose
- **1st order kinetics** – drug eliminated proportional to dose
- **Takes 5 half-lives** for a drug to reach steady state
- **Volume of distribution** = amount of drug in the body divided by amount of drug in plasma or blood
  - Drugs with a high volume of distribution have higher concentrations in the **extravascular compartment** (eg fat tissue) compared with intravascular concentrations.
- **Bioavailability** – fraction of unchanged drug reaching the systemic circulation
  - Assumed to be 100% for intravenous drugs, less for other routes (ie oral)
- **ED_{50}** – drug level at which <u>desired effect</u> occurs in 50% of patients
- **LD_{50}** – drug level at which <u>death</u> occurs in 50% of patients
- **Tolerance** – decline in potency with continued use
- **Hyperactive** – effect at an unusually low dose
- **Tachyphylaxis** – tolerance after only a few doses
- **Potency** – dose required for effect
- **Efficacy** – ability to achieve result without untoward effect
- **Drug metabolism** (hepatocyte smooth endoplasmic reticulum, P-450 system)
  - **Phase I** – demethylation, oxidation, reduction, hydrolysis reactions (mixed function oxidases, requires NADPH/oxygen)
  - **Phase II** – **glucuronic acid** (**#1**) and sulfates attached (forms **water-soluble metabolite**); usually inactive and ready for excretion. Biliary excreted drugs may become deconjugated in intestines with reabsorption, some in active form (termed entero-hepatic recirculation; eg cyclosporine).
  - **Inhibitors of P-450** – cimetidine, isoniazid, ketoconazole, erythromycin, Cipro, Flagyl, allopurinol, verapamil, amiodarone, MAOIs, disulfiram
  - **Inducers of P-450** – cruciform vegetables, ETOH, cigarette smoke, phenobarbital (barbiturates), Dilantin, theophylline, warfarin
- **Kidney** – most important organ for eliminating most drugs (glomerular filtration and tubular secretion); #2 biliary system
- **Polar drugs** (ionized) – <u>water</u> soluble; more likely to be eliminated in unaltered form
- **Nonpolar drugs** (nonionized) – <u>fat</u> soluble; more likely metabolized before excretion
- **Gout** – caused by high **uric acid** in blood (negatively birefringent crystals); end product of purine metabolism; causes exquisite pain, swelling, and redness
  - **Podagra** – when it affects the big toe joint space (1st MTP joint); MC area affected (50% of cases)
  - **Colchicine** – anti-inflammatory; binds **tubulin** and inhibits migration (chemotaxis) of WBCs
  - **Indomethacin** – NSAID; inhibits prostaglandin synthesis (reversible cyclooxygenase inhibitor)
  - **Allopurinol** – xanthine oxidase inhibitor, blocks uric acid formation from xanthine
  - **Probenecid** – increases renal secretion of uric acid

- **Lipid-lowering agents**
  - **Cholestyramine** – binds bile acids in gut, forcing body to resynthesize bile acids from cholesterol, thereby lowering body cholesterol; can bind vitamin K and cause bleeding tendency
  - **HMG-CoA reductase inhibitors** (statin drugs) – can cause liver dysfunction, rhabdomyolysis
  - **Niacin** (inhibits cholesterol synthesis) – can cause flushing. Tx: **ASA**
- **GI drugs**
  - **Metoclopramide** (Reglan, prokinetic) – **inhibits dopamine receptors**; can be used to increase gastric and gut motility
  - **Erythromycin** (prokinetic) – binds and activates motilin receptor
  - **Alvimopan** (prokinetic) – **antagonist to mu-opioid receptor**; used for postop ileus and to improve bowel recovery
  - **Loperamide** – slows gut motility; agonist to **mu-opioid receptors**
  - **Lomotil** (diphenoxylate/atropine) – slows gut; agonist to **opioid receptors**
  - **Promethazine** (Phenergan, antiemetic) – **inhibits dopamine receptors**; S/E: **tardive dyskinesia** (Tx: **diphenhydramine** [Benadryl])
  - **Ondansetron** (Zofran, antiemetic) – central-acting **serotonin receptor inhibitor**
  - **Omeprazole** – proton pump inhibitor; **blocks H/K ATPase** in stomach parietal cells
  - **Cimetidine/ranitidine** – histamine **H₂ receptor blockers**; decrease acid in stomach
  - **Octreotide** – long-acting **somatostatin analogue**; decreases gut secretions
- **Cardiac drugs**
  - **Digoxin**
    - **Inhibits Na/K ATPase** and increases myocardial **calcium**
    - **Slows atrial-ventricular conduction**
    - Also acts as an **inotrope**
    - Decreases **blood flow** to intestines – has been implicated in causing **mesenteric ischemia**
    - **Hypokalemia** increases sensitivity of heart to digitalis; can precipitate arrhythmias or AV block
    - Is **not** cleared with dialysis
    - Other side effects: visual changes (yellow hue), fatigue, arrhythmias
  - **Amiodarone** – good for acute atrial and ventricular arrhythmias
    - S/Es: **pulmonary fibrosis** w/ prolonged use; can also cause **hypo-** and **hyperthyroidism**
  - **Magnesium** – used to treat torsades de pointes (ventricular tachycardia)
  - **Adenosine** – causes transient interruption of the AV node
  - **ACE inhibitors** (angiotensin-converting enzyme inhibitors) – captopril
    - Best single agent shown to improve survival in patients with <u>CHF</u>
    - Can prevent CHF after myocardial infarction
    - Can prevent progression of renal dysfunction in patients with hypertension and DM
    - Can precipitate renal failure in patients with renal artery stenosis
  - **Beta-blockers** – may prolong life in patients with severe LV failure
    - Reduce risk of **MI** and **atrial fibrillation** postoperatively
    - Best single agent shown to improve survival after <u>myocardial infarction</u>
  - **Atropine** – acetylcholine antagonist; increases heart rate
- **Metyrapone** and **aminoglutethimide** – inhibit adrenal steroid synthesis
  - Used in patients with adrenocortical CA
- **Leuprolide** – analogue of GnRH and LHRH
  - Inhibits release of LH and FSH from pituitary when given continuously (paradoxic effect); used in patients with metastatic prostate CA
- **Tamsulosin** (Flomax) – alpha-adrenergic receptor antagonist used for BPH

- **NSAIDs**: nonselective COX inhibitors (indomethacin, ibuprofen)
  - Inhibit prostaglandin synthesis and lead to $\downarrow$ mucus and HCO_3^- secretion and $\uparrow$ acid production (mechanism of **gastritis, ulcer formation**, and **GI bleeding**)
  - Decreased prostaglandin synthesis also leads to constriction of renal afferent arterioles, leading to **renal insufficiency**.
- **NSAIDs**: selective COX-2 inhibitors (celecoxib)
  - Only binds inducible cyclooxygenase 2
  - Fewer GI side effects compared to nonselective agents
  - Increased risk of cardiovascular events (stroke, myocardial infarction)
- **Misoprostol** – a PGE_1 derivative; a **protective prostaglandin** used to prevent peptic ulcer disease; consider use in patients on chronic NSAIDs
- **Haldol** – antipsychotic, inhibits dopamine receptors
  - Can cause **extrapyramidal** (tardive dyskinesia) manifestations (Tx: Benadryl)
  - Can cause **prolonged QT syndrome** and **ventricular tachycardia** (Tx: amiodarone or DC cardioversion if unstable)
- **Furosemide** (Lasix) – loop diuretic
  - Side effects (over-diuresis) – metabolic alkalosis, hypokalemia, ototoxicity
- **Spironolactone** – inhibits aldosterone
  - Side effects (over-diuresis) – metabolic acidosis, hyperkalemia
- **Infliximab** (Remicade) – antibody to TNF-alpha (given IV)
  - Used in inflammatory bowel disease
  - Most significant Cx is infection risk (TB reactivation or new infection).
  - CHF can also occur.
  - Should not be used in patients with an active infection
- **ASA poisoning** – tinnitus, headaches, nausea, and vomiting
  - 1st – respiratory alkalosis
  - 2nd – metabolic acidosis
- **Gadolinium** – MC side effect: nausea
  - Do <u>not</u> use with renal insufficiency; can cause acute renal failure and nephrogenic systemic fibrosis
- **Iodine contrast**
  - MC side effect – **nausea**
  - MC side effect requiring medical Tx – **dyspnea**
- **Tylenol overdose** – Tx: *N*-acetylcysteine

8 Anesthesia

ANESTHESIA INDUCTION
- Results in loss of consciousness, lack of sensation, and anesthesia
- Can use inhalational (MC – sevoflurane) or intravenous agent (MC – propofol)

INHALATIONAL INDUCTION AGENTS
- **MAC** – minimum alveolar concentration = smallest concentration of inhalational agent at which 50% of patients will not move with incision
  - Small MAC → more lipid soluble = more potent
  - Speed of induction is inversely proportional to solubility.
  - Nitrous oxide is fastest but has high MAC (low potency).
- Inhalational agents cause unconsciousness, amnesia, and some analgesia (pain relief).
- Blunt hypoxic drive
- Most have some **myocardial depression**, ↑ cerebral blood flow, and ↓ renal blood flow.
- **Nitrous oxide** (NO_2) – fast, minimal myocardial depression; tremors at induction
  - Diffuses into closed spaces (avoid in patients with small bowel obstruction or pneumothorax)
- **Halothane** – slow onset/offset, highest degree of cardiac depression and arrhythmias; least pungent, which is good for children
  - Halothane hepatitis – fever, eosinophilia, jaundice, ↑ LFTs
- **Sevoflurane** – fast, less laryngospasm and less pungent; good for mask induction
- **Isoflurane** – good for neurosurgery (lowers brain O_2 consumption; no increase in ICP)
  - Pungent (not used for induction)
- **Enflurane** – can cause seizures
- MCC intraop **bradycardia** – inhalational anesthesia (Tx: atropine)

INTRAVENOUS INDUCTION AGENTS
- **Propofol** – very rapid distribution and on/off; provides anesthesia and amnesia; sedative
  - Side effects: hypotension, respiratory depression, metabolic acidosis (avoid prolonged use in children)
  - **Not an analgesic**
  - Do not use in patients with egg allergy, pregnancy, or Parkinson's.
  - Metabolized in liver and by plasma cholinesterases
- **Ketamine** – dissociation of thalamic/limbic systems; places patient in a cataleptic state (amnesia, analgesia)
  - No respiratory depression
  - Side effects: **hallucinations**, catecholamine release (↑ CO_2, tachycardia, HTN), ↑ airway secretions
  - _Considered safe_ with **head injury**
  - Good for **children**
- **Etomidate** – fewer hemodynamic changes; fast acting
  - Fewest cardiac side effects (good for patients with CHF or angina)
  - Not analgesic
  - Continuous infusions can lead to adrenocortical suppression.
- **Rapid sequence intubation** – can be indicated for recent oral intake, GERD, delayed gastric emptying, pregnancy, bowel obstruction (pre-oxygenate, etomidate, succinylcholine typical sequence), cricoid pressure

- **Dexmedetomidine (Precedex)** – sedation agent for intubated patients (<u>not</u> an induction agent)
  - Provides **anesthesia** and **analgesia** without blunting hypoxic drive
  - Good for early extubation protocols (eg cardiac surgery)
  - Use not recommended for more than 24 hours
  - Is a CNS alpha-2 receptor agonist

MUSCLE RELAXANTS (PARALYTICS)

- **Diaphragm** – last muscle to go down and 1st muscle to recover from paralytics
- **Neck muscles and face** – 1st to go down and last to recover from paralytics
- **Depolarizing agents** – only one is **succinylcholine**; depolarizes neuromuscular junction
- **Succinylcholine** – fast, short acting; causes fasciculations, ↑ ICP; degraded by plasma pseudocholinesterases (can <u>not</u> be reversed); many side effects →
  - **Malignant hyperthermia**
    - Caused by a defect in calcium metabolism
    - Calcium released from sarcoplasmic reticulum causes **muscle excitation – contraction syndrome** (ryanodine receptor defect)
    - Side effects: 1st sign is ↑ **end-tidal CO$_2$**, then fever, tachycardia, rigidity, acidosis, hyperkalemia, rhabdomyolysis.
    - Tx: **dantrolene** (10 mg/kg) inhibits Ca release and decouples excitation complex; cooling blankets, HCO$_3$, glucose, supportive care
  - **Hyperkalemia** – depolarization releases K
    - **Do not use** in patients with severe burns, neurologic injury, neuromuscular disorders, spinal cord injury, massive trauma, or acute renal failure (all have up-regulation of acetylcholine receptors which can release significant amounts of K).
  - **Open-angle glaucoma** can become closed-angle glaucoma.
  - **Atypical pseudocholinesterases** – cause prolonged paralysis (Asians)
- **Nondepolarizing agents**
  - Inhibit neuromuscular junction by competing with acetylcholine
  - Can get prolongation of these agents with myasthenia gravis
  - **Cis-atracurium** – undergoes **Hoffman elimination**
    - Can be used in **liver** and **renal failure** (drug is broken down in the blood)
    - Histamine release (hypotension)
  - **Rocuronium** – fastest, intermediate duration; hepatic metabolism
  - **Vecuronium** – fast; intermediate duration; hepatic metabolism
  - **Pancuronium** – slow acting, long-lasting; renal metabolism
    - Most common side effect – ***tachycardia*** *(no hypotension)*
  - **Reversing drugs for nondepolarizing agents**
    - **Sugammadex** – selective relaxant binding agent (binds the paralytic drug)
      - Used to reverse Rocuronium and Vecuronium only
      - Does <u>not</u> require glycopyrrolate or atropine (although atropine given if bradycardia occurs)
    - **Neostigmine** – blocks **acetylcholinesterase**, increasing acetylcholine
    - **Edrophonium** – blocks **acetylcholinesterase**, increasing acetylcholine
    - **Glycopyrrolate** or **Atropine** should be given with <u>neostigmine or edrophonium</u> to counteract effects of generalized acetylcholine overdose.

LOCAL ANESTHETICS

- Work by **increasing action potential threshold**, preventing Na influx
- Sensory block > motor block
- Can use 0.5 cc/kg of 1% lidocaine
- Maximum dosing
  - **Lidocaine** 4 mg/kg (7 mg/kg with epi)
  - **Bupivacaine** 2 mg/kg (3 mg/kg with epi)
- Can re-administer after 2 hours

- **Infected tissues** are hard to anesthetize secondary to **acidosis**.
- **Length of action** – bupivacaine $>$ lidocaine $>$ procaine
- Side effects: perioral paresthesias (1st sign), tremors, seizures, tinnitus, arrhythmias (CNS symptoms occur before cardiac)
- **Epinephrine** allows higher doses to be used, stays locally.
  - **No epinephrine** with arrhythmias, unstable angina, uncontrolled hypertension, poor collaterals (penis and ear), uteroplacental insufficiency
- **Amides** (all have an "i" in first part of the name) – lidocaine, bupivacaine, mepivacaine; rarely cause allergic reactions
- **Esters** – tetracaine, procaine, cocaine; $\uparrow$ allergic reactions due to PABA analogue

NARCOTICS (OPIOIDS)

- Morphine, fentanyl, Demerol (meperidine), codeine, hydromorphone (Dilaudid)
- Are all CNS **mu-opioid receptor agonists**
- Profound analgesia, respiratory depression ($\downarrow CO_2$ drive), no cardiac effects, blunt sympathetic response; overdose – pinpoint pupils, somnolent
- Metabolized by the liver and excreted via kidney
- Overdose of narcotics – Tx: **Narcan** (naloxone; works for all; mu-opioid receptor antagonist)
- Avoid use of narcotics (especially Demerol) in patients on **MAOIs** → can cause **hyperpyrexic coma** (serotonin release syndrome – fever, tachycardia, seizures, coma)
- **Morphine** – analgesia, euphoria, respiratory depression, miosis, constipation, histamine release (causes hypotension), $\downarrow$ cough
- **Demerol** – analgesia, euphoria, respiratory depression, miosis, tremors, fasciculations, convulsions
  - **No histamine release**
  - Can cause **seizures** (buildup of **normeperidine** analogues) – *avoid in patients with renal failure* and be careful with total amount given for other patients
- **Methadone** – simulates morphine, less euphoria; agonist to CNS mu-opioid receptor
- **Fentanyl** – fast acting; 80× strength of **morphine** (does not cross-react in patients with morphine allergy); no histamine release
- **Sufentanil** and **remifentanil** – *very* fast-acting narcotics with short half-lives
- Most potent narcotic – *sufentanil*
- Careful with combining opioids and benzodiazepines (synergistic effect)

BENZODIAZEPINES

- Anticonvulsant, amnesic, anxiolytic, **respiratory depression**; not analgesic; liver metabolism
- Agonist to the GABA receptor in the CNS (most prevalent inhibitory brain receptor)
- **Versed** (midazolam) – short acting; contraindicated in pregnancy, crosses placenta
- **Valium** (diazepam) – long acting
- **Ativan** (lorazepam) – long acting
- Overdose of these drugs – Tx: **flumazenil** (competitive inhibitor; may cause seizures and arrhythmias; contraindicated in patients with elevated ICP or status epilepticus)

EPIDURAL AND SPINAL ANESTHESIA

- **Epidural anesthesia** – allows analgesia by **sympathetic denervation** (sensory blockade); vasodilation
  - Has been shown to decrease respiratory Cx and cardiac events; no change in mortality
  - **Morphine** in epidural can cause **respiratory depression** (use Dilaudid to avoid this).
  - **Lidocaine** in epidural can cause **decreased heart rate** and **blood pressure**.
  - Dilute concentrations allow sparing of motor function.
  - Tx for **acute hypotension** and **bradycardia**: turn epidural down; fluids, phenylephrine, atropine

- T-5 epidural can affect cardiac accelerator nerves.
- Epidural contraindicated with <u>hypertrophic cardiomyopathy</u> or <u>cyanotic heart disease</u> → **sympathetic denervation** causes decreased afterload, which worsens these conditions
- **Thoracotomy** insertion level: T6–T9
- **Laparotomy** insertion level: T8–T10
- **Spinal anesthesia** – injection into subarachnoid space, spread determined by baricity and patient position
  - Inject below L2 to avoid hitting the spinal cord.
  - Can perform any surgery below the umbilicus with spinal anesthesia alone
  - Neurologic blockade is above motor blockade.
  - Spinal contraindicated with hypertrophic cardiomyopathy, cyanotic heart disease
- **Caudal block** – through sacrum, good for pediatric hernias and perianal surgery
- **Epidural and spinal complications** – hypotension, headache, urinary retention (MC complication; need urinary catheter in these patients), abscess/hematoma formation, respiratory depression (with high spinal)
- **Spinal headaches** – caused by CSF leak after spinal/epidural; headache gets worse sitting up; Tx: rest, fluids, caffeine, analgesics; **blood patch** to site if it persists > 24 hours

PERIOPERATIVE COMPLICATIONS

- Preop **renal failure** (#1) and **CHF** – associated with most postop hospital **mortality**
- **Postop MI** – may have no chest pain; can have hypotension, arrhythmias, ↑ filling pressures, oliguria, bradycardia; can happen intraop or postop (usually 2–3 days after surgery)
  - **Dx** – EKG and troponins (best test)
  - Initial Tx (BMOAN) – beta-blocker, morphine, oxygen, ASA, sublingual nitrates
  - **ST elevation MI (STEMI)** – emergently go to the cardiac cath lab for percutaneous coronary intervention (PCI)
- **Patients who need cardiology workup preop** – aortic stenosis, angina, previous MI, shortness of breath, CHF, walks < 2 blocks due to shortness of breath or chest pain, FEV_1 < 70% predicted, severe valvular disease, PVCs > 5/min, high-grade heart block, age > 70, DM, renal insufficiency, patients undergoing major vascular surgery (peripheral and aortic)

ASA Physical Status (PS) Classes

Class	Description
1	Healthy
2	Mild disease without limitation (controlled hypertension, obesity, diabetes mellitus, significant smoking history, older age)
3	Severe disease (angina, previous MI, poorly controlled hypertension, diabetes mellitus with complications, moderate COPD)
4	Severe constant threat to life (unstable angina, CHF, renal failure, liver failure, severe COPD)
5	Moribund (ruptured AAA, saddle pulmonary embolus)
6	Donor
E	Emergency

- Most **aortic** and **peripheral vascular surgeries** are considered <u>high</u> risk.
- **Carotid endarterectomy** (CEA) is considered <u>moderate</u> risk surgery.
- **Biggest risk factors for postop MI**: uncompensated CHF (#1, S3 gallop, JVD), recent MI, age > 70, DM, previous MI, unstable angina, Cr > 2, stroke/TIA
- **Beta-blocker** – most effective agent to prevent intraop and postop cardiovascular events
- Wait **6–8 weeks** after MI before elective surgery.
- Best determinant of esophageal vs. tracheal intubation – **end-tidal CO2** ($ETCO_2$)

Cardiac Risk[a] Stratification for Noncardiac Surgical Procedures

High (cardiac risk > 5%) – emergent operations (especially in elderly); aortic, peripheral, and other major vascular surgery (_except_ CEA); long procedure with large fluid shifts

Intermediate (cardiac risk < 5%) – CEA; head and neck surgery; intraperitoneal and intrathoracic surgery; orthopedic surgery; prostate surgery

Low[b] (cardiac risk < 1%) – endoscopic procedures; superficial procedures; cataract surgery; breast surgery

[a]Combined incidence of cardiac death and nonfatal myocardial infarction.
[b]Do not generally require further preoperative cardiac testing.

- Intubated patient undergoing surgery with **sudden transient rise in ETCO$_2$**
  - Dx: most likely **hypoventilation**
  - Tx: ↑ tidal volume or ↑ respiratory rate
  - Could also be due to **CO$_2$ embolus** (would have associated hypotension, followed by a massive drop in **ETCO$_2$** from lack of blood flow to lungs)
  - Could also be due to **malignant hyperthermia**
  - Could also be due to **capnothorax**
- **Capnothorax** (CO$_2$ pneumothorax)
  - From upper GI laparoscopic procedure (eg Nissen) with CO$_2$ pneumothorax due to **pleural tear**
  - Causes **trouble ventilating**; may see **bulging diaphragm**; elevated **ETCO$_2$**
  - If **hypotensive**, likely **tension capnothorax** – enlarge pleural tear to decompress
  - Tx: **Stop insufflation** and add **PEEP** (generally resolves in 30 minutes).
    - If it doesn't resolve – **thoracentesis** to remove CO$_2$
    - If it resolves – resume procedure at **lower insufflation**
    - If **lung** was injured when pleura was entered – place **chest tube** at end of procedure
  - **Small PTX** noticed after laparoscopic Nissen (< 2 cm) – observe (repeat CXR in 8 hours)
- Intubated patient with **sudden drop in ETCO$_2$** – likely became **disconnected from the vent**
  - Could also be due to pulmonary embolism, air embolism, cardiac arrest, or some other massive drop in cardiac output (patient would also have **hypotension**)
- **Air embolus**
  - MC occurs with air sucking through a central line or central line site.
  - CO$_2$ embolus can occur with laparoscopic procedures.
  - Sx's: sudden drop in **ETCO$_2$**, hypotension, tachycardia, mill wheel murmur (air lock prevents venous return)
  - Tx: Stop CO$_2$ insufflation if laparoscopic procedure.
    - Trendelenburg (head down) and left lateral decubitus position (keeps air in right ventricle)
    - Hyperventilate with 100% oxygen (helps reabsorb air embolus faster).
    - Aspirate central line if present (try to remove air).
    - Pressors and inotropes
    - Prolonged CPR
- **Endotracheal tube** – should be placed 2 cm above the carina
- MC **PACU complication** – _nausea and vomiting_
- MCC postop **hypoxemia** – **atelectasis** (alveolar hypoventilation)
- MCC postop **hypercarbia** – **poor minute ventilation** (need to take bigger breaths or increase tidal volumes)
- **Safest surgical setting** – bipolar cautery (only affects area between circuit)
- **Adequate pain control** – 3/10 or less
  - Signs of inadequate pain control – tachycardia, diaphoresis, splinting, hypertension
- **Visceral pain** Tx: opioids
- **Somatic pain** Tx: NSAIDs and opioids
- **Higher volume hospitals** are associated with lower mortality for abdominal aortic aneurysm repair and for pancreatic resection.

9 Fluids and Electrolytes

TOTAL BODY WATER

- Roughly ⅔ of the total body weight is water (men).
  - **Infants** have a little more body water; **women** have a little less.
- ⅔ of water weight is intracellular (mostly muscle).
- ⅓ of water weight is extracellular.
  - ⅔ of extracellular water is interstitial.
  - ⅓ of extracellular water is intravascular.
- Third space fluid is **interstitial fluid**.
- **Proteins** – determine <u>plasma/interstitial</u> compartment oncotic pressures
- **Na** – determines <u>intracellular/extracellular</u> osmotic pressure
- **Volume overload** – most common cause is iatrogenic; first sign is **weight gain**
- **Cellular catabolism** – can release a significant amount of H_2O
- **0.9% normal saline**: Na 154 and Cl 154; **3% normal saline**: Na 513 and Cl 513
- **Lactated Ringer's** (LR; ionic composition of plasma): Na 130, K 4, Ca 2.7, Cl 109, lactate 28 (lactate is converted to HCO_3^- in the body)
- **Serum osmolality**: $(2 \times Na) + (glucose/18) + (BUN/2.8)$
  - Normal: 280–295
- **Water** shifts from areas of low solute concentration (low osmolarity) to areas of high solute concentration (high osmolarity) to achieve **osmotic equilibration**.

MAINTENANCE IV FLUIDS

- 4 cc/kg/h for 1st 10 kg
- 2 cc/kg/h for 2nd 10 kg
- 1 cc/kg/h for each kg after that
- **IV maintenance fluids** after **major adult gastrointestinal surgery**
  - During operation and 1st 24 hours, use **LR**.
  - After 24 hours, switch to **D5 ½ NS with 20 mEq K^+**.
    - 5% dextrose will stimulate **insulin release** and **prevent protein breakdown** (prevents protein catabolism).
    - D5 ½ NS @ 125/h provides 150 g glucose per day (525 kcal/day).
- During open abdominal operations, fluid loss is **0.5–1.0 L/h** unless there are measurable blood losses.
- Usually do not have to replace blood lost unless it is **> 500 cc**
- Best indicator of adequate volume replacement is **urine output**.
- **Urine output** – should be kept at least 0.5 cc/kg/h; should not be replaced, usually a sign of normal postoperative diuresis
- **Insensible fluid losses** – 10 cc/kg/day; 75% **skin** (#1; sweat), 25% respiratory, pure water
  - Increases in insensible losses – fever, burns, large open wounds, ventilated patients

FLUID RESUSCITATION (FOR SIGNIFICANT DEHYDRATION)

- **Sweat** loss (eg marathon runner) – Tx: normal saline
- **Gastric fluid** loss (eg gastric outlet obstruction) – Tx: normal saline
- **Pancreas**, **biliary**, or **small bowel** fluid loss – Tx: lactated ringers (may need extra HCO_3^-)
- **Large bowel** (eg massive diarrhea) – Tx: lactated ringers (may need extra K^+)
- **GI fluid losses** should generally be replaced **cc/cc**.
- *Avoid* albumin unless special circumstances such as large volume paracentesis replacement or hepatorenal syndrome.
  - Concern over **leakage of colloid** into interstitial space due **to increased capillary permeability** resulting in **interstitial/pulmonary edema**

GI FLUID SECRETION

- Stomach   1-2 L/day
- Biliary system   500-1,000 mL/day
- Pancreas   500-1,000 mL/day
- Duodenum   500-1,000 mL/day

GI ELECTROLYTE LOSSES

- Sweat – hypotonic (Na concentration 35-65)
- Saliva – K^+ (*highest concentration of K^+ in body*)
- Stomach – H^+ and Cl^-
- Pancreas – HCO_3^-
- Bile – HCO_3^-
- Small intestine – HCO_3^-, some K^+
- Large intestine – K^+
- Dialysis can remove K, Ca, Mg, PO_4, urea, and creatinine.
- **Normal body K^+ requirement**: 0.5-1.0 mEq/kg/day
- **Normal body Na^+ requirement**: 1-2 mEq/kg/day

POTASSIUM (NORMAL 3.5–5.0)

- **Hyperkalemia** – peaked T waves on EKG (arrhythmias); often occurs with **renal failure**
  - Tx: **calcium gluconate** (1st drug to give; membrane stabilizer for heart)
  - **Sodium bicarbonate** (causes alkalosis, K enters cell in exchange for H)
  - **10 U insulin** and **1 ampule of 50% dextrose** (K driven into cells with glucose)
  - **Kayexalate**
  - **Lasix**
  - **Albuterol**
  - **Dialysis** if refractory
- **Hypokalemia** – T waves disappear (usually from **over-diuresis** [eg too much Lasix])
  - Can also occur with **diarrhea**
  - Fatigue, weakness, muscle cramps/twitches
  - May need to replace Mg^+ before you can correct K^+
- **Pseudohyperkalemia** – hemolysis of blood sample

SODIUM (NORMAL 135–145)

- **Hypernatremia** – usually from **poor fluid intake** (concentrated urine)
  - Restlessness, irritability, seizures
  - If <u>dehydrated</u>, replace volume loss with **D5 ½ normal saline**.
  - If using **D5 water, give slowly** to avoid **brain swelling**.
- **Hyponatremia** – usually from **fluid overload** (dilute urine)
  - Headaches, nausea, vomiting, seizures
  - **Water restriction** is first-line treatment for <u>fluid overload</u> hyponatremia, then **diuresis**.
  - Correct Na slowly to avoid **central pontine myelinolysis** (no more than 1 mEq/h).
  - **Hyperglycemia** (eg DKA) and **hyperlipidemia** (eg from acute pancreatitis) can cause **pseudohyponatremia**.
  - **Hyponatremia** can occur from **isotonic fluid loss** (usually from GI tract) compensated by water retention – treatment is isotonic fluids (lactated Ringer's if pH is normal/acidotic or normal saline if pH is alkalotic).
- **Diabetes insipidus** (low ADH) – **hypernatremia** and **increased urine output** (low urine specific gravity [dilute urine]), high serum osmolality
  - Can occur with ETOH, head injury
  - First line Tx: **free water**
  - Tx if refractory and severe: **DDAVP** (synthetic analogue of ADH)

- **SIADH** (high ADH) – **hyponatremia** and **low urine output** (high urine osmolality [concentrated urine]), low serum osmolality
  - Can occur with head injury
  - First line Tx: **fluid restriction** and **diuresis** (slowly)
  - Tx if refractory and severe: **conivaptan, tolvaptan** (competitive antagonist for kidney V2 receptor)

CALCIUM (NORMAL 8.5–10.0; NORMAL IONIZED CA 1.0–1.5)

- **Hypercalcemia** (Ca usually > 13 for symptoms)
  - Acute hypercalcemia causes lethargic state, N/V, hypotension.
  - **Breast cancer** most common malignant cause
  - **Hyperparathyroidism** most common benign cause (also MCC overall)
  - **MCC hypercalcemic crisis** – undiagnosed **hyperparathyroidism** with stressor (eg surgery); as a group, **hypercalcemia of malignancy** is likely #1
  - No lactated Ringer's (contains Ca^{2+})
  - No thiazide diuretics (these retain Ca^{2+})
  - Tx: **Fluids** (normal saline at 200–300 cc/h) and **Lasix** (start after patient is euvolemic)
  - For **malignant disease** → calcitonin, alendronic acid (bisphosphonates; inhibit osteoclasts), glucocorticoids, dialysis
- **Hypocalcemia** (Ca usually < 8 or ionized Ca < 1 for symptoms) – perioral tingling and numbness (1st symptom), hyperreflexia, Chvostek's sign (tapping on facial nerve produces twitching), Trousseau's sign (carpopedal spasm with blood pressure cuff), prolonged QT interval
  - Can occur after **parathyroidectomy**
  - May need to replace Mg^+ before you can correct Ca
  - **Albumin adjustment for calcium** – for every 1 g/dL decrease in albumin (normal is 4 g/dL), add 0.8 to Ca
  - **MCC** – previous **thyroidectomy** (injured the parathyroid glands at surgery)

MAGNESIUM (NORMAL 2.0–2.7)

- **Hypermagnesemia** – causes lethargic state; usually occurs in **renal failure** patients taking magnesium containing products (laxatives, antacids)
  - Tx: **calcium**
- **Hypomagnesemia** – causes irritability, confusion, hyperreflexia, seizures; usually occurs with **massive diuresis**, **chronic TPN** without magnesium replacement, or **ETOH abuse**; signs similar to hypocalcemia

PHOSPHATE (NORMAL 2.5–4.5)

- **Hyperphosphatemia** – most often associated with **renal failure**
  - Tx: sevelamer hydrochloride (Renagel), low-phosphate diet (avoid dairy), dialysis
- **Hypophosphatemia** – most often associated with **refeeding syndrome**; usually from PO_4 shift from extracellular to intracellular
  - Sx's: failure to wean from the ventilator, muscle weakness, confusion
  - Tx: **potassium phosphate**

RESPIRATORY ACIDOSIS

- **High CO_2** from low tidal volumes (TV) or low respiratory rate (RR; eg narcotic overdose)
- Tx: Increase minute ventilation (Narcan if overdose).

RESPIRATORY ALKALOSIS

- **Low CO_2** from hyperventilation (high TV and/or high RR; eg anxiety, high altitudes)
- Tx: lower minute ventilation; acetazolamide can be used for altitude sickness

METABOLIC ACIDOSIS

- **Anion gap = Na − (HCO_3 + Cl)**; Normal is < 10–15
- **High anion gap acidosis** – excessive production of fixed acids; **"MUDPILES"** = **m**ethanol, **u**remia, **d**iabetic ketoacidosis, **p**ar-aldehydes, **i**soniazid, **l**actic acidosis, **e**thylene glycol, **s**alicylates
- **Normal anion gap acidosis** – usually loss of Na/HCO_3^- (ileostomies, small bowel fistulas, lactulose), rapid infusion of HCO_3^--deficient fluids, primary hyperparathyroidism, diarrhea, mafenide acetate (Sulfamylon; inhibits carbonic anhydrase), acetazolamide (Diamox; inhibits carbonic anhydrase)
- Tx: underlying cause; keep pH > 7.20 with bicarbonate; severely ↓ pH can affect myocardial contractility
- Correction of acidosis can lead to **hypokalemia.**

METABOLIC ALKALOSIS

- Usually a contraction alkalosis (loss of fluid [eg NG tube suction, overdiuresis with Lasix])
  - **Nasogastric suction** – results in **hypochloremic, hypokalemic, metabolic alkalosis,** and **paradoxical aciduria** →
  - Loss of Cl^- and H ion from stomach secondary to nasogastric tube (hypochloremia and alkalosis)
  - Loss of water causes kidney to reabsorb Na in exchange for K^+ (Na/K ATPase), thus losing K^+ (hypokalemia).
  - Na^+/H^- exchanger activated in an effort to reabsorb water along with K^+/H^- exchanger in an effort to reabsorb K^+ → results in paradoxical aciduria
  - Tx: **normal saline** (most important to correct the Cl^- deficit)
- **Respiratory compensation** (CO_2 regulation) for acidosis/alkalosis takes **minutes.**
- **Renal compensation** (HCO_3^- regulation) for acidosis/alkalosis takes **hours to days.**

Acid–Base Balance			
Condition	pH (7.4)	CO_2 (40)	HCO_3 (24)
Respiratory acidosis	↓	↑	↑
Respiratory alkalosis	↑	↓	↓
Metabolic acidosis	↓	↓	↓
Metabolic alkalosis	↑	↑	↑

ACUTE RENAL FAILURE

- **FeNa** = (urine Na/Cr)/(plasma Na/Cr) − fractional excretion of Na; *best test for azotemia*
- **Prerenal** – FeNa < 1%, urine Na < 20, BUN/Cr ratio > 20, urine osmolality > 500 mOsm
  - 70% of renal mass must be damaged before ↑ Cr and BUN.
- **Contrast dyes** – prehydration best prevents renal damage; HCO_3^- and *N*-acetylcysteine
- **Myoglobin** – converted to ferrihemate in acidic environment, which is toxic to renal cells; Tx: hydration, alkalinize urine

TUMOR LYSIS SYNDROME

- Release of purines and pyrimidines leads to ↑ **PO_4, K,** and **uric acid,** leads to ↓ Ca.
- Can ↑ BUN and Cr (from renal damage; can lead to acute renal failure), EKG changes
- RFs – leukemias, lymphomas
- Tx: **hydration** (*best*), rasburicase (converts uric acid in inactive metabolite allantoin), allopurinol (↓ uric acid production), diuretics, alkalinization of urine

VITAMIN D (CHOLECALCIFEROL)

- Made in skin (UV sunlight converts 7-dehydrocholesterol to cholecalciferol)
- Goes to **liver** for **(25-OH)**, then **kidney** for **(1-OH)**. This creates the active form of vitamin D.
- **Active form of vitamin D** – increases **calcium-binding protein**, leading to increased **intestinal Ca absorption**

CHRONIC RENAL FAILURE

- ↑ K, Mg, PO_4, BUN, and creatinine
- ↓ Na and Ca
- ↓ **Active vitamin D** (↓ 1-OH hydroxylation) → ↓ Ca reabsorption from gut (↓ Ca-binding protein)
- **Anemia** – from low erythropoietin

Transferrin – transporter of iron
Ferritin – storage form of iron

10 Nutrition

INTRODUCTION

- **Caloric need** – approximately 20–25 calories/kg/day
- **Calories**:

Fat (lipids)	9 calories/g
Protein	4 calories/g
Oral carbohydrates	4 calories/g
Dextrose	3.4 calories/g

- **Nutritional requirements for average healthy adult male (70 kg)**
  - **20% protein** calories (**1 g protein/kg/day**; 20% should be essential amino acids)
  - **20% fat** calories – important for essential fatty acids
  - **60% carbohydrate** calories
  - 1,500–1,700 calories/day
- **Trauma**, **surgery**, or **sepsis** stress can increase kcal requirement 20%–40%.
- **Pregnancy** increases kcal requirement 300 kcal/day.
- **Lactation** increases kcal requirement 500 kcal/day.
- **Protein requirement** also increases with above.
- **Burns**
  - Calories: 25 kcal/kg/day + (30 kcal/day × % burn)
  - Protein: 1–1.5 g/kg/day + (3 g/day × % burn)
  - Don't exceed 3,000 kcal/day.
- Much of **energy expenditure** is used for **heat production**.
- **Fever** increases **basal metabolic rate** (10% for each degree above 38.0°C).
- If overweight and trying to calculate caloric need, use equation: weight = [(actual weight − ideal body weight) × 0.25] + IBW.
- **Harris–Benedict equation** calculates basal energy expenditure based on **weight, height, age**, and **gender**.
- **Central line TPN** – glucose based; maximum glucose administration −3 g/kg/h
- **Peripheral line parenteral nutrition** (PPN) – fat based
- **Short-chain fatty acids** (eg butyric acid) – fuel for **colonocytes**
- **Glutamine** – fuel for **small bowel enterocytes**
  - Most common amino acid in **bloodstream** and **tissue**
  - Most common amino acid released from **muscle** with **catabolism**
  - Releases NH_4 in kidney, thus helping with **nitrogen excretion**
  - Can be used for **gluconeogenesis**, as an **energy source**, or in the **urea cycle**
  - Enhances **immune function** by inhibiting small bowel mucosal breakdown and preventing bacterial translocation
- **Primary fuel for most neoplastic cells** – glutamine

PREOPERATIVE NUTRITIONAL ASSESSMENT

- **Approximate half-lives**
  - Albumin – 18 days
  - Transferrin – 8 days
  - Prealbumin – 2 days
- Normal **protein** level: 6.0–8.5
- Normal **albumin** level: 3.5–5.5
- Normal **prealbumin** level: 15–35
- **Acute indicators of nutritional status** – prealbumin (#1), retinal binding protein, transferrin
- **Ideal body weight** (IBW)
  - Men = 106 lb + 6 lb for each inch over 5 ft
  - Women = 100 lb + 5 lb for each inch over 5 ft

- **Preoperative signs of severe malnutrition**
  - Acute weight loss > 20% in 3 months
  - Albumin < 3.0
  - Transferrin < 200
  - Anergy to skin antigens
- **Low albumin** (< 3.0) – strong risk factor for **morbidity** and **mortality** after surgery
- **Preop nutrition** is indicated *only* for patients with **severe malnutrition** undergoing **major abdominal or thoracic procedures**.
- **Early enteral feeding** increases survival with **sepsis, pancreatitis,** and **burns**.

RESPIRATORY QUOTIENT (RQ; METABOLIC CART/INDIRECT CALORIMETRY)

- Ratio of CO_2 produced / O_2 consumed – is a measurement of energy expenditure
- **RQ > 1** = lipogenesis (overfeeding)
  - Tx: ↓ carbohydrates and caloric intake
  - High carbohydrate intake can lead to CO_2 buildup and difficulty weaning from ventilator.
  - CO_2 is produced when excess carbohydrates are converted to fats.
  - Too many **carbohydrates** can also cause **hyperglycemia** and **immunosuppression**.
  - Too many **fat calories** can cause excessive **inflammation** (omega 3 fatty acids [eg linolenic acid] have less inflammation).
- **RQ < 0.7** = ketosis and fat oxidation (starving)
  - Tx: ↑ carbohydrates and caloric intake
- Pure **fat utilization** – RQ = 0.7
- Pure **protein utilization** – RQ = 0.8
- Pure **carbohydrate utilization** – RQ = 1.0
- Balanced nutrition – RQ = 0.825

POSTOPERATIVE PHASES

- **Diuresis phase** – postoperative days 2–5
- **Catabolic phase** – postoperative days 0–3 (negative nitrogen balance)
- **Anabolic phase** – postoperative days 3–6 (positive nitrogen balance)

STARVATION OR MAJOR STRESS (SURGERY, TRAUMA, SYSTEMIC ILLNESS)

Metabolic Differences Between the Responses to Simple Starvation and to Injury		
	Starvation	Injury
Basal metabolic rate	−	+ +
Presence of mediators (eg TNF-α, IL-1)	−	+ + +
Major fuel oxidized	Fat	Mixed (fat, protein)
Ketone body production	+ + +	±
Gluconeogenesis	+	+ + +
Protein metabolism	+	+ + +
Negative nitrogen balance	+	+ + +
Hepatic ureagenesis	+	+ + +
Muscle proteolysis	+	+ + +
Hepatic protein synthesis	+	+ + +

- The magnitude of metabolic response is proportional to the degree of injury.
- **Glycogen stores**
  - Depleted after **24–36 hours** of starvation (⅔ in **skeletal muscle**, ⅓ in liver) → body then switches to **fat**
  - Skeletal muscle lacks **glucose-6-phosphatase** (found only in **liver**).
  - Glucose-6-phosphate stays in muscle after breakdown from glycogen and is utilized there.
  - The **liver** is the source of systemic glucose during stress times or starvation.

- **Gluconeogenesis precursors** – amino acids (especially **alanine**, **#1**), lactate, pyruvate, glycerol; occurs in the **liver**
  - **Alanine** is the simplest amino acid precursor for gluconeogenesis.
    - Is the **primary substrate** for gluconeogenesis
  - **Alanine** and **phenylalanine** – only amino acids to increase during times of stress
  - **Late starvation** – gluconeogenesis occurs in <u>kidney</u>
- **Starvation**
  - Protein-conserving mechanisms **do <u>not</u> occur after trauma** (or surgery) secondary to catecholamines and cortisol.
  - Protein-conserving mechanisms do occur with **starvation**.
  - **Fat** (ketones) is the main source of energy in **starvation** and in **trauma**; however, with trauma the energy source is more mixed (fat and protein).
  - Fat is the body's largest potential energy source.
  - Most patients can tolerate a 15% weight loss without major complications.
  - Start **enteral nutrition** within **24–48 hours** after event (after resuscitation and stabilization) in **severely ill patients** (eg trauma, pancreatitis).
  - Patients can tolerate about **5–7 days** without eating; **start TPN** at that point if not able to start enteral nutrition.
  - Enteral nutrition *preferred* to avoid **bacterial translocation** (bacterial overgrowth, increased permeability due to starved enterocytes, bacteremia) and **TPN complications**
  - **PEG tube** – consider when regular feeding not possible (eg CVA) or predicted to not occur for **> 4 weeks**
  - **Tube feeds**
    - **Diarrhea** – slow rate, add fiber, less-concentrated feeds
    - **High gastric residuals** – Tx: Reglan, erythromycin
    - **Renal formulation** – contains low concentrations of K, PO_4, and protein
  - **Brain** – utilizes <u>ketones</u> with progressive starvation (normally uses **glucose**)
  - **Peripheral nerves**, **adrenal medulla**, **red blood cells**, and **white blood cells** are all **obligate glucose users**.
  - **Refeeding syndrome**
    - Occurs when feeding after prolonged starvation/malnutrition
    - **ETOH abuse** often present
    - Shift from fat to carbohydrate metabolism
    - Symptoms usually occur on **day 4** following re-feeding.
    - Results in decreased **K**, **Mg**, and **PO_4**; causes cardiac dysfunction, profound weakness, encephalopathy, CHF, failure to wean from the ventilator
    - Decreased ATP, the most significant problem
    - Prevent this by starting to re-feed at a **low rate** (10–15 kcal/kg/day).
  - **Cachexia** – anorexia, weight loss, wasting
    - Thought to be mediated by **TNF-α**
    - Glycogen breakdown, lipolysis, protein catabolism
  - **Kwashiorkor** – protein deficiency
  - **Marasmus** – starvation
- **Major stress**
  - Causes an increase in **catecholamines**, **cortisol**, and **cytokines** (eg TNF-α, IL-1)
  - Results in significant **protein breakdown** (negative nitrogen balance)
  - **Hepatic urea formation** occurs at high levels.

NITROGEN BALANCE

- Based on 24-hour urine nitrogen collection
- **6.25 g of protein** contains **1 g of nitrogen**.
- **N balance** = (N in − N out) = ([protein/6.25] − [24-hour urine N + 4 g])
  - **Positive N balance** – more protein ingested than excreted (anabolism)
  - **Negative N balance** – more protein excreted than taken in (catabolism)

- Total protein synthesis for a healthy, normal 70-kg male is **250 g/day**.
- **Liver**
  - Responsible for amino acid production and breakdown
  - Majority of protein breakdown from skeletal muscle is **glutamine** (#1) and **alanine**.
  - **Urea production** is used to get rid of **ammonia** (NH_3) from amino acid breakdown.
- **Urea cycle – glutamine** is the primary NH_3 donor; reactions occur in the **liver** and urea is removed by the **kidney**; accounts for 90% of all N loss

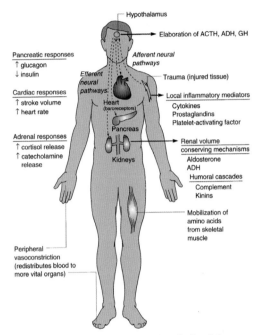

Homeostatic adjustments initiated after injury.

FAT DIGESTION

- **Triacylglycerides** (TAGs), **cholesterol**, and **lipids**
  - Broken down by pancreatic lipase, cholesterol esterase, and phospholipase to micelles and free fatty acids
  - **Micelles** – aggregates of bile salts, **long-chain free fatty acids**, and monoacylglycerides
    - Enter enterocyte by fusing with membrane
    - **Bile salts** – increase absorption area for fats, helping form **micelles**
    - **Cholesterol** – used to synthesize bile salts
    - **Fat-soluble vitamins** (A, D, E, K) – absorbed in micelles
  - **Medium-** and **short-chain fatty acids** – enter enterocyte by simple diffusion
- **Micelles and other fatty acids enter enterocytes.**
  - **Chylomicrons** are formed (90% TAGs, 10% phospholipids/proteins/cholesterol) which enter **lymphatics** (thoracic duct).
  - **Long-chain fatty acids** – enter **lymphatics** (terminal villous lacteals) along with chylomicrons
  - **Medium-** and **short-chain fatty acids** – enter **portal system** (same as amino acids and carbohydrates)
- **Lipoprotein lipase** – on endothelium in liver and adipose tissue; clears <u>chylomicrons and TAGs</u> from the blood, breaking them down to <u>fatty acids</u> and <u>glycerol</u>

- **Free fatty acid–binding protein** – on endothelium in the liver and adipose tissue; binds short- and medium-chain fatty acids
- **Saturated fatty acids** – used for **fuel** by **cardiac** and **skeletal muscles**
  - **Fatty acids** (ketones – acetoacetate, beta-hydroxybutyrate) – preferred source of energy for **colonocytes**, **liver**, **heart**, and **skeletal muscle**
- **Unsaturated fatty acids** – used as **structural components** for cells
- **Hormone-sensitive lipase** (HSL) – in fat cells; breaks down **TAGs** (storage form of **fat**) to **fatty acids** and **glycerol**, which are released into the bloodstream (HSL is sensitive to growth hormone, catecholamines, glucocorticoids)
- **Essential** fatty acids – linolenic, linoleic
  - Needed for prostaglandin synthesis (long-chain fatty acids)
  - Important for immune cells

CARBOHYDRATE DIGESTION

- Begins with **salivary amylase**, then pancreatic amylase and disaccharidases
- **Glucose** and **galactose** – absorbed by secondary active transport (Na gradient formed by ATPase); released into **portal vein**
- **Fructose** – facilitated diffusion; released into **portal vein**
- **Sucrose** = fructose + glucose
- **Lactose** = galactose + glucose
- **Maltose** = glucose + glucose
- Carbohydrates are the body's main energy source.
- Glucose enters glycolysis or is stored as glycogen.

PROTEIN DIGESTION

- Begins with **stomach pepsin**, then trypsin, chymotrypsin, and carboxypeptidase
- **Trypsinogen** released from pancreas and activated by **enterokinase**, which is released from the duodenum
  - Other pancreatic protein enzymes are then activated by trypsin.
  - Trypsin can then also autoactivate other trypsinogen molecules.
- **Protein** broken down to amino acids, dipeptides, and tripeptides by proteases
- Absorbed by secondary active transport; released as free amino acids into portal vein
- Amino acids are taken up by cells under the influence of insulin.
- During stress, amino acids are shunted to the **liver** for **gluconeogenesis**.
- Limit protein intake in patients with **liver failure** and **renal failure** to **avoid ammonia** and **urea buildup** (respectively) and possible worsening encephalopathy.
- **Branched-chain** amino acids – leucine, isoleucine, valine ("LIV")
  - Metabolized in **muscle**
  - Possibly important source of protein in patients with liver failure
  - Are **essential amino acids**
- **Essential** amino acids – leucine, isoleucine, valine, histidine, lysine, methionine, phenylalanine, threonine, and tryptophan
- **Non-essential amino acids** – those that start with A, G, or C plus serine, tyrosine, and proline

CENTRAL VENOUS TPN (GENERAL COMPOSITION)

- **10% amino acid solution**
- **25% dextrose solution**
- **Electrolytes** (Na [need 2 mg/kg/day], Cl, K [need 1 mg/kg/day], Ca, Mg, PO$_4$, acetate)
- **Mineral** and **vitamins**
- Makes 2–3 L solution, given at 100–150 cc/hr
- **Lipids** – given separately from TPN
  - 10% lipid solution contains 1.1 kcal/cc; 20% lipid solution contains 2 kcal/cc.

- **Acetate** – buffer to increase pH of the solution
- Need to add **Vit K** separately
- ETOH abuse – add thiamine, folate, and multivitamin
- Long-term TPN Cx – cirrhosis
- Short-term TPN Cx – line issues (pneumothorax, infection)

Mineral and Vitamin Deficiencies	
Deficiency	**Effect**
Chromium	Hyperglycemia, encephalopathy, neuropathy
Selenium	Cardiomyopathy, weakness
Copper	Pancytopenia
Zinc	Poor wound healing; alopecia, rash
Phosphate	Weakness (failure to wean off ventilator), encephalopathy, decreased phagocytosis
Thiamine (B_1)	Wernicke's encephalopathy, cardiomyopathy (Beri Beri)
Pyridoxine (B_6)	Sideroblastic anemia, glossitis (beefy tongue), peripheral neuropathy
Cobalamin (B_{12})	Megaloblastic anemia, peripheral neuropathy, glossitis
Folate	Megaloblastic anemia, glossitis
Ascorbic acid (C)	Scurvy, poor wound healing
Niacin	Pellagra (diarrhea, dermatitis, dementia)
Essential fatty acids	Dermatitis, hair loss, thrombocytopenia
Vitamin A	Night blindness
Vitamin K	Coagulopathy
Vitamin D	Rickets, osteomalacia, osteoporosis
Vitamin E	Neuropathy

CORI CYCLE

- Glucose is utilized and converted to **lactate** in muscle.
- Lactate then goes to the **liver** and is converted back to **pyruvate** and eventually **glucose** via gluconeogenesis.
- Glucose is then transported back to muscle.

METABOLIC SYNDROME (NEED 3)

- Waist circumference (> 40 inches in men, > 35 inches in women)
- Insulin resistance (fasting glucose > 100)
- High TAGs (> 150)
- Low HDL (< 40 in men, < 50 in women)
- Hypertension ($> 130/85$)

11 Oncology

INTRODUCTION

- **Cancer #2 cause of death in the United States**
- **MC CA in women** – breast CA
- **MC cause of CA-related death in women** – lung CA
- **MC CA in men** – prostate CA
- **MC cause of CA-related death in men** – lung CA
- Most important prognostic indicator for **lung CA** and **breast CA** devoid of systemic metastases – **nodal status**
- Most important prognostic indicator for **sarcoma** devoid of systemic metastases – **tumor grade**
- **PET** (positron emission tomography) – used to identify **metastases**; detects **fluorodeoxyglucose** (FDG) molecules
  - **False positives** (5–10%) – **inflammatory disease** (eg histoplasmosis, TB, sarcoid)
  - **False negatives** (5–10%) – **slow-growing tumors** (carcinoid, bronchoalveolar lung CA)
  - Accuracy low in the head due to increased glucose uptake by the brain
  - Test may not work well in patients with diabetes (glucose competes) or hyper-insulinemia (insulin drives FDG into normal cells).
- **Cytotoxic T cells** need MHC complex to attack tumor.
- **Natural killer cells** can independently attack tumor cells.
- Tumor antigens are random unless viral-induced tumor.
- **Hyperplasia** – increased number of cells
- **Metaplasia** – replacement of one tissue with another (GERD squamous epithelium in esophagus changed to columnar gastric tissue; eg Barrett's esophagus)
- **Dysplasia** – altered size, shape, and organization (eg Barrett's dysplasia)
- **Core needle biopsy** – gives architecture
- **Fine-needle aspiration** – gives cytology (just cells)

TUMOR MARKERS

- CEA – colon CA
- AFP – liver CA
- CA 19-9 – pancreatic CA
- CA 125 – ovarian CA
- Beta-HCG – testicular CA, choriocarcinoma
- PSA – prostate CA (thought to be the tumor marker with the **highest sensitivity**, although specificity is low)
- NSE – small cell lung CA, neuroblastoma
- BRCA I and II – breast CA
- Chromogranin A – carcinoid tumor
- Ret oncogene – thyroid medullary CA
- **Half-lives** – CEA: 18 days; PSA: 18 days; AFP: 5 days

ONCOGENESIS

- **Cancer transformation**:
  1. Heritable alteration in genome *and*;
  2. Loss of growth regulation
- **Latency period** – time between exposure and formation of clinically detectable tumor
  - **Initiation** – carcinogen acts with DNA
  - **Promotion** of cancer cells then occurs
  - **Progression** of cancer cells to clinically detectable tumor

- Neoplasms can arise from **carcinogenesis** (eg smoking), **viruses** (eg EBV), or **immunodeficiency** (eg HIV).
- **Retroviruses** contain **oncogenes**.
  - Epstein-Barr virus – associated with Burkitt's lymphoma (8:14 translocation) and nasopharyngeal CA (c-myc)
- **Proto-oncogenes** are **human genes** with **malignant potential**.

Malignancy	Associated Infectious Agent
Cervical cancer	*Human papillomavirus*
Gastric cancer	*Helicobacter pylori*
Hepatocellular carcinoma	Hepatitis B and hepatitis C viruses
Nasopharyngeal carcinoma	EBV
Burkitt's lymphoma	EBV
Various lymphomas	HIV

EBV, Epstein-Barr virus; HIV, human immunodeficiency virus.

RADIATION THERAPY (XRT)

- **M phase** (mitosis) – most vulnerable stage of cell cycle for XRT
- Most damage done by formation of **oxygen radicals** → maximal effect with **high oxygen levels**
- Main target is **DNA** – oxygen radicals and XRT itself damage DNA and other molecules
- **Higher-energy radiation** has **skin-preserving effect** (maximal ionizing potential not reached until deeper structures).
- **Fractionate XRT doses**
  - Allows **repair** of normal cells
  - Allows **re-oxygenation** of tumor
  - Allows **redistribution** of tumor cells in cell cycle
- Very radiosensitive tumors (high mitotic rate) – **seminomas, lymphomas**
- Very radioresistant tumors (low mitotic rate) – **epithelial, sarcomas**
- **Large tumors** – less responsive to XRT due to <u>lack of oxygen in the tumor</u>
- XRT can be used for painful bony metastases.
- **Brachytherapy** – source of radiation in or next to tumor (Au-198, I-128); delivers high, concentrated doses of radiation
- **Gamma knife** – cobalt XRT

CHEMOTHERAPY AGENTS

- **Cell cycle–specific agents** (5FU, methotrexate) – exhibit plateau in cell-killing ability
- **Cell cycle–nonspecific agents** – linear response to cell killing
- **Tamoxifen** (blocks estrogen receptor) – decreases short-term (5-year) risk of breast CA 45% (1% risk of blood clots, 0.1% risk of endometrial CA)
- **Taxane** (docetaxel) – promotes microtubule formation and stabilization that cannot be broken down; cells are ruptured; side effects – peripheral neuropathy
- **Bleomycin** and **busulfan** – can cause pulmonary fibrosis
- **Cisplatin** (platinum alkylating agent) – nephrotoxic, neurotoxic, ototoxic
- **Carboplatin** (platinum alkylating agent) – **bone** (myelo) suppression
- **Vincristine** (microtubule inhibitor) – peripheral neuropathy, neurotoxic
- **Vinblastine** (microtubule inhibitor) – **bone** (myelo) suppression
- **Alkylating agents** – transfer alkyl groups; form covalent bonds to DNA
  - **Cyclophosphamide** – **acrolein** is the active metabolite
    - Side effects: gonadal dysfunction, SIADH, hemorrhagic cystitis
    - **Mesna** can help with hemorrhagic cystitis.

- **Levamisole** – **anthelmintic drug** thought to stimulate immune system against cancer
- **Methotrexate** – inhibits <u>dihydrofolate reductase</u> (DHFR), which inhibits purine and DNA synthesis
  - Side effects: renal toxicity, radiation recall
  - **Leucovorin rescue** (folinic acid) – reverses effects of methotrexate by re-supplying folate
- **5-Fluorouracil (5FU)** – inhibits <u>thymidylate synthetase</u>, which inhibits purine and DNA synthesis
  - **Leucovorin** (folinic acid) – increases toxicity of 5FU
- **Doxorubicin** (Adriamycin) – DNA intercalator, O_2 radical formation
  - **Cardiomyopathy** – **heart toxicity** secondary to O_2 **radicals** at total doses > 500 mg/m^2
- **Etoposide** (VP-16) – inhibits topoisomerase (which normally unwinds DNA)
- **Least myelosuppression** – bleomycin, vincristine, busulfan, cisplatin
- **GCSF** (granulocyte colony–stimulating factor) – used for **neutrophil recovery** after chemo; side effects – **Sweet's syndrome** (acute febrile neutropenic dermatitis)

MISCELLANEOUS

- Three main groups of CA – epithelial tumors (ectoderm), sarcomas (mesoderm), and adenocarcinoma (endoderm)
- **Resection of a normal organ to prevent cancer**
  - Breast – BRCA I or II with strong family history
  - Thyroid – RET proto-oncogene with family history thyroid CA
- **Tumor suppressor genes** (usually inhibit cell cycle or induce apoptosis)
  - **Retinoblastoma** (Rb1) – chromosome 13; involved in **cell cycle** regulation
  - **p53** – chromosome 17; involved in **cell cycle** (normal gene induces cell cycle arrest and **apoptosis**; abnormal gene allows unrestrained cell growth)
  - **APC** – chromosome 5; involved with **cell cycle** regulation and movement
  - **DCC** – chromosome 18; involved in **cell adhesion**
  - **bcl** – involved in **apoptosis** (programmed cell death)
  - **BRCA** – involved in DNA damage/repair; also cell cycle regulation
- **Proto-oncogenes**
  - **ras** proto-oncogene – G protein defect (GTPase)
  - **src** proto-oncogene – tyrosine kinase defect
  - **sis** proto-oncogene – platelet-derived growth factor receptor defect
  - **erb B** proto-oncogene – epidermal growth factor receptor defect
  - **myc** (c-myc, n-myc, l-myc) proto-oncogenes – transcription factors
- **Li–Fraumeni syndrome** – defect in **p53 gene** → patients get childhood sarcomas, breast CA, brain tumors, leukemia, adrenal CA
- **Cowden syndrome** – defect in **PTEN** gene; get <u>benign</u> **hamartomas** (skin, mucus membranes, GI tract); increased risk for CA (usually thyroid, breast, and endometrial CA)
- **Hereditary diffuse gastric cancer** – defect in **CDH1**; also at risk for other cancers (breast, colorectal, thyroid, and ovarian)
- **Colon CA**
  - Genes involved in development include **APC**, **p53**, **DCC**, and **K-ras**.
  - **APC** thought to be the **initial step** in the evolution of colorectal CA
  - **Colon CA usually does not go to bone.**
- **Carcinogens**
  - **Coal tar** – larynx, skin, bronchial CA
  - **Beta-naphthylamine** – urinary tract CA (bladder CA)
  - **Benzene** – leukemia
  - **Asbestos** – mesothelioma

- **Cancer spread**
  - Suspicious supraclavicular nodes – neck, breast, lung, stomach (Virchow's node), pancreas
  - Suspicious axillary node – **lymphoma** (#1), breast, melanoma
  - Suspicious periumbilical node – pancreas (Sister Mary Joseph's node)
  - Ovarian metastases – stomach (Krukenberg tumor), colon
  - Bone metastases – **breast** (#1), prostate
  - Skin metastases – breast, melanoma
  - Small bowel metastases – **melanoma** (#1)
- **Clinical trials**
  - Phase I – is it **safe** and at what dose? (examines side effects)
  - Phase II – is it **effective** and at what dose?
  - Phase III – is it **better** than existing therapy? (randomized control trial)
  - Phase IV – studies **long-term** side effects and efficacy
- **Types of therapy**
  - **Induction** – initial treatment
  - **Primary** (neoadjuvant) – administration of an agent before another main Tx: eg chemo-XRT given 1st, followed by surgery
  - **Adjuvant** – combined with another modality; given after other therapy is used
  - **Salvage** – for tumors that fail to respond to initial chemotherapy
- **Lymph nodes** have poor barrier function → better to view them as signs of **probable metastasis**
- **En bloc multiorgan resection** can be attempted for some tumors (eg colon into uterus, adrenal into liver, gastric into spleen); aggressive local invasiveness is different from metastatic disease.
- **Palliative surgery** – tumors of hollow viscus causing obstruction or bleeding (colon CA), breast CA with skin or chest wall involvement
- **Sentinel lymph node biopsy** – no role in patients with clinically palpable nodes; you need to go after and sample these nodes
- **Colon metastases to the liver** – 35% 5-year survival rate if successfully resected
- **Prognostic indicators for survival after resection of hepatic colorectal metastases** – disease-free interval > 12 months, tumor number < 3, CEA < 200, size < 5 cm, negative nodes
- **Most successfully cured metastases with surgery** – germ cell tumor (#1 seminoma; 75% 5-YS)
- **Ovarian CA** – one of the few tumors for which **surgical debulking** improves chemotherapy (not seen in other tumors)
- **Curable solid tumors with chemotherapy only** – Hodgkin's and non-Hodgkin's lymphoma
- **T-cell lymphomas** – HTLV-1 (skin lesions), mycosis fungoides (Sézary cells)
- **HIV-related malignancies** – Kaposi's sarcoma, non-Hodgkin's lymphoma
- **V-EGF** (vascular epidermal growth factor) – causes angiogenesis; involved in tumor metastasis

12 Transplantation

TRANSPLANT IMMUNOLOGY

- **HLA-A**, **B**, and **DR** – most important in recipient/donor matching (human leukocyte antigens)
  - **HLA-DR** – most important overall (HLA = human leukocyte antigen)
  - HLA is the major histocompatibility complex (MHC) in humans.
- Time on the list and HLA matching are the primary determinants of organ allocation in the U.S.
- **ABO blood compatibility** – generally required for all transplants (except liver)
  - **Type O** – universal donor
  - **Type AB** – universal recipient
- **Crossmatch** – detects **preformed recipient antibodies** to the donor organ by mixing recipient serum with donor lymphocytes → if these antibodies are present, it is termed a **positive crossmatch** and **hyperacute rejection** would likely occur with TXP
- **Panel reactive antibody** (PRA)
  - Technique identical to crossmatch; detects preformed recipient antibodies using a panel of HLA typing cells
  - Get a percentage of cells that the recipient serum reacts with → a **high PRA** ($> 50\%$) is often a contraindication to TXP (increased risk of hyperacute rejection)
  - Transfusions, pregnancy, previous transplant, and autoimmune diseases can all increase PRA.
- **Mild rejection** – pulse steroids
- **Severe rejection** – steroid and antibody therapy (ATG or thymoglobulin)
- **Skin cancer** – #1 malignancy following any transplant (squamous cell CA #1)
- **Posttransplant lympho-proliferative disorder** (PTLD) – next most common malignancy following transplant (**Epstein-Barr virus** related)
  - Sx's: small bowel obstruction, mass, adenopathy
  - RFs: cytolytic drugs
  - Tx: withdrawal of immunosuppression; rituximab (anti-CD20; decreases B cells); may need chemotherapy and XRT for aggressive tumor
- Risks of long-term immunosuppression – CA, cardiovascular disease, infection, osteopenia
- Donors with hepatitis or HIV can be matched with recipients having the same disease.

DRUGS

- **Mycophenolate** (MMF, CellCept)
  - Inhibits de novo purine synthesis, which **inhibits growth of T cells**
  - Side effects: GI intolerance (#1, N/V/D), myelosuppression
  - Need to keep WBCs > 3
  - Used as maintenance therapy to prevent rejection
  - Azathioprine (Imuran) has similar action.
- **Steroids** (prednisone, Solu-Medrol) – inhibit **inflammatory cells** (macrophages) and **genes for cytokine synthesis** (IL-2 most important); used for induction after TXP, maintenance, and acute rejection episodes
- **Cyclosporin** (CSA)
  - Binds **cyclophilin protein**; CSA-cyclophilin complex then inhibits **calcineurin**, which results in decreased **cytokine synthesis** (**IL-2** most important); used for maintenance therapy
  - Side effects: nephrotoxicity, hepatotoxicity, tremors, seizures, hemolytic-uremic syndrome

- Need to keep trough 200–300
- Undergoes **hepatic metabolism** and **biliary excretion** (reabsorbed in the gut, get entero-hepatic recirculation)
- **FK-506** (Prograf, tacrolimus)
  - Binds **FK-binding protein**; actions similar to CSA but more potent
  - Side effects: nephrotoxicity, more GI symptoms, mood changes, and diabetes than CSA, much less entero hepatic recirculation compared to CSA
  - Less rejection episodes in kidney TXP's w/ FK-506 compared to CSA
  - Need to keep trough 10–15
- **Sirolimus** (Rapamycin)
  - Binds FK-binding protein like FK-506 but **inhibits mammalian target of rapamycin (mTOR)**; result is that it **inhibits T and B cell response to IL-2**
  - Used as maintenance therapy
  - Is <u>not</u> nephrotoxic (unlike CSA and tacrolimus)
  - Side effect – interstitial lung disease
- **Anti-thymocyte globulin** (ATG)
  - Equine (ATGAM) or rabbit (Thymoglobulin) **polyclonal antibodies** against T-cell antigens (CD2, CD3, CD4)
  - Used for induction and acute rejection episodes
  - Is **cytolytic** (complement dependent)
  - Need to keep WBCs > 3
  - Side effects: **cytokine release syndrome** (fever, chills, pulmonary edema, shock) – steroids and Benadryl given before drug to try to prevent this; PTLD; myelosuppression

TYPES OF REJECTION

- **Hyperacute rejection** (occurs within minutes to hours)
  - Caused by **preformed antibodies** that should have been picked up by the crossmatch (type II hypersensitivity reaction)
  - MCC – ABO incompatibility
  - Activates the **complement** cascade and thrombosis of vessels occurs
  - Tx: **emergent retransplant** (or just removal of organ if kidney)
- **Accelerated rejection** (occurs < 1 week)
  - Caused by sensitized **T cells** to donor HLA
  - Tx: ↑ immunosuppression, pulse steroids, and possibly antibody Tx
- **Acute cellular rejection** (occurs after 1st week)
  - Caused by **T cells** (cytotoxic and helper T cells; cell-mediated) to HLA antigens
  - Tx: ↑ immunosuppression, pulse steroids, and possibly antibody Tx
- **Acute humeral rejection** (occurs after 1st week)
  - Caused by antibodies to donor antigens
  - Tx: pulse steroids, antibody therapy, plasmapheresis
- **Chronic rejection** (occurs months to years after TXP)
  - Partially a type IV hypersensitivity reaction (sensitized **T cells**)
  - **Antibody formation** also plays a role.
  - Leads to graft fibrosis
  - RF – increased number of acute rejection episodes
  - MCC – HLA incompatibility
  - Tx: ↑ immunosuppression – no really effective treatment; retransplant

KIDNEY TRANSPLANTATION

- Can store kidney for 48 hours
- Need ABO type compatibility and crossmatch
- **UTI** – can still use kidney
- **Acute ↑ in creatinine** (1.0–3.0) – can still use kidney

- HIV is <u>not</u> a contraindication.
- Mortality primarily from **stroke** and **MI**
- Attach to **iliac vessels**
- **Complications**
  - **Urine leaks** (#1) – Tx: drainage and stenting best
  - **Renal artery stenosis** – diagnose with ultrasound (flow acceleration occurs at level of stenosis)
    - Tx: PTA with stent
  - **Lymphocele** – most common cause of external ureter compression
    - MC occurs **3 weeks** after TXP (late decreased urine output with hydronephrosis and fluid collection).
    - Tx: 1st try **percutaneous drainage**; if that fails, then need **peritoneal window** (make hole in peritoneum, lymphatic fluid drains into peritoneum and is reabsorbed – 95% successful)
  - **Postop oliguria** – usually due to **ATN** (pathology shows hydrophobic changes [dilation and loss of tubules])
  - **Postop diuresis** – usually due to **urea** and **glucose**
  - **New proteinuria** – suggestive of **renal vein thrombosis**
  - **Postop diabetes** – side effect of CSA, FK, steroids
  - **Viral infections** – **CMV** – Tx: ganciclovir; **HSV** – Tx: acyclovir
  - **Acute rejection** – usually occurs in 1st 6 months; pathology shows tubulitis (vasculitis with more severe form)
  - **Kidney rejection workup** – usually for ↑ in Cr or poor urine output
    - **Ultrasound with duplex** (to rule out vascular problem and ureteral obstruction) and **biopsy**
    - Empiric **decrease in CSA** or **FK** (these can be nephrotoxic)
    - Empiric **pulse steroids**
    - Empiric **fluid/Lasix** challenge
  - **Chronic rejection** – usually do not see until after 1 year; no good treatment
  - **5-year graft survival overall** – 70% (cadaveric 65%, living donors 75%)
  - Extends life by **15 years**
  - **MCC mortality** – myocardial infarction
- **Living kidney donors**
  - Dual-collecting systems is not a contraindication.
  - Most common complication – wound infection (1%)
  - Most common cause of death – fatal PE
  - The remaining kidney hypertrophies.

LIVER TRANSPLANTATION

- Can store for 24 hours
- Contraindications to liver TXP – **current ETOH abuse, acute ulcerative colitis**
- Chronic **hepatitis C** – most common reason for liver TXP in adults
- **MELD score** uses **creatinine, INR,** and **bilirubin** to predict if patients with cirrhosis will benefit more from liver TXP than from medical therapy (MELD > 15 benefits from liver TXP).
- Criteria for **urgent TXP** – fulminant hepatic failure (**encephalopathy** – stupor, coma)
- Patients with hepatitis B antigenemia can be treated with **HBIG** (hepatitis B immunoglobulin) and **lamivudine** (protease inhibitor) after liver TXP to help prevent reinfection.
- **Hepatitis B** – reinfection rate is reduced to 20% with the use of HBIG and lamivudine
- **Hepatitis C** – disease most likely to recur in the new liver allograft; reinfects essentially all grafts

- **Hepatocellular CA** – if no vascular invasion, extra-hepatic spread, or metastases can still consider TXP (_not_ if cholangiocarcinoma)
  - Usually get **neoadjuvant chemo** prior to TXP along with **tumor ablation** or **TACE** (see Liver chapter)
  - **Resectable** liver CA and **Child's A** – proceed with **resection**
  - **Resectable** liver CA and **Child's B/C** – **Liver TXP evaluation**
- **Portal vein thrombosis** – not a contraindication to TXP
- **ETOH** – 20% will start drinking again (recidivism)
- **Macrosteatosis** – extracellular fat globules in the liver allograft
  - Risk factor for **primary non-function** – if 50% of cross-section is macrosteatotic in potential donor liver, there is a 50% chance of primary non-function
- Duct-to-duct anastomosis is performed.
  - Hepaticojejunostomy in kids
- Right subhepatic, right, and left subdiaphragmatic drains are placed.
- **Biliary system** (ducts, etc.) depends on **hepatic artery** blood supply.
- Most common arterial anomaly – **right hepatic coming off SMA**
- **Liver problems postop** – get liver duplex U/S with biopsy
- **Complications**
  - **Bile leak** (#1) – Tx: place **drain**, then **ERCP with stent** across leak
  - **Primary nonfunction**
    - **1st 24 hours** – total bilirubin > 10, bile output < 20 cc/12 h, elevated PT and PTT; **after 96 hours** – mental status changes, ↑ LFTs, renal failure, respiratory failure
    - Usually requires **retransplantation**
  - **Hepatic artery stenosis** – place stent
  - **Early hepatic artery thrombosis**
    - MC early vascular Cx
    - → LFTs, ↓ bile output, **fulminant hepatic failure**
    - Tx: MC will need **emergent retransplantation** for ensuing fulminant hepatic failure (can try to stent or revise anastomosis).
  - **Late hepatic artery thrombosis**
    - Results in biliary strictures and abscesses (not fulminant hepatic failure)
  - **Abscesses** – most commonly from **late** (chronic) **hepatic artery thrombosis**
  - **IVC stenosis/thrombosis** (rare) – edema, ascites, renal insufficiency; Tx: thrombolytics, IVC stent; heparin
  - **Portal vein thrombosis** (rare): _early_ – abdominal pain; _late_ – UGI bleeding, ascites, may be asymptomatic; Tx – if _early_, **re-op thrombectomy** and **revise anastomosis**
  - **Cholangitis** – get **PMNs** around portal triad (_not_ mixed infiltrate)
  - **Acute rejection** – T cell mediated against blood vessels
    - Clinical – fever, jaundice, ↓ bile output
    - Labs – leukocytosis, eosinophilia, ↑ LFTs, ↑ total bilirubin, and ↑ PT
    - Pathology – shows **portal triad lymphocytosis**, **endotheliitis** (mixed infiltrate), and **bile duct injury**
    - Usually occurs in 1st 2 months
    - **Chronic rejection** – after liver TXP; get disappearing bile ducts (antibody and cellular attack on bile ducts); gradually get bile duct obstruction with ↑ in alkaline phosphatase, portal fibrosis
- **Retransplantation rate** – 20%
- **5-year survival rate** – 70%
- **Living donor**
  - For **adult** transplant – take **right lobe**
  - For **child** transplant – take **left lateral lobe** (segments 2 + 3)
  - Liver is regenerated 100% in 6–8 weeks.

PANCREAS TRANSPLANTATION

- MC indication – DM w/ renal failure
- Need both **donor celiac artery** and **SMA** for arterial supply
- Need **donor portal vein** for venous drainage
- Attach to iliac vessels
- Most use **enteric drainage** for pancreatic duct. Take second portion of duodenum from donor along with ampulla of Vater and pancreas, then perform anastomosis of donor duodenum to recipient bowel.
- **Successful pancreas/kidney TXP** results in stabilization of retinopathy, ↓ neuropathy, ↑ nerve conduction velocity, ↓ autonomic dysfunction (gastroparesis), ↓ orthostatic hypotension.
  - *No reversal of vascular disease*
- **Complications**
  - **Venous thrombosis** (#1) – hard to treat
  - **Rejection** – hard to diagnose if patient does not also have a kidney transplant
    - Can see ↑ glucose or amylase; fever, leukocytosis

HEART TRANSPLANTATION

- Can store for 6 hours
- Need ABO compatibility and crossmatch
- For patients with life expectancy < 1 year
- Persistent **pulmonary hypertension** after heart transplantation
  - Associated with <u>early mortality</u> after heart TXP
  - Tx: inhaled nitric oxide, ECMO if severe
- Routine right ventricular biopsies (to check for rejection) are performed at set intervals.
- **Acute rejection** – shows <u>perivascular lymphocytic infiltrate</u> with varying grades of <u>myocyte inflammation and necrosis</u>
- **MCC early mortality** – infection
- *Chronic allograft vasculopathy* (progressive diffuse coronary atherosclerosis) – MCC of late death and death overall following heart TXP
- Median: 10-year survival

LUNG TRANSPLANTATION

- Can store for 6 hours
- Need ABO compatibility and crossmatch
- For patients with life expectancy < 1 year
- #1 cause of <u>early mortality</u> – **reperfusion injury** (Tx: similar to ARDS)
- Indication for double-lung TXP – **cystic fibrosis**
- Exclusion criteria for using lungs – aspiration, moderate to large contusion, infiltrate, purulent sputum, $PO_2 < 350$ on 100% FiO_2 and PEEP 5
- **Acute rejection** – perivascular lymphocytosis
- **Chronic rejection** – *bronchiolitis obliterans*; MCC of late death and death overall following lung TXP
- Median: 5-year survival

OPPORTUNISTIC INFECTIONS

- **Viral** – CMV, HSV, VZV
- **Fungal** – *Pneumocystis jiroveci* pneumonia (reason for **Bactrim** prophylaxis), *Aspergillus*, *Candida*, *Cryptococcus*

Hierarchy for Permission for Organ Donation from Next of Kin – 1) spouse, 2) adult son or daughter, 3) either parent, 4) adult brother or sister, 5) guardian, 6) any other person authorized to dispose of the body

13 Inflammation and Cytokines

INFLAMMATION PHASES
- **Injury** – leads to exposed collagen, platelet-activating factor release, and tissue factor release from endothelium
- **Platelets bind collagen** – release growth factors (platelet-derived growth factor [PDGF]); leads to PMN and macrophage recruitment
- **Macrophages** – *dominant role in wound healing*; release important **growth factors** (PDGF) and **cytokines** (IL-1 and TNF-α)

GROWTH AND ACTIVATING FACTORS
- **PDGF**
  - *Key growth factor in wound healing*
  - Chemotactic and activates **inflammatory cells** (PMNs and macrophages)
  - Chemotactic and activates **fibroblasts** → collagen and ECM proteins
  - **Angiogenesis**
  - **Epithelialization**
  - Chemotactic for smooth muscle cells
  - Has been shown to accelerate wound healing
- **EGF** (epidermal growth factor)
  - Chemotactic and activates **fibroblasts**
  - **Angiogenesis**
  - **Epithelialization**
- **FGF** (fibroblastic growth factor)
  - Chemotactic and activates **fibroblasts** → collagen and ECM proteins
  - **Angiogenesis**
  - **Epithelialization**
- **PAF** (platelet-activating factor) – is not stored, generated by **phospholipase** in endothelium; is a **phospholipid**
  - Chemotactic for inflammatory cells; ↑ adhesion molecules
  - Activates platelets
- **Chemotactic factors**
  - For inflammatory cells – PDGF, IL-8, LTB-4, C5a and C3a, PAF; TNF-α, IL-1
  - For fibroblasts – PDGF, EGF, FGF
- **Angiogenesis factors** – hypoxia (#1), PDGF, EGF, FGF, IL-8
- **Epithelialization factors** – PDGF, EGF, FGF
- **PMNs** – last 1–2 days in tissues (7 days in blood)
- **Platelets** – last 7–10 days
- **Lymphocytes** – involved in chronic inflammation (T cells) and antibody production (B cells)
- **TXA$_2$ and PGI$_2$** – see Chapter 2 (Hematology)
- **TGF-beta** – immunosuppressive

TYPE I HYPERSENSITIVITY REACTIONS
- **Mast cells** – primary cell in **type I hypersensitivity reactions**
  - Main source of histamine in **tissues**
- **Basophils**
  - Main source of histamine in **blood**; not found in tissue
- **Histamine** – vasodilation, tissue edema, postcapillary leakage
  - Primary effector in **type I hypersensitivity reactions** (allergic reactions)

- **Bradykinin** – peripheral vasodilation, increased permeability, pain, pulmonary vasoconstriction, bronchoconstriction; involved in **angioedema**
  - **Angiotensin-converting enzyme** (ACE) – inactivates bradykinin; located in **lung**

NITRIC OXIDE (NO)

- Has **arginine** precursor (substrate for nitric oxide synthase)
- NO activates **guanylate cyclase** and increases **cGMP**, resulting in vascular smooth muscle **dilation**.
- Is also called endothelium-derived relaxing factor
- **Endothelin** – causes vascular smooth muscle **constriction** (opposite effect of nitric oxide)

IMPORTANT CYTOKINES

- Main initial cytokine response to injury and infection is release of **TNF-α** and **IL-1**
- Initiates the inflammatory cascade
- **Tumor necrosis factor-alpha** (TNF-α)
  - **Macrophages** – largest producers of TNF
  - Increases adhesion molecules
  - Overall, a procoagulant
  - Causes cachexia in patients with cancer
  - Activates neutrophils and macrophages → more cytokine production, cell recruitment
  - High concentrations of TNF-α can cause systemic inflammatory response syndrome (SIRS), shock, and multisystem organ failure (MSOF).
- **IL-1**
  - Main source also macrophages; effects similar to TNF-α and synergizes TNF-α
  - Responsible for **fever** (PGE_2 mediated in hypothalamus)
    - Raises thermal set point, causing fever
    - **NSAIDs** decrease fever by reducing PGE_2 synthesis.
  - **Alveolar macrophages** – cause fever with **atelectasis** by releasing **IL-1**
- **IL-6** – increases **hepatic acute phase proteins** (C-reactive protein, amyloid A)
- **IL-8** – PMN chemotaxis, angiogenesis
- **IL-10** – decreases the inflammatory response

INTERFERONS

- Released by **lymphocytes** in response to <u>viral infection</u> or other stimulants
- Activate macrophages, natural killer cells, and cytotoxic T cells
- **Inhibit viral replication**

HEPATIC ACUTE PHASE RESPONSE PROTEINS

- **IL-6** – most potent stimulus
- *Increased* – **C-reactive protein** (an opsonin, activates complement), **amyloid A and P**, fibrinogen, haptoglobin, ceruloplasmin, alpha-1 antitrypsin, and C3 (complement)
- *Decreased* – **albumin**, **prealbumin**, and **transferrin**

CELL ADHESION MOLECULES

- **Selectins** – <u>L-selectins</u>, located on leukocytes, bind to <u>E- (endothelial)</u> and <u>P- (platelets) selectins</u>; **rolling adhesion**
- **Beta-2 integrins** (CD 11/18 molecules) – on leukocytes; bind ICAMs, etc., **anchoring adhesion**
- **ICAM, VCAM, PECAM, ELAM** – on endothelial cells, bind beta-2 integrin molecules located on leukocytes and platelets. These are also involved in **transendothelial migration** (diapedesis).

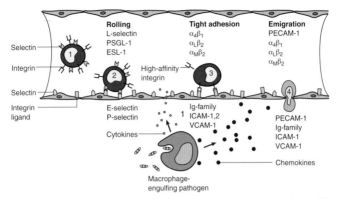

Leukocyte recruitment. (1) Circulating leukocytes express integrins in a low-affinity conformation. (2) Exposure to activated endothelium leads to rolling, which is mediated by L-selectin and P-selectin on the neutrophil and E-selectin on the endothelium. (3) Leukocyte exposure to cytokines released by macrophages phagocytosing pathogens induces a high-affinity integrin conformation. Tight leukocyte—endothelial adhesion involves integrin engagement with counter-ligand expressed on the endothelium. (4) Subsequent exposure to chemokines leads to diapedesis, which is further mediated by the family of β_1- and β_2-integrins.

COMPLEMENT

- **Classic pathway** (IgG or IgM) – antigen–antibody complex activates
  - **Factors C1, C2**, and **C4** – found only in the classic pathway
- **Alternative pathway** – endotoxin, bacteria, other stimuli activate
  - **Factors B, D**, and **P** (properdin) – found only in the alternate pathway
- **C3** – common to and is the convergence point for both pathways
- **Mg** – required for both pathways
- **Anaphylatoxins** – C3a, C4a, C5a; ↑ vascular permeability, bronchoconstriction; activate mast cells and basophils
- **Membrane attack complex** – C5b, C6b, C7b, C8b, C9b; causes **cell lysis** (usually bacteria) by creating a hole in the cell membrane
- **Opsonization** (targets antigen for immune response) – **C3b** and C4b
- **Chemotaxis** for inflammatory cells – **C3a** and C5a

PROSTAGLANDINS

- Cyclooxygenase pathway (platelets and endothelium-derived)
- Produced from arachidonic precursors
- **PGI$_2$** and **PGE$_2$** – vasodilation, bronchodilation, ↑ permeability; inhibit platelets
- **NSAIDs** – inhibit cyclooxygenase (reversible)
- **Aspirin** – inhibits cyclooxygenase (irreversible), inhibits platelet adhesion by decreasing TXA$_2$
- **Steroids** – inhibit phospholipase, which converts phospholipids to arachidonic acid → inhibits inflammation

LEUKOTRIENES

- Lipoxygenase pathway (leukocyte-derived)
- Produced from arachidonic precursors
- **LTC$_4$, LTD$_4$, LTE$_4$** – slow-reacting substances of anaphylaxis; bronchoconstriction, vasoconstriction followed by increased permeability (wheal and flare)
- **LTB$_4$** – chemotactic for inflammatory cells

CATECHOLAMINES

- Peak **24–48 hours** after injury
- Norepinephrine released from sympathetic postganglionic neurons
- Epinephrine and norepinephrine released from adrenal medulla (neural response to injury)

MISCELLANEOUS

- **Neuroendocrine response to injury** – afferent nerves from site of injury stimulate CRF, ACTH, ADH, growth hormone, epinephrine, and norepinephrine release
- **Thyroid hormone** – does _not_ play a major role in injury or inflammation
- **CXC chemokines** – chemotaxis, angiogenesis, wound healing
  - **IL-8** and **platelet factor 4** are CXC chemokines
  - C = cysteine; X = another amino acid
- Oxidants generated in inflammation (oxidants/main producer oxidase):
  Superoxide anion radical (O_2^-)   NADPH oxidase
  Hydrogen peroxide (H_2O_2)   Xanthine oxidase
- Cellular defenses against oxidative species (oxidants/defense):
  Superoxide anion radical   _**Superoxide dismutase**_
  Hydrogen peroxide   _Glutathione **peroxidase**, **catalase**_
- **Reperfusion injury** – **PMNs** are the primary mediator
- **Chronic granulomatous disease** – NADPH-oxidase system enzyme defect in PMNs
  - Results in ↓ superoxide radical (O_2^-) formation
- Primary mechanism of injury for oxygen radicals – DNA damage
- Respiratory burst (macrophages and PMNs) – release of superoxide anion and hydrogen peroxide

14 Wound Healing

WOUND HEALING

- **Inflammation** (days 1–10) – PMNs, macrophages: TNF-alpha, IL-1, PDGF
- **Proliferation** (5 days–3 weeks) – fibroblasts (deposit **collagen**), neovascularization, **granulation tissue** formation; type III collagen replaced with type I; **epithelialization** (1–2 mm/day); PDGF, FGF, EGF
- **Remodeling** (3 weeks–1 year) – decreased vascularity
  - Net amount of collagen does not change with remodeling, although significant production and degradation occur.
  - Collagen **cross-linking** occurs.
- **Peripheral nerves** regenerate at **1 mm/day**.
- **Order of cell arrival in wound**
  - **Platelets**
  - **PMNs**
  - **Macrophages**
  - **Lymphocytes** (recent research shows arrival before fibroblasts)
  - **Fibroblasts**

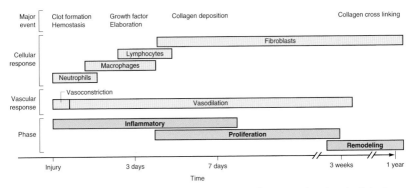

Timeline of phases of wound healing with dominant cell types and major physiologic events.

- *Macrophages are essential for wound healing (release of growth factors, cytokines, etc.).*
- **Fibronectin** – produced by fibroblasts; chemotactic for macrophages; anchors fibroblasts
- **Provisional matrix** – mostly fibronectin and **hyaluronic acid**
- **Fibroblasts** – replace fibronectin-fibrin with **collagen**
- **Predominant cell type by day**
  - **Days 0–2** – PMNs
  - **Days 3–4** – macrophages
  - **Days 5 and on** – fibroblasts
- **Platelet plug** – platelets and fibrin
- **Accelerated wound healing** – reopening a wound results in quicker healing the 2nd time (as healing cells are already present there)

- **Epithelial integrity** – most important factor in healing **open wounds** (secondary intention)
  - Migration from **hair follicles** (#1 site), wound edges, and sweat glands
  - Dependent on **granulation tissue** in wound
  - Unepithelialized wounds leak serum and protein, promote bacteria.
- **Tensile strength** – most important factor in healing **closed incisions** (primary intention)
  - Depends on collagen deposition and cross-linking of collagen
- **Suture removal**
  - Face – 1 week
  - Other areas – 2 weeks
- **Delayed primary closure** – thought to prevent wound infection; risk of abscess formation after closure
- **Submucosa** – strength layer of bowel
  - Weakest time point for small bowel anastomosis – 3–5 days
- **Myofibroblasts** (smooth muscle cell–fibroblast; communicate by **gap junctions**)
  - Involved in **wound contraction** and healing by **secondary intention**
  - Perineum has better wound contraction than leg.

Collagen Subtypes

Type	Description
I	Most common type of collagen: **skin**, **bone**, and **tendons**
	Primary collagen in a **healed wound**
II	**Cartilage**
III	Increased in **healing wound**, also in **blood vessels** and **skin**
IV	**Basement membranes**
V	Widespread, particularly found in the **cornea**

- **Alpha-ketoglutarate**, **vitamin C**, **oxygen**, and **iron** are required for collagen synthesis; includes hydroxylation (prolyl hydroxylase) and subsequent **cross-linking of proline residues** in collagen
  - Collagen has proline every 3rd amino acid.
  - Proline cross-linking improves **wound tensile strength**.
- **Scurvy** – vitamin C deficiency
- **Zinc** – important for many enzyme reactions involved in wound healing
- **Tensile strength never equal to pre-wound** (80%)
  - **Type III collagen** – predominant collagen type synthesized during proliferation
  - **Type I collagen** – predominant collagen type synthesized during remodeling
  - Type III replaced by type I collagen by 3 weeks
    - **At 8 weeks**, wound reaches maximum tensile strength, which is 80% of its original strength.
    - Maximum collagen accumulation at **3 weeks** → after that the amount of collagen stays the same, but continued **cross-linking** improves strength
    - **D-Penicillamine** – inhibits collagen cross-linking
- **Essentials for wound healing**
  - **Moist** environment (avoid desiccation)
  - **Oxygen delivery** – optimize fluids, no smoking, pain control, arterial revascularization, supplemental oxygen
    - Want transcutaneous oxygen measurement (TCOM) > 25 mm Hg
  - **Avoid edema** – leg elevation
  - **Remove necrotic tissue.**

- **Impediments to wound healing**
  - **Bacteria > $10^5/cm^2$** – ↓ oxygen content, collagen lysis, prolonged inflammation
  - **Devitalized tissue** and **foreign bodies** – retards granulation tissue formation and wound healing
  - **Cytotoxic drugs** – 5FU, methotrexate, cyclosporine, FK-506, etc. can impair wound healing in 1st 14 days after injury
  - **Diabetes** – can contribute to poor wound healing by impeding the early-phase inflammation response (hyperglycemia causes poor leukocyte chemotaxis)
  - **Albumin < 3.0** – risk factor for poor wound healing
  - **Steroids** – prevent wound healing by inhibiting macrophages, PMNs, and collagen synthesis by fibroblasts; ↓ wound tensile strength as well
  - **Vitamin A** (25,000 IU qd) – counteracts effects of steroids on wound healing
  - **Wound ischemia** (hypoxia) – can be caused by fibrosis, pressure (sacral decubitus ulcer, pressure sores), poor arterial inflow (atherosclerosis), poor venous outflow (venous stasis), smoking, radiation, edema, vasculitis
- **Diseases associated with abnormal wound healing**
  - **Osteogenesis imperfecta** – type I collagen defect
  - **Ehlers–Danlos syndrome** – 10 types identified, all collagen disorders
  - **Marfan's syndrome** – fibrillin defect (connective tissue protein)
  - **Epidermolysis bullosa** – excessive fibroblasts. Tx: phenytoin
  - **Scurvy** – vitamin C deficiency
  - **Pyoderma gangrenosum – Tx: steroids**
- **Wound dehiscence** – leakage of large amounts of pink "salmon-colored" fluid from wound; if left alone, can result in evisceration
  - **Risk factors** – deep wound infection (#1); poor nutrition, COPD, DM, coughers
  - Tx: place retention sutures
- **Diabetic foot ulcers** – usually at **Charcot's joint** (2nd MTP joint); secondary to **neuropathy** (can't feel feet, pressure from walking leads to ischemia); also on **heel**
- **Leg ulcers** – 90% due to **venous insufficiency**; Tx: Unna boot (elastic wrap), **pentoxifylline, ASA**
- **Scars** – contain a lot of proteoglycans, **hyaluronic acid**, and water
  - **Scar revisions** – wait for 1 year to allow maturation; may improve with age
  - **Infants** heal with **little or no scarring**.
- **Cartilage** – contains no blood vessels (get nutrients and oxygen by **diffusion**)
- **Denervation** – has no effect on wound healing
- **Chemotherapy** – has no effect on wound healing after 14 days
- **Keloids** – autosomal dominant; dark skinned
  - **Collagen goes beyond original scar**; from failure of collagen breakdown
  - Tx: intra-lesion steroid injection; silicone, pressure garments, XRT
- **Hypertrophic scar tissue** – dark skinned; **flexor surfaces** of upper torso
  - **Collagen stays within confines of original scar.**
  - Often occurs in burns or wounds that take a long time to heal
  - Tx: **steroid injection**, silicone, pressure garments

PLATELET GRANULES

- **Alpha granules**
  - **Platelet factor 4** – aggregation
  - **Coagulation factors V and VIII**
  - **vWF**
  - **Fibrinogen**
  - **Beta-thrombomodulin** – binds thrombin
  - **Platelet-derived growth factor** (PDGF) – chemoattractant
  - Transforming growth factor beta (TGF-beta) – modulates above responses
- **Dense granules** – contain **adenosine, serotonin**, and **calcium**
- Platelet aggregation factors – **TXA_2, thrombin, platelet factor 4**

15 Trauma

TRAUMA STATISTICS/EARLY ISSUES

- **1st peak** for trauma deaths (0–30 minutes) – deaths due to lacerations of heart, aorta, brain, brainstem, or spinal cord; cannot really save these patients; death is too quick
- **2nd peak** for trauma deaths (30 minutes–4 hours) – deaths due to head injury (#1) and hemorrhage (#2); these patients can be saved with rapid assessment (golden hour)
- **3rd peak** for trauma deaths (days to weeks) – deaths due to multisystem organ failure and sepsis
- **Blunt injury** – 80% of all trauma; <u>liver</u> most commonly injured (some texts say spleen)
  - Kinetic energy $= \frac{1}{2} MV^2$, where M = mass, V = velocity
  - **Falls** – age and body orientation biggest predictors of survival. LD_{50} is 4 stories.
- Start with **primary survey** after patient arrives (ABCDEs).
- **Penetrating injury** – <u>small bowel</u> most commonly injured (some texts say liver)
- **Head injury** – most common cause of death after reaching the ER alive
- **Infection** – most common cause of death in the long term
- **Tongue** – most common cause of upper airway obstruction → perform jaw thrust
- **Seat belt sign** – concern for small bowel perforations, pancreatic injury, lumbar spine fractures, sternal fractures
- **Saphenous vein** at ankle – best cutdown site for venous access if large bore IV and central access not possible
- **Intra-osseous proximal tibia cannulation** – preferred alternative route in children < 6
- **Hemorrhage** – most common cause of death in 1st hour
  - **Blood pressure** is usually OK until 30% of total blood volume is lost.
  - Resuscitate with **2 L Lactated Ringers**, then switch to **blood**.
- **Hemorrhagic shock – tachycardia** (HR > 100) and **narrowed pulse pressure** are first signs
  - SBP < 90; pale, shivering, cold, clammy, anxious, poor urine output (< 0.5 cc/kg/hr)
- **Single patient with visible bleeding source** – apply local pressure (gloved finger/hand) until definitive management
- **Massive civilian casualties with visible bleeding sources** – apply tourniquets until definitive management (health care provider can treat multiple patients)
- **Acute traumatic coagulopathy/hemostatic resuscitation**
  - **Coagulopathy** occurs in **severely injured** trauma patients <u>*prior*</u> to resuscitation and arriving at the hospital; **hypothermia** and **acidosis** also occur.
    - Can result in **massive transfusion**; increases morbidity and mortality
    - **Hemostatic resuscitation** is indicated for patients receiving ≥ **4 units** pRBCs in the *first hour or* ≥ **10 units pRBCs** within 24 hours (approximate indications).
  - **Hemostatic resuscitation** – give **RBCs:FFP:platelets** in a ratio of **1:1:1**
  - Also early correction of **hypothermia/acidosis/hypocalcemia**
  - Consider **tranexamic acid** (decreases fibrinolysis and reduces bleeding; 1 g load then 1 g over 8 hours).
- **Damage control surgery** (for severely injured trauma patients)
  - Early control of **bleeding** (surgical and/or interventional) and **contamination** with *delay* in definitive surgery until patient is stabilized
  - Give **blood products** (hemostatic resuscitation) to ensure <u>oxygenation</u> and correct <u>coagulopathy</u> (*not give continued lactated Ringers*).
  - <u>*Limit*</u> *crystalloid solutions* to avoid hemodilution (initial 2 L LR *only*).
  - Allow **permissive hypotension** (SBP > 80) until hemorrhage controlled (after that want SBP > 90).
  - <u>*Exceptions*</u> – traumatic brain injury patients (want SBP > 90 initially)

- Prolonged abdominal surgery, multiple transfusions, now coagulopathic with hypothermia and acidosis – Tx: pack off bleeders, temporary abdominal closure, to ICU for resuscitation, warming, and correction of coagulopathy
- **Diagnostic peritoneal lavage** (DPL; generally not used **anymore**)
  - Used in hypotensive patients (SBP < 90) with blunt trauma
  - Positive if > 10 cc blood, > 100,000 RBCs/cc, food particles, bile, bacteria, > 500 WBC/cc
  - Need laparotomy if DPL is positive
  - DPL needs to be supraumbilical if pelvic fracture present.
  - **DPL misses** – retroperitoneal bleeds, contained hematomas
- **FAST scan** (focused abdominal sonography for trauma)
  - Ultrasound scan used in lieu of DPL
  - Checks for **fluid** (ie blood, urine, succus) in peri-hepatic fossa, peri-splenic fossa, pelvis, and pericardium
  - Examiner dependent; less sensitivity/specificity compared to CT scan
  - Obesity can obstruct view.
  - May not detect free fluid < 50–80 mL
  - Need laparotomy if FAST scan is positive
  - **FAST scan misses** (false negatives) – retroperitoneal bleed, hollow viscous injury, pancreatic injury
- In hypotensive patients with a **negative FAST scan** (or negative DPL), you need to find the source of bleeding (**pelvic fracture, chest,** or **extremity**).
- **Need abdominal CT scan with contrast following blunt trauma in patients** with: abdominal pain, need for general anesthesia, closed head injury, intoxicants on board, paraplegia, distracting injury, or hematuria
  - Patients requiring DPL that turned out negative will need an abdominal CT scan.
  - **CT scan misses** – hollow viscous injury, diaphragm injury
- **Need exploratory laparotomy** with peritonitis, evisceration, positive DPL, uncontrolled visceral hemorrhage (unstable patient), free air, diaphragm injury, intraperitoneal bladder injury, contrast extravasation from hollow viscus, specific renal, pancreas, biliary tract, and spleen and liver injuries, positive FAST scan
- **Penetrating abdominal gunshot wound** (GSW) – requires exploratory laparotomy
  - Any entrance or exit wound below nipple considered to involve abdomen (includes flank)

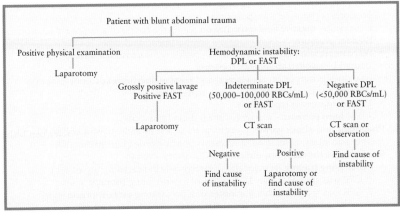

Diagnosis of blunt abdominal trauma.

- **Anterior abdominal stab wounds**
  - If patient **unstable** – laparotomy
  - If patient is **stable** – need local exploration in ED to check **fascia** (anterior rectus sheath or superior abdominal oblique fascia)
    - If fascia <u>not</u> violated – can **observe** and **discharge** from ED
    - If fascia violated – **diagnostic laparoscopy** to see if peritoneum entered (some suggest CT scan and serial exams)
- **Flank stab wounds** – possible injury to **retroperitoneal contents** (eg colon, kidney, ureter)
  - Dx: abdominal CT scan with oral, rectal, and IV contrast (triple contrast)
- **Thoracoabdominal stab wound** – difficulty diagnosing a **diaphragm injury** even with CT
  - Dx: diagnostic laparoscopy

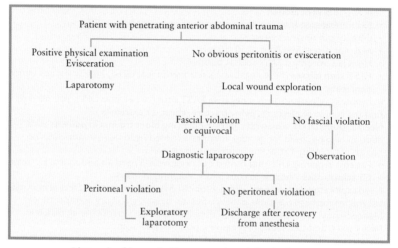

Diagnosis of low-velocity penetrating abdominal trauma.

- **Abdominal compartment syndrome**
  - Sx's – hypotension, distended abdomen, low urine output, increased airway pressures, prolonged transport time
  - Occurs after **massive fluid resuscitation** during the course of a prolonged laparotomy
  - **Bladder pressure** > 25–30 suggests compartment syndrome.
  - **IVC compression** is the final common pathway for *decreased cardiac output*.
  - Caused by **swollen abdominal contents**
  - Low cardiac output causes **visceral** and **renal malperfusion** ($\downarrow$ urine output).
  - Upward displacement of diaphragm causes hypoxia.
  - Tx: decompressive laparotomy
    - For **burn patients** – place peritoneal drain for ascites
- **Pneumatic anti-shock garment** – controversial; use in patients with SBP < 50 and no thoracic injury. Release compartments one at a time after reaching ER.
- **Resuscitative thoracotomy indications** (ED thoracotomy)
  - **Penetrating trauma** (resuscitative thoracotomy indicated for <u>any</u> below):
    1. CPR was started within **15 minutes** of a penetrating **thoracic** injury.
    2. CPR was started within **5 minutes** of a penetrating **extra-thoracic** injury (eg penetrating abdominal trauma).
    3. Patient had **signs of life** and pulse or pressure was lost (SBP < 60) on **way to ED** or **in ED**.

- **Blunt trauma** – resuscitative thoracotomy only if pressure or pulse lost **in ED** (CPR started within 5 minutes)
- Tx: anterolateral thoracotomy, rib spreader, open pericardium anterior to phrenic nerve, control any cardiac injury (digital compression), cross-clamp aorta (watch for esophagus anterior to aorta; feel for NG tube), control bleeding source if not already identified, cardiac massage, resuscitation
- **Catecholamines** – peak 24–48 hours after injury
- **ADH, ACTH**, and **glucagon** – also ↑ after trauma (fight or flight response)
- Thyroid hormone <u>not</u> involved

BLOOD TRANSFUSION

- <u>Type O blood</u> (universal donor) – contains no A or B antigens; males can receive Rh-positive blood; females who are prepubescent or of childbearing age should receive Rh-negative blood
- <u>Type-specific blood</u> (nonscreened, non-cross-matched) – can be administered relatively safely, but there may be effects from antibodies to HLA minor antigens in the donated blood

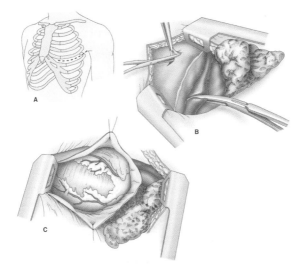

(A) Emergency department thoracotomies are performed through the fourth and fifth intercostal spaces using the anterolateral approach. **(B)** If the thoracotomy is performed for abdominal injury, the descending thoracic aorta is clamped. If blood pressure improved to > 70 mm Hg, the patient is transported to the operating room for laparotomy. For patients in whom blood pressure does not reach 70 mm Hg, further treatment is futile. If the thoracotomy is performed for a cardiac injury, the pericardium is opened longitudinally and anterior to the phrenic nerve. **(C)** The heart can then be rotated out of the pericardium for repair.

HEAD INJURY

- **Glasgow Coma Scale (GCS)**
  - **Motor**
    - **6** – follows commands
    - **5** – localizes pain
    - **4** – withdraws from pain

- **3** – flexion with pain (decorticate)
- **2** – extension with pain (decerebrate)
- **1** – no response
- **Verbal**
  - **5** – oriented
  - **4** – confused
  - **3** – inappropriate words
  - **2** – incomprehensible sounds
  - **1** – no response
- **Eye opening**
  - **4** – spontaneous opening
  - **3** – opens to command
  - **2** – opens to pain
  - **1** – no response
- **GCS score** – ≤ **14** – head CT; ≤ **8** – intubation and (with head injury) ICP monitor
- Most important prognostic indicator – **motor score**

Indications for Head CT

- Suspected skull penetration by a foreign body
- Discharge of cerebrospinal fluid (CSF), blood, or both from the nose
- Hemotympanum or discharge of blood or CSF from the ear
- Head injury with alcohol or drug intoxication
- Altered state of consciousness at the time of examination
- Focal neurologic signs or symptoms
- Any situation precluding proper surveillance (eg going to the OR)
- Head injury plus additional trauma
- Loss of consciousness at any point

- **Penetrating injury** has worst survival of all head injuries.
- Intubated patients get a score of 1T for verbal.
- Neurologic damage in trauma can be caused by the **initial blow**, subsequent **hematoma**, and later **brain swelling**.
- **Epidural hematoma** – most commonly due to arterial bleeding from the **middle meningeal artery**
  - Head CT – shows lenticular (lens-shaped) deformity
  - Patients often have loss of consciousness (LOC) → then lucid interval (awake) → then sudden deterioration (vomiting, restlessness, LOC)
  - Craniotomy for significant neurologic deterioration or shift > 5 mm
- **Subdural hematoma** – most commonly from tearing of **venous plexus** (bridging veins) that cross between the dura and arachnoid
  - **Head CT** – shows crescent-shaped deformity
  - Craniotomy for significant neurologic deterioration or shift > 5 mm
  - **Chronic subdural hematomas** – usually in elderly after minor fall or severe alcoholics; mental status deteriorates over days to weeks as hematoma forms
- **Intracerebral hematoma** (intraparenchymal hemorrhage) – usually **frontal** or temporal
  - Most common brain injury in trauma (occurs with blunt trauma)
  - Can cause significant mass effect requiring operation
- **Cerebral contusions** – can be coup or contrecoup
- **Traumatic intraventricular hemorrhage** – need **ventriculostomy** if causing hydrocephalus
- **Diffuse axonal injury** – shows up better on **MRI** than CT scan
  - **MRI** – blurring of gray-white matter; multiple small punctate hemorrhages
  - Tx: supportive; may need craniectomy if refractory ICP elevation
  - Very poor prognosis

- **Cerebral perfusion pressure** (CPP = MAP − ICP; indicates cerebral blood flow)
  - **CPP** = mean arterial pressure (MAP) *minus* intracranial pressure (ICP)
  - **Signs of elevated ICP** − ↓ ventricular size, loss of sulci, loss of cisterns
  - Reduced CPP results in **secondary traumatic brain injury**.
  - **ICP monitors** (intraparenchymal bolt) – indicated for GCS ≤ 8 with head injury, suspected ↑ ICP, or patient with moderate to severe head injury and inability to follow clinical exam (eg is intubated)
- **Supportive treatment for elevated ICP**
  - Normal ICP is 10; > 20 needs treatment (want ICP < 20)
  - Want CPP > 60 (give volume and pressors [eg phenylephrine] to improve MAP)
  - **Sedation** and **paralysis** (decrease brain activity and oxygen demand)
  - **Raise head of bed** (lowers ICP).
  - **Relative hyperventilation** for modest cerebral vasoconstriction (keep CO_2 30–35); do not want to over-hyperventilate and cause cerebral ischemia from too much vasoconstriction
  - Keep **Na 140–150, serum Osm 295–310** – may need to use <u>hypertonic saline</u> at times (draws fluid out of brain)
  - **Mannitol** – load 1 g/kg, give 0.25 mg/kg q4h after that (draws fluid from brain)
  - Consider **removing C collar** (improves cerebral perfusion).
  - **Barbiturate coma** – consider if above not working
  - **Ventriculostomy w/ CSF drainage** (keep ICP < 20)
  - **Craniotomy decompression** – if not able to get ICP down medically (can also perform burr hole)
  - **Fosphenytoin** or **Keppra** (for 1 week) – given prophylactically to prevent seizures with moderate to severe head injury
  - **Peak ICP** (max brain swelling) – occurs **48–72 hours** after injury
  - **Cushing's reflex** (triad) – bradycardia, HTN, low/altered respirations (Cheyne-Stokes breathing); late sign that indicates impending brain herniation
  - **Secondary brain injury** – from hypotension and/or hypoxia (try to avoid)
- **Dilated pupil (blown pupil)**
  - Possible **ipsilateral temporal lobe pressure** on **CN III** (oculomotor)
  - Blown pupil and patient **stable** – get head CT (patient may have baseline anisocoria)
  - Blown pupil and patient **unstable** – address hypotension before getting head CT (eg go to the OR for significant abdominal bleeding; angiography for significant pelvic bleeding); consider burr hole if not able to make it to head CT for a while
- **Basal skull fractures**
  - **Raccoon eyes** (peri-orbital ecchymosis) – anterior fossa fracture
  - **Battle's sign** (mastoid ecchymosis) – middle fossa fracture; can injure **facial nerve** (CN VII)
    - If acute facial nerve injury, need exploration and repair
    - If delayed, likely secondary to edema and exploration not needed
  - Can also have hemotympanum and CSF rhinorrhea/otorrhea with basal skull fractures
  - *Avoid* nasotracheal intubation in these patients.
- **Temporal skull fractures** – can injure CN VII and VIII (vestibulocochlear nerve)
  - Most common site of **facial nerve injury** – *geniculate ganglion*
  - Temporal skull fractures most commonly associated with lateral skull or orbital blows
- **Most skull fractures do <u>not</u> require surgical treatment.**
  - Operate if **significantly depressed** (> 1 cm), **contaminated** (open fracture), or **persistent CSF leak** not responding to conservative therapy (close dura).
- **CSF leaks** after skull fracture – treat expectantly; can use **lumbar CSF drainage** if persistent

- **Coagulopathy** with **traumatic brain injury** – due to release of **tissue thromboplastin**
- **Head trauma and on Coumadin/NOAC**
  - If head CT is **abnormal** – reverse with PCC or NOAC reversal agent
  - If head CT is **normal** – repeat head CT in 8 hours (can have delayed bleeds)
- **Hypovolemic shock cannot occur from intracranial bleeding alone** – need to look for another source or the patient has neurogenic shock

SPINE TRAUMA

- The higher the spine injury, the greater the morbidity and mortality.
- Screening for spine injury – CT scan
- Significant head injury – need to assess C-spine
- Best indication for steroids with spine injury – worsening deficit
- **Cervical spine** (MC spine injury)
  - **C-1 burst** (Jefferson fracture) – caused by axial loading
    - Tx: rigid collar
  - **C-2 hangman's fracture** – caused by distraction and extension
    - Tx: traction and halo
  - **C-2 odontoid fracture**
    - Type I – above base, stable
    - Type II – at base, unstable (will need fusion or halo)
    - Type III – extends into vertebral body (will need fusion or halo)
  - **Facet** fractures or dislocations – can cause cord injury; usually associated with hyperextension and rotation with ligamentous disruption
  - **Dens = odontoid process**
  - **Clinical clearance of C spine** – must have no other injuries, GCS 15, not intoxicated, no neck tenderness, and no neuro deficits
- **Thoracolumbar spine**
  - 3 columns of the thoracolumbar spine:
    - <u>Anterior</u> – anterior longitudinal ligament and anterior ½ of the vertebral body
    - <u>Middle</u> – posterior ½ of the vertebral body and posterior longitudinal ligament
    - <u>Posterior</u> – facet joints, lamina, spinous processes, interspinous ligament
  - If **more than 1 column** is disrupted, the spine is considered **unstable** and needs **operative fixation**.
    - **Compression** (wedge) **fractures** usually involve the anterior column only and are considered stable (Tx: TLSO brace).
    - **Burst fractures** are considered unstable (anterior and middle; > 1 column) and require spinal fusion.
  - **Upright fall** – at risk for calcaneus, lumbar, and wrist/forearm fractures
- Need **MRI** for neurologic deficits without bony injury to check for ligamentous injury
- MRI also indicated for prevertebral soft tissue swelling without bony injury
- **Indications for emergent surgical spine decompression**
  - Fracture or dislocation not reducible with distraction
  - Open fractures
  - Soft tissue or bony compression of the cord
  - Progressive neurologic dysfunction
- **Spinal shock** – refers to sensory/motor deficits (<u>not</u> hypotension)

MAXILLOFACIAL TRAUMA

- Fracture of **temporal bone** is the most common cause of <u>facial nerve injury</u> (at the geniculate ganglion).
- Try to preserve skin and not trim edges with facial lacerations.

Le Fort Classification of Facial Fractures

Type	Description	Treatment
I	Maxillary fracture straight across (−)	Reduction, stabilization, intramaxillary fixation (IMF) ± circumzygomatic and orbital rim suspension wires
II	Lateral to nasal bone, underneath eyes, diagonal toward maxilla (/ \)	Same as Le Fort I
III	Lateral orbital walls (- -)	Suspension wiring to stable frontal bone; may need external fixation

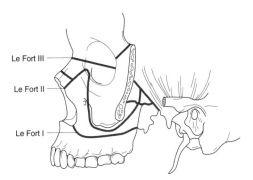

Le Fort classification system of maxillofacial fractures.

- **Nasoethmoidal orbital fractures** – 70% have a CSF leak (tau protein)
  - Conservative therapy for up to **2 weeks**
  - Can try epidural catheter to ↓ CSF pressure and help it close CSF leak
  - May need surgical closure of **dura** to stop leak
- **Nosebleeds**
  - **Anterior** – packing
  - **Posterior** – can be hard to deal with; try balloon tamponade 1st
    - May need angioembolization of **internal maxillary artery** or ethmoidal artery
- **Orbital blowout fractures** – patients with impaired upward gaze or diplopia with upward vision need repair; perform restoration of orbital floor with bone fragments or bone graft
- **Mandibular injury** – malocclusion #1 indicator of injury
  - Diagnosis – fine-cut facial CT scans with reconstruction to assess injury
  - Most repaired with IMF (metal arch bars to upper and lower dental arches, 6–8 weeks) or open reduction and internal fixation (ORIF)
- **Tripod fracture** (zygomatic bone) – ORIF for cosmesis
- Patients w/ maxillofacial fractures are at high risk for **cervical spine injuries.**
- **Scalp lacerations** – hair removal is generally <u>not</u> necessary

NECK TRAUMA

- **Asymptomatic blunt** – neck CTA (include C-spine assessment)
- **Asymptomatic penetrating** – neck CTA; need **EGD** or **esophagram** for zone I and II injuries; include **chest** in neck CTA for zone I injuries

Neck Zones

Zone	Surgical Approach
I	Clavicle to cricoid cartilage – **median sternotomy** is needed to reach these lesions
II	Cricoid to angle of mandible – **lateral neck incision**
III	Angle of mandible to the base of skull – **lateral neck incision**; may need jaw subluxation, digastric and sternocleidomastoid muscle release, and/or mastoid sinus resection to reach vascular injuries in this location

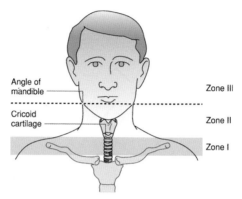

Zones of the neck. Zone I is the cricoid cartilage to the top of the clavicles.
The important implication of a zone I injury is the greater potential for intrathoracic great vessel injury.

- **Symptomatic blunt** or **penetrating neck trauma** (Sx's – shock, bleeding, expanding hematoma, losing or lost airway, subcutaneous air, stridor, dysphagia, hemoptysis, neurologic deficit) → **all need exploration** (use approaches listed above)
- **Blunt cerebrovascular injury** (have low threshold for imaging) – need **neck CTA** for any significant blunt head/neck injury (eg Le Fort II and III, basilar skull Fx, DAI, cervical spine Fx), any hyperflexion/hyperextension/rotation mechanism (eg attempted hanging), neuro finding not explained by brain imaging, epistaxis from suspected arterial source, or GCS < 8 with head injury
  - Isolated neck skin seatbelt sign (without soft tissue injury) _not_ considered a risk factor
  - **Distal internal carotid artery** most common site (can have dissection, transection, arterio-venous fistula, or pseudoaneurysm)
  - **Completely occluded** carotid Tx: **Plavix** or **heparin** to prevent clot propagation
  - **Partially occluded** carotid and **symptomatic** Tx: **covered stent** (open repair if that fails)
  - **Partially occluded** carotid and **asymptomatic** Tx: **Plavix** or **heparin**; repeat CTA before discharge
  - Carotid **AV fistula, pseudoaneurysm, or symptomatic partially occluded dissection** Tx: **covered stent**
  - Isolated cervical seat belt sign without symptoms is _not_ enough to warrant neck CTA.
- **Esophageal injury**
  - *Hardest neck injury to find*
  - **Esophagoscopy** and **esophagogram** – best combined modality (find essentially 95% of injuries when using both methods)
  - **Contained injuries** – can be observed

- **Noncontained injuries:**
  - If **small** injury and **minimal contamination** → <u>primary closure</u> (see Esophagus chapter)
  - If **extensive** injury or significant **contamination** (ie can't repair) →
    - **Neck** esophageal injuries – just place drains for wide drainage (will heal on its own; also used it you can't find injury)
    - **Chest** esophageal injuries – chest tubes to drain injury and place spit fistula in neck (will eventually need esophagectomy)
- Always drain esophageal and hypopharyngeal repairs – 20% leak rate
- Approach to esophageal injuries
  - Neck – **left side**
  - Upper ½ of thoracic esophagus – **right thoracotomy** (avoids aorta)
  - Lower ⅓ of thoracic esophagus – **left thoracotomy** (left-sided course)
- **Laryngeal fracture** and **tracheal injuries**
  - These are **airway emergencies** (addressed in **primary survey**).
  - Symptoms: **crepitus, stridor, respiratory compromise**
  - Need to **secure airway emergently in ER** (Tx: cricothyroidotomy)
  - Tx: primary repair, can use strap muscle for airway support; tracheostomy necessary for most to allow edema to subside and to check for stricture (need to convert cricothyroidotomy to tracheostomy)
- **Thyroid gland injuries** – control bleeding (suture ligate) and drain (<u>not</u> thyroidectomy)
- **Recurrent laryngeal nerve injury** – can try to repair or can reimplant in <u>cricoarytenoid muscle</u> (Sx – hoarseness)
- **Shotgun injures to neck** – need angiogram and neck CT; esophagus/trachea evaluation
- **Vertebral artery bleeds** (posterior neck arterial bleeding) – can embolize or ligate (no sequela in majority)
- **Common/internal carotid artery bleeds** – ligation will cause stroke in 20%
- **External carotid artery** – can be ligated for extensive facial fracture bleeding
- **Expanding neck hematoma** – can compromise airway
- **Cricothyroidotomy** – indicated if usual intubation cannot be accomplished (eg severe maxillofacial trauma, airway foreign body, severe laryngospasm) and patient has impending loss of airway

CHEST TRAUMA

- **Chest tube placement** (for hemothorax)
  - > 1,500 cc after initial insertion, > 200 cc/h for 4 hours, > 2,500 cc/24 h, or bleeding with instability → all indications for **thoracotomy in OR** (anterolateral on side of injury; keep patient supine)
  - Need to drain all of the blood (in < 48 hours) to prevent fibrothorax, pulmonary entrapment, infected hemothorax, and empyema
  - **Unresolved hemothorax** (retained hemothorax) after 2 well-placed chest tubes → Tx: VATS drainage
  - Most important RF for empyema – **retained hemothorax**
- **Persistent pneumothorax** despite 2 well-placed chest tubes – Dx: bronchoscopy (look for mucus plug or tracheobronchial injury)
- **Multiple painful rib fractures** – consider local nerve block and thoracic epidural to prevent splinting and hypoxia (especially in elderly; also prevents atelectasis and pneumonia)
- **Sucking chest wound** (open pneumothorax)
  - Needs to be at least ⅔ the diameter of the trachea to be significant
  - Cover wound with dressing that has tape on three sides → prevents development of <u>tension pneumothorax</u> while allowing lung to expand with inspiration
- **Flail chest** – ≥ 2 consecutive ribs broken at ≥ 2 sites → results in paradoxical motion
  - Underlying **pulmonary contusion** – biggest pulmonary impairment (cause of hypoxia)
  - Tx: pain control (consider epidural), BiPAP (intubation if severe), consider rib plating

- **Pulmonary contusion** – very sensitive to fluid overload; need judicious use of fluids/diuretics after resuscitation period to prevent further pulmonary dysfunction
  - Deteriorating blood gases and lung opacities can occur up to 48 hours after initial trauma.
- **Tracheobronchial injury**
  - MC with blunt trauma
  - Sx's – large continuous air-leak; large pneumomediastinum, persistent pneumothorax, subcutaneous air
  - Patient may have worse oxygenation after chest tube placement.
  - One of the very few indications in which clamping the chest tube may be indicated
  - Bronchus injuries are more common on the **right**.
  - May need to **mainstem intubate** patient on unaffected side
  - Dx: bronchoscopy (90% are within 1 cm of the carina)
  - Tx: repair if <u>large air leak and respiratory compromise</u>, after <u>2 weeks of persistent air leak</u>, if you <u>can't get the lung up</u>, or if the <u>injury is > ⅓ the diameter of the trachea</u>
  - Intubate with long, single-lumen tube to the unaffected side (*avoid* dual-lumen tube which can worsen injury).
  - **Right thoracotomy** for <u>right mainstem, trachea, and proximal *left* mainstem injuries</u> (avoids the aorta)
  - **Left thoracotomy** for <u>distal left mainstem injuries (rare injury)</u>
  - **Bubbles** seen in heart after thoracotomy – likely **air embolism** through **pulmonary veins**
    - Could also be air in an intravenous line with patent foramen ovale (PFO)
- **Esophageal injury** – see section "Neck Trauma"; esophageal injuries are the hardest to Dx
- **Diaphragm**
  - Injuries are more likely to be found on **left** and to result from **blunt trauma.**
  - CXR – see **air–fluid level** in chest from <u>stomach herniation</u> through hole (diagnosis can be made essentially with CXR)
  - **Transabdominal** approach if **< 1 week**
  - **Chest** approach if **> 1 week** (need to take down adhesions in the chest)
  - May need PTFE mesh (Gore-Tex)

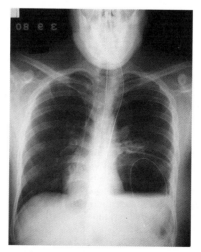

Chest roentgenogram demonstrating a nasogastric tube within the left chest.

- **Aortic transection** (blunt aortic injury)
  - **Signs** – widened mediastinum ($\geq$ 8 cm), 1st or 2nd rib fractures, apical capping, loss of aortopulmonary window, loss of aortic contour, left hemothorax, trachea deviation to right, NG tube deviation to the right, sternal fracture, scapular fracture, thoracic outlet hematoma, thoracic spine fracture
  - **Tear** is usually in the **proximal descending thoracic aorta** at the **ligamentum arteriosum** (just distal to left subclavian takeoff).
    - Other areas – near aortic valve and where aorta traverses diaphragm
  - Due to shearing from **sudden deceleration** (eg MVA, fall)
  - If the patient reaches hospital alive, the **adventitial layer** contained the hemorrhage (hematoma; considered partial transection), although this can potentially rupture leading to exsanguination.
  - CXR normal in 5% of patients with aortic tears (need high index of suspicion) – get aortic evaluation if significant mechanism (eg head on car crash > 45 mph, fall > 15 ft, other severe deceleration injuries)
  - Dx: CT angiogram of chest
  - Initial Tx: Maintain blood pressure between **100 and 120 mm Hg** (use esmolol if hypertensive; Nipride after that) until definitive repair.
  - **Important to identify and treat _other_ life-threatening injuries 1st** → (eg patient with positive DPL, pelvic fracture with shock, significant head bleed) – all addressed _before_ the aortic transection
  - Operative approach – place a **covered stent endograft** (distal transections only); if that fails – need **left thoracotomy and open repair** using partial left heart bypass
  - Significant intracerebral hemorrhage is a contraindication to open repair.
  - **Left hand ischemia** following endograft placement (ie graft covered left subclavian artery) Tx – **carotid to subclavian bypass**
- **Approach for specific injuries**
  - **Median sternotomy** – for injuries to ascending aorta, innominate artery, proximal right subclavian artery, innominate vein, proximal left common carotid, proximal left subclavian artery (use trap-door incision through the left 2nd intercostal space)
    - **Innominate vein** covers take-off of arch vessels
  - **Left thoracotomy** – for injuries to distal left subclavian artery, descending aorta
  - **Distal right subclavian artery** – midclavicular incision, resection of medial clavicle
- **Myocardial contusion** (blunt cardiac injury) – **sternal fracture** is highest risk factor
  - V-tach and V-fib most common causes of death; risk highest in 1st 24 hours
  - Dx: EKG and troponins
  - **Supra-ventricular tachycardia** (SVT; sinus tachycardia) – most common arrhythmia overall in these patients
  - **Normal EKG** and **normal troponin** rules out injury.
  - If **EKG abnormal**, **troponin abnormal**, or **patient unstable** despite usual trauma workup – need **echocardiogram**
  - Need **telemonitoring** for 24–48 hours
- **Aspiration** – may not produce CXR findings immediately
- **Penetrating chest injury** – start with a **CXR** if the patient is **stable** (place chest tube on side of injury for pneumothorax or hemothorax)
  - **Penetrating "box" injuries** – borders are clavicles, xiphoid process, nipples
  - Need pericardial window, bronchoscopy, esophagoscopy, barium swallow
  - Possible angiogram for high chest or low zone I neck injuries
  - **Penetrating chest wound outside "box"** without pneumothorax or hemothorax
    - Need chest tube if patient requires intubation
    - Otherwise follow patient's serial CXRs
  - **Pericardial window** – if you find blood, need **median sternotomy** to fix possible injury to heart or great vessels; place pericardial drain

- **Penetrating injuries anterior-medial to midaxillary line and below nipples**
  - Need laparotomy or laparoscopy
  - May also need evaluation for **penetrating "box" injury** depending on the exact location
  - Some are using FAST scan of the pericardium instead of pericardial window for "box" injuries.
- **Traumatic causes of cardiogenic shock** – cardiac tamponade, cardiac contusion, tension pneumothorax
- **Tension pneumothorax** (one way valve effect causes air entry and pressure build up)
  - Hypotension, tachycardia, ↑ airway pressures, ↓ breath sounds, bulging neck veins, tracheal shift
  - BP can worsen with intubation.
  - Can see bulging diaphragm during laparotomy
  - Cardiac compromise secondary to ↓ venous return to the right atrium (IVC, SVC compression)
  - Tx: chest tube (needle decompression through 2nd intercostal space an option if chest tube not available)
- **Sternal fractures** – these patients are at high risk for **cardiac contusion**
- **1st** and **2nd rib fractures** – high risk for aortic transection

PELVIC TRAUMA

- Pelvic fractures can be a major source of **blood loss**.
- If hemodynamically unstable with pelvic fracture and negative DPL, negative CXR, and no other signs of blood loss or reasons for shock →
  - Stabilize pelvis (C-clamp, external fixator, or sheet) and go to angio for **embolization**.
  - Some groups go to OR for **pre-peritoneal packing** if unstable patient, followed by angio.
- These patients are at high risk for **genitourinary** and **rectal injuries**.
- **Anterior pelvic fractures** – more likely to have venous bleeding; MC source of bleeding (pelvic venous plexus); pelvic fixation will tamponade most pelvic venous bleeding
- **Posterior pelvic fractures** – more likely to have arterial bleeding
- May need **diverting colostomy** for open pelvic fractures with rectal tears and perineal lacerations
- Pelvic fracture repair itself may need to be delayed until other associated injuries are repaired.
- Intraop **penetrating injury pelvic hematomas** – <u>open</u> (some suggest going to angiography for these)

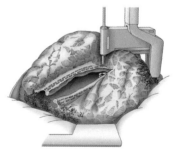

Pulmonary tractotomy. Dividing the pulmonary parenchyma between adjacent staple lines permits rapid direct access to injured vessels or bronchi along the tract of a penetrating injury.

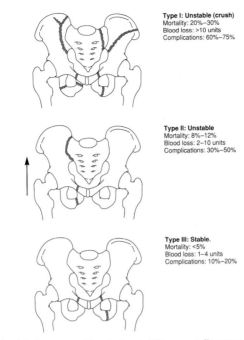

Type I: Unstable (crush)
Mortality: 20%–30%
Blood loss: >10 units
Complications: 60%–75%

Type II: Unstable
Mortality: 8%–12%
Blood loss: 2–10 units
Complications: 30%–50%

Type III: Stable.
Mortality: <5%
Blood loss: 1–4 units
Complications: 10%–20%

Classification of pelvic fractures with relative stability, mortality rates, and blood loss indicated.

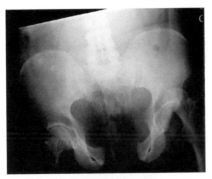

Wide pubic diastasis, characteristic of "open book" horizontally unstable pelvis (type B), with associated femoral head fracture and hip dislocation.

- Intraop **blunt injury pelvic hematomas** – <u>leave</u>; if expanding or patient unstable → stabilize pelvic fracture, pack pelvis if in OR, and go to angiography for **embolization**; if packs are placed intraop, remove after 24–48 hours when patient is stable
- Severe pelvic trauma requires proctoscopy and retrograde cystourethrogram to look for injuries; also need vaginal exam in women
- Isolated anterior ring fracture with minimal sacral-iliac displacement – Tx: weight bearing as tolerated
- MC associated injury with pelvic fracture – **head injury**

DUODENAL TRAUMA

- Usually from blunt trauma (crush or deceleration injury)
- Children can get duodenal hematoma from bicycle handle bar trauma.
- **2nd portion of the duodenum** (descending portion, near ampulla of Vater) – most common area of injury
- Can also get tears near ligament of Treitz
- 80% of injuries requiring surgery can be treated with **debridement** and **primary closure** (or primary anastomosis); residual bowel circumference should be ≥ 50% normal.
- **Segmental resection** with primary end-to-end closure possible with **all segments** *except* **second portion of the duodenum**.
- 25% mortality in these patients because of associated **shock**
- **Fistulas** are the major source of morbidity.
- **Intraop duodenal hematomas** (≥ **2 cm** considered significant; usually in third portion of duodenum overlying spine in blunt injury) – need to open for both blunt and penetrating injuries
- **Duodenal hematomas on CT scan** (or missed on initial CT scan)
  - Can present with high **small bowel obstruction** (SBO) 12–72 hours after injury
  - UGI study will show "**stacked coins**" or "**coiled spring**" appearance (make sure there is no extravasation of contrast).
  - Tx: **conservative** (NGT and TPN) – cures 90% over 2–3 weeks (hematoma is reabsorbed)

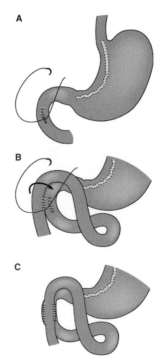

Jejunal serosal patch.

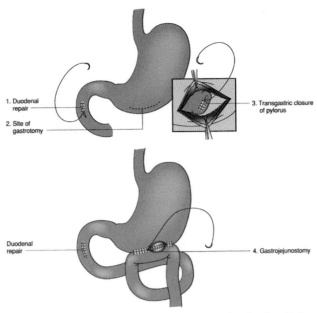

1. Duodenal repair
2. Site of gastrotomy
3. Transgastric closure of pylorus

Duodenal repair
4. Gastrojejunostomy

Gastro-jejunostomy and pyloric exclusion for complex duodenal injury.

- If at laparotomy and duodenal, biliary system, or pancreas injury suspected, perform **Kocher maneuver** and **open lesser sac** through the omentum; check for <u>hematoma</u>, <u>bile</u>, <u>succus</u>, and <u>fat necrosis</u> → if found, need formal inspection of the entire duodenum (also need to check for pancreatic/biliary system injury)
- **Diagnosing suspected duodenal injury** – abdominal CT with contrast initially. UGI contrast study best. CT scan may show bowel wall thickening, hematoma, free air, contrast leak, or retroperitoneal fluid/air.
  - If CT scan is worrisome for injury but nondiagnostic, can repeat the CT in 8-12 hours to see if the finding is getting worse
  - Free **intraperitoneal air** or **contrast leak** – Tx: go to the OR
- Tx: Try to get **primary repair** or **anastomosis**; may need to divert with <u>pyloric exclusion</u> and <u>gastrojejunostomy</u> to allow healing. Place a distal feeding jejunostomy and possibly a proximal draining jejunostomy tube that threads back to duodenal injury site. **Place drains.**
  - If **2nd portion of duodenum** and can't get primary repair
    - Place **jejunal serosal patch** over hole; may need Whipple in future
    - Need pyloric exclusion and gastrojejunostomy
    - Consider feeding and draining jejunostomies; leave drains.
    - Trauma Whipple is rarely if ever indicated (very high mortality).
  - **Drains** – remove when patient tolerating diet without an increase in drainage
  - **Fistulas** – often close with time; Tx: bowel rest, TPN, octreotide, conservative management for 4-6 weeks

SMALL BOWEL TRAUMA
- Most common organ injured with penetrating injury (some texts say liver)
- These injuries can be hard to diagnose early if associated with blunt trauma.

- **Free fluid** and <u>no</u> solid organ injury – considered a hollow viscous injury until proven otherwise
- **Occult small bowel injuries**
  - Abdominal CT scan showing **intra-abdominal fluid not associated with a solid organ injury, bowel wall thickening**, or a **mesenteric hematoma** is suggestive of injury.
  - **Need close observation and possibly repeat abdominal CT** after 8–12 hours or so to make sure finding is not getting worse
  - Need to make sure patients with these nonconclusive findings can **tolerate a diet before discharge**
- **Small lacerations** → repaired **transversely** (avoids **stricture)**
- **Large lacerations** (> **50% of bowel circumference** or results in **lumen diameter** < ⅓ **normal**) or if bowel is devascularized → perform resection and anastomosis
- **Multiple close lacerations** – just resect that segment
- Intra-op **mesenteric hematomas** – open if expanding or large (> 2 cm)
- **If damage control surgery** – just staple off and resect bowel <u>without</u> anastomosis

COLON TRAUMA (SIGMOID COLON CONSIDERED LEFT COLON HERE)

- Most associated with **penetrating** injury
- **Right** and **transverse colon** injuries Tx: 1) primary repair <u>or</u> 2) resection and anastomosis (for <u>destructive injuries</u> [ie > 50% circumference or associated with significant colon devascularization]); all are essentially treated like small bowel injuries.
  - *<u>No</u> diversion needed for right and transverse colon injuries*
- **Left colon** – perform *primary repair <u>without diversion</u> for all injuries if < 50% circumference and not associated with colon devascularization (treats <u>majority</u>)*
  - If **left-sided colectomy** is performed (ie for <u>destructive</u> lesions [> 50% circumference or colon devascularization]), *diverting ileostomy* is indicated for **gross contamination** (eg peritonitis), ≥ **6 hours** has elapsed between injury and repair, significant **comorbidities,** *or* ≥ **6 units pRBCs** have been given.
  - If patient is in **shock** and can't perform primary repair → just bring up **end colostomy** and leave **Hartmann's pouch** after resection (avoids left sided anastomosis in a sick patient and diverts stool)
- Intra-op **paracolonic hematomas** – <u>open</u> both blunt and penetrating

RECTAL TRAUMA

- Most associated with **penetrating** injury
- *Intraperitoneal* *injuries*
  - *Perform primary repair <u>without diversion</u> for all injuries if nondestructive* (< 50% circumference and <u>not</u> associated with devascularization) – *treats <u>majority</u>*
  - If **low anterior resection** (LAR) is performed (ie for destructive lesions [> 50% circumference or for rectal devascularization]), *a diverting loop colostomy is <u>always indicated</u> (different than above)*; if in **shock**, place end colostomy <u>only</u>.
- *Extraperitoneal* *injuries*
  - *High rectal* (proximal ⅓) – **primary repair** usual (**laparotomy,** mobilize rectum); if LAR needed, place diverting loop colostomy (follow LAR pathway above)
  - *Middle rectal* (middle ⅓) – often inaccessible due to location (too low for laparotomy, too high for transanal repair); if repair not easily feasible, there is extensive damage, or if you can't find it → *place end colostomy <u>only</u>* (<u>not</u> APR); this area will heal after 6–8 weeks, take down colostomy at that time
  - *Low rectal* (distal ⅓) – most repaired **primarily** with **transanal approach**; if repair not easily feasible, there is extensive damage, or if you can't find it → *place end colostomy <u>only</u>* (<u>not</u> APR)
- Presacral drains and rectal washout are generally <u>not</u> recommended.

LIVER TRAUMA

- Most common organ injury with blunt abdominal trauma (some texts say spleen)
- Lobectomy rarely necessary
- **Common hepatic artery** – can be ligated with collaterals through gastroduodenal artery
- **Pringle maneuver** (clamping **portal triad**) does not stop bleeding from **hepatic veins** or **retro-hepatic IVC.**
- **Damage control peri-hepatic packing** – can pack severe penetrating liver injuries if patient becomes unstable in the OR and the injury is not easily fixed (eg retro-hepatic IVC injury). Go to the ICU and get the patient resuscitated and stabilized. Live to fight another day.
- **Atriocaval shunt** – for retrohepatic IVC injury, allows for control while performing repair
- Intra-op **portal triad hematomas** – need to be explored
- Intra-op **contained subcapsular hematomas** – leave alone
- **Common bile duct injury** (Kocher maneuver and dissect out portal triad)
  - < 50% of circumference – **repair over stent**
  - > 50% circumference or complex injury – go with **choledochojejunostomy**
  - May need intraoperative cholangiogram to define injury
  - 10% of duct anastomoses leak – place drains intraop
- **Portal vein injury** – need to repair (lateral venorrhaphy)
  - May need to transect through the pancreas to get to the injury in the portal vein
  - Will need to perform **distal pancreatectomy** with that maneuver
  - Ligation of portal vein associated with 50% mortality
- **Omental graft** – can be placed in liver laceration to help with bleeding and prevent bile leaks
- **Leave drains** with **liver injuries.**
- **Unstable patients** (SBP < 90 despite 2 L LR) with blunt liver injuries should **go to the OR** (may need angioembolization later).

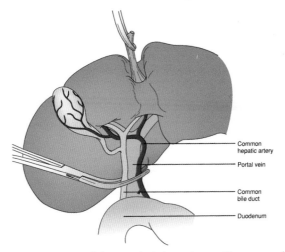

Common hepatic artery

Portal vein

Common bile duct

Duodenum

Pringle maneuver compression of the portal triad structures with a noncrushing vascular clamp for hepatic inflow control. If possible, clamp times should be limited to 15- to 20-minute intervals.

- **Nonoperative management** of **blunt liver** injuries (only in **stable** patients)
  - If the patient becomes **unstable** (SBP < 90) or is a **transient responder** despite aggressive resuscitation including ≥ **4 units** of pRBCs or requires ≥ **4 units** of pRBCs to keep Hct > 25 → **go to OR** (if unstable) _or_ **angioembolization** (if transient responder)
  - **Active contrast extravasation** (ie blush) or **pseudoaneurysm** on CT scan and patient is **stable** or **transient responder** → **angioembolization**
  - With nonoperative management requires bed rest for **5 days**
  - The higher the injury grade, the more likely an intervention is needed (highest is **grade VI** – hepatic avulsion, likely not compatible with life).

SPLEEN TRAUMA

- Fully healed after 6 weeks
- Postsplenectomy sepsis greatest risk **within 2 years** of splenectomy
- Need vaccines to pneumococcus, meningococcus, and H. influenzae 2 weeks after splenectomy
- Threshold for splenectomy in **children** is high (unusual to have to remove spleen in children)
- Splenic salvage is associated with increased transfusions.
- Intra-op **subcapsular hematomas** – leave alone
- **Unstable patients** (SBP < 90 despite 2 L LR) with blunt splenic injuries → **go to OR for splenectomy**
- **Nonoperative management** of **blunt splenic** injuries (only in **stable patients**)
  - If the patient becomes **unstable** (SBP < 90) or is a **transient responder** despite aggressive resuscitation including ≥ **2 units** of pRBCs or requires ≥ **2 units** of pRBCs to keep Hct > 25 → **go to OR** (if unstable) _or_ **angioembolization** (if transient responder)
  - **Active contrast extravasation** (ie blush), **pseudoaneurysm**, or **AV fistula** on CT scan and patient is **stable** or **transient responder** → **angioembolization**
  - With nonoperative management need bed rest for **5 days**
  - The higher the injury grade, the more likely an intervention will be needed (highest **grade V** – completely shattered spleen or complete hilar disruption that devascularizes spleen).

PANCREATIC TRAUMA

- **Penetrating injury** – accounts for 80% of all pancreatic injuries
- **Blunt injury** – can result in pancreatic duct fractures, usually perpendicular to the duct
  - Most common **missed injury** with blunt trauma
- Edema or necrosis of peripancreatic fat usually indicative of injury
- Can have associated duodenal injury
- **Pancreatic contusion** – leave if stable, place drains if in OR
- 80% of all injuries are treated with just drains.
- Primary concern is figuring out if the **pancreatic duct** is involved.
- **Distal pancreatic duct injury** – distal pancreatectomy, can take up to 80% of the gland
- **Pancreatic head duct injury and not reparable** – place drains only (_not_ trauma Whipple)
  - Delayed Whipple or possible ERCP w/ stent may eventually be necessary.
- Whipple vs. distal pancreatectomy based on duct injury in relation to the **SMV** (superior mesenteric vein)

- Kocher maneuver helps evaluate the pancreas operatively.
- **Leave drains** with pancreatic injury.
- Intra-op **pancreatic hematoma** – both penetrating and blunt need to be opened
- Persistent or rising **amylase** may indicate missed pancreatic injury.
- CT scans poor at diagnosing pancreatic injuries initially
  - Delayed signs – fluid, edema, necrosis
- **ERCP** good at finding duct injuries and may be able to treat with temporary stent

VASCULAR TRAUMA

- **Vascular repair** (or vascular shunt) performed _before_ **orthopedic repair**
- Pulse deficit or distal ischemia with orthopedic injury → reduce fracture or dislocation 1st, then reassess pulse/ABIs (ankle brachial index)
- **Major signs** of extremity vascular injury (hard signs):
  - Active hemorrhage
  - Pulse deficit
  - Expanding or pulsatile hematoma
  - Distal ischemia
  - Bruit or thrill
    - → **Go to OR for exploration for any of above** (may need angio in OR to define injury)
- **Minor signs** of extremity vascular injury (soft signs):
  - History of hemorrhage
  - Large stable/nonpulsatile hematoma
  - ABI < 0.9
  - Unequal pulses
    - → **Get CT angio for any of above** (formal angiogram if vascular injury found)
- **Arterial injures** – reversed saphenous vein graft will be needed if arterial segment > **2 cm** missing
  - Use vein from the contralateral leg when fixing lower extremity arterial injuries.
  - Consider prophylactic fasciotomy for superficial femoral or popliteal artery injuries.
  - Transection of single artery in the calf in an otherwise healthy patient → ligate
- **Vein injuries** that need usually need **primary repair** – vena cava, femoral, popliteal, brachiocephalic, subclavian, and axillary
  - If not able to repair or in damage control surgery – can simply ligate (consider **prophylactic fasciotomy** for iliac, femoral, or popliteal vein ligation)
  - The closer the ligation to the supra-renal IVC, the higher the morbidity.
  - _Avoid_ ligation of supra-renal IVC (high risk of renal failure).
- Cover site of anastomosis with viable tissue and muscle.
- Consider **prophylactic fasciotomy** for any ischemia > 4–6 hours (prevents compartment syndrome).
- **Compartment syndrome** – consider if compartment pressures are > 20 mm Hg or if clinical exam suggests elevated pressures (see Vascular chapter)
  - Pain with passive motion → paresthesia → poikilothermia → pallor → paralysis → pulselessness (late finding)
  - Most commonly occurs after supracondylar humeral fractures, tibial fractures, crush injuries, knee dislocations, or other injuries that result in a disruption and then restoration of blood flow after 4–6 hours
  - Compartment syndrome can lead to **rhabdomyolysis** and subsequent **renal failure.**
  - Tx: **fasciotomy**
  - Can also occur in patients found "**down**" due to muscle crush injury

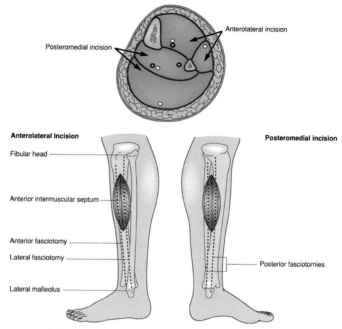

Surgical approach for four compartment fasciotomies through incisions on the medial and lateral aspects of the calf.

- **IVC** – primary repair if residual stenosis is < 50% the diameter of the IVC; otherwise, place saphenous vein or synthetic patch
  - Bleeding of IVC best controlled with proximal and distal pressure, <u>not</u> clamps → can tear it
  - Repair posterior wall injury through the anterior wall (may need to cut through the anterior IVC to get to posterior IVC injuries).
  - May have to consider ligation if damage control scenario

ORTHOPEDIC TRAUMA

- Can have > **2 L blood** loss from a **femur fracture**
- Orthopedic emergencies – pelvic fractures in unstable patients, spine injury with deficit, open fractures, dislocations or fractures with vascular compromise, compartment syndrome
- Femoral neck fractures and hip dislocations – high risk for **avascular necrosis**
- Long bone fracture or dislocations with loss of pulse (or weak pulse) → immediate reduction of fracture or dislocation and reassessment of pulse:
  - If pulse does not return → go to OR for vascular bypass or repair (may need angiography in OR to define injury)
  - If pulse is weak → CT angio
  - Exception – all *knee dislocations* need to go for **formal angiogram**, unless pulse is absent, in which case you would just go to OR (may need angio in OR to define injury)
  - **Upright falls** are associated with **calcaneus, lumbar,** and **distal forearm** (radius/ulnar) fractures.

Orthopedic Trauma	Concomitant Nerve/Artery Injury
UPPER EXTREMITY	
Anterior shoulder dislocation	Axillary nerve
Posterior shoulder dislocation	Axillary artery
Proximal humerus Fx	Axillary nerve
Midshaft humerus Fx (or spiral humerus Fx)	Radial nerve
Distal (supracondylar) humerus Fx	Brachial artery
Elbow dislocation	Brachial artery
Distal radius Fx	Median nerve
LOWER EXTREMITY	
Anterior hip dislocation	Femoral artery
Posterior hip dislocation	Sciatic nerve
Distal (supracondylar) femur Fx	Popliteal artery
Posterior knee dislocation	Popliteal artery
Fibula neck Fx	Common peroneal nerve
OTHER FRACTURES	
Temporal or parietal bone Fx	Epidural hematoma; facial nerve
Maxillofacial Fx	Cervical spine Fx
Sternal Fx	Cardiac contusion
First or second rib Fx	Aortic transection
Scapula Fx	Pulmonary contusion, aortic transection
Rib Fx's (left, 8–12)	Spleen laceration
Rib Fx's (right, 8–12)	Liver laceration
Pelvic Fx	Bladder rupture, urethral transection

RENAL TRAUMA

- MCC – blunt trauma (often associated with lower rib fractures)
- **Hematuria** is the best indicator of renal trauma.
- All patients with hematuria need an abdominal CT scan.
- IVP can be useful if going immediately to OR without abdominal CT scan → will identify presence of functional contralateral kidney, which could affect intraoperative decision making
- **Left renal vein** – can be ligated near IVC; has **adrenal** and **gonadal vein collaterals**; right renal vein does not have these collaterals
- **Anterior → posterior** renal hilum structures – **vein, artery, pelvis** (VAP)
- 95% of injuries are treated nonoperatively.
- Not all urine extravasation injuries require operation.
- **Kidney cortical injuries** – Tx: primary repair
- **Indications for operation**
  - **Acutely** – ongoing hemorrhage with instability
  - **After acute phase** – major collecting system disruption, non-resolving urine extravasation, severe hematuria
- With exploration, try to get control of the **vascular hilum 1st**.
- Place **drains** intraop, especially if collecting system is injured.
- **Methylene blue dye** (given IV) can be used at the end of the case to check for leak.
- **When at exploration for another blunt injury or penetrating trauma:**
  - **Blunt renal injury with hematoma** – leave unless preop CT/IVP shows no function or significant urine extravasation
  - **Penetrating renal injury with hematoma** – open unless preop CT/IVP shows good function without significant urine extravasation
- **Trauma to flank and IVP (or CT scan) shows no uptake in stable patient** – Tx: angiogram; can stent if flap present

BLADDER TRAUMA

- **Hematuria** best indicator of bladder trauma
- Blood at the meatus or scrotal/sacral hematoma – suspect bladder or urethral injury
- > 95% associated with **pelvic fractures** (blunt trauma)
- Signs and symptoms – meatal blood, sacral or scrotal hematoma
- Dx: **cystogram** (include post-void films)
- **Extraperitoneal bladder rupture** – cystogram shows starbursts
  - Tx: Foley 7–14 days
- **Intraperitoneal bladder rupture** – more likely in kids, cystogram shows leak
  - Tx: operation and repair of defect, followed by Foley drainage

URETERAL TRAUMA

- MCC – penetrating injury
- Hematuria unreliable → multiple shot **IVP** and **retrograde urethrogram** (RUG) best tests
- If **large ureteral segment** is missing (> 2 cm) and cannot perform reanastomosis:
  - **Upper ⅓ injuries** and **middle ⅓ injuries that won't reach bladder** (above pelvic brim)
    - Temporize with **percutaneous nephrostomy** (tie off both ends of the ureter); can go with <u>ileal interposition</u> or <u>trans-ureteroureterostomy</u> later
  - **Lower ⅓ injuries** – reimplant in the bladder; may need psoas (bladder) hitch procedure
- If **small ureteral segment** is missing (< 2 cm):
  - **Upper ⅓ injuries** and **middle ⅓ injuries** – mobilize ends of ureter and perform **primary repair** over double-J stent (fine, absorbable suture)
  - **Lower ⅓ injuries** – reimplant in the bladder (easier anastomosis than primary repair)
- One-shot IVP does not evaluate the ureters sufficiently.
- IV indigo carmine or IV methylene blue can be used to check for leaks.
- Blood supply is medial in the upper ⅔ of the ureter and lateral in the lower ⅓ of the ureter.
- **Leave drains** for all ureteral injuries.

URETHRAL TRAUMA

- **Hematuria** or **blood at meatus best signs**; free-floating (high riding) prostate gland; scrotal/perineal hematoma; usually associated with pelvic fractures (blunt trauma)
- <u>No Foley</u> if this injury is suspected
- **Retrograde urethrogram** (RUG) best test
- Membranous portion at risk for transection
- **Significant tears** – Tx: **suprapubic cystostomy** and repair in 2–3 months (*safest method* – high stricture and impotence rate if repaired early)
- **Small, partial tears** – Tx: may get away with bridging urethral catheter across tear area and repair in 2–3 months
- **Genital trauma** – can get fracture in erectile bodies from vigorous sex
  - Need to repair the tunica albuginea and Buck's fascia
- **Testicular trauma** – get ultrasound to see if tunica albuginea is violated, then repair if necessary

TRAUMA DURING PREGNANCY

- At all costs, **save the mother** (follow resuscitation pathway).
- Roll patient to the **left** to get pressure off IVC.
- Pregnant patients can have up to a ⅓ total blood volume loss without signs.

- Estimate pregnancy based on **fundal height** (20 cm = 20 weeks = umbilicus).
- Place **fetal monitor** if pregnancy ≥ **24 weeks** gestation.
- Try to avoid CT scan with early pregnancy. If life-threatening and needed, get CT scan.
- Ultrasound (FAST scan) may have a role in pregnant patients.
- Check for vaginal discharge – blood, amnion; check for effacement, dilation, fetal station.
- **Indicators of fetal maturity** – lecithin:sphingomyelin (LS) ratio > 2:1; positive **phosphatidylcholine** in amniotic fluid
- **Placental abruption** – > 50% results in almost 100% fetal death rate
  - > 50% of all traumatic placental abruptions result in fetal demise.
  - Signs of abruption – uterine tenderness, contractions, fetal HR < 120
  - Can be caused by **shock** (most common mechanism) or **mechanical forces**
  - **Kleihauer-Betke test** – looks for fetal blood cells in maternal circulation (fetal-maternal hemorrhage); if positive, give **Rhogam** if Rh− mother
- **Uterine rupture** – more likely to occur in the <u>posterior fundus</u>
  - If occurs after delivery of child, aggressive resuscitation even in the face of shock leads to the best outcome. The uterus will eventually clamp down after delivery; just have to aggressively resuscitate until then (fluids, blood)
- **Indications for C-section during exploratory laparotomy for trauma**
  - Persistent maternal shock or severe injuries and pregnancy near term (> 34 weeks)
  - Pregnancy a threat to the mother's life (hemorrhage, DIC)
  - Mechanical limitation to life-threatening vessel injury
  - Risk of fetal distress exceeds risk of immaturity
  - Direct intra-uterine trauma

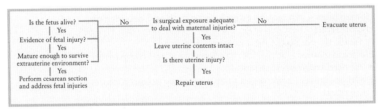

Assessment of the pregnant uterus during celiotomy.

Management of Intra-op Hematomas		
Hematoma (≥ 2 cm Considered Significant)	**Penetrating Trauma**	**Blunt Trauma**
Pelvic	Open	Leave
Paraduodenal	Open	Open
Portal triad	Open	Open
Retrohepatic	Leave if stable	Leave
Midline supramesocolic	Open	Open
Midline inframesocolic	Open	Open
Pericolonic	Open	Open
Perirenal	Open[a]	Leave[b]

[a]Unless preoperative CT scan or IVP shows no injury.
[b]Unless preoperative CT scan or IVP shows injury.

Retroperitoneum Zones and Intra-op Management

Zone	Location	Associated Injuries
1	Central retroperitoneum	Pancreaticoduodenal or major abdominal vascular injury (<u>open</u> hematomas in these areas for <u>both</u> penetrating and blunt trauma)
2	Flank or perinephric area	Injuries to genitourinary tract or colon (<u>open</u> hematomas if penetrating trauma; usually <u>leave alone</u> if blunt unless expanding/pulsatile hematoma)
3	Pelvis	Pelvic fractures, iliac vessel/rectal/urological injuries (<u>open</u> hematomas if penetrating trauma; <u>leave alone</u> if blunt - may need angioembolization)

OTHER

- Patients with penetrating injuries require a tetanus shot.
- **Drains** – leave drains with pancreatic, liver, biliary system, urinary, and duodenal injuries
- **Snakebites** (symptoms depend on species) – shock, bradycardia, and arrhythmias can result; Tx: stabilize patient, anti-venin (different types for different species; eg rattlesnake, coral snake), tetanus shot
- **Beestings** – kill many more people in US than snake bites due to anaphylaxis; wheezing, rash, hypotension (vasomotor shock); Tx for anaphylaxis – epinephrine (EpiPen)
- **Black widow spider bites** – nausea, vomiting, muscle cramps; Tx – IV calcium gluconate, muscle relaxants
- **Brown recluse spider bites** – skin ulcer with necrotic center and surrounding erythema; Tx: Dapsone; skin grafting may be needed but wait at least a week to see full extent of damage
- **Wild animal bites** – need rabies prophylaxis unless the animal can be found, killed, and brain examined
- **Human bites** – can require extensive irrigation and debridement
- **Hypothermia** – best initial Tx: warm air conduction (Bair Hugger); also give warm IV fluids; do not stop CPR until warm and dead
- **Electrical injuries** – at risk for rhabdomyolysis and compartment syndrome
  - All need volume resuscitation
  - Other injuries – solid organ fracture, hollow viscous rupture, quadriplegia, cataracts
  - MCC of immediate death – **cardiac arrest** from ventricular fibrillation

16 Critical Care

CARDIOVASCULAR SYSTEM

Normal Values

Parameter	Value
Cardiac output (CO) (L/min)	4–8
Cardiac index (CI) (L/min)	2.5–4
Systemic vascular resistance (SVR, afterload)	$1{,}100 \pm 300$
Pulmonary capillary wedge pressure (wedge pressure)	11 ± 4
Central venous pressure (CVP)	7 ± 2
Pulmonary artery pressure (PAP)	$25/10 \pm 5$
Mixed venous oxygen saturation (SvO_2)	75 ± 5

- CO = stroke volume $\times$ heart rate
- $MAP = CO \times SVR$, $CI = CO/BSA$
- Kidney gets 25% of CO, brain gets 15%, heart gets 5%.
- **Cardiac performance** (left ventricle) is determined by **preload, afterload, contractility,** and **HR**.
- Preload – linearly related to left ventricular end-diastolic pressure (LVEDP); **wedge pressure = preload = LVEDP** (LVEDP is a surrogate for LV end-diastolic **volume**)

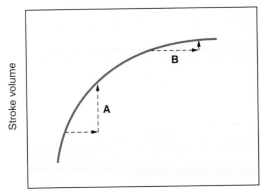

Preload

The concept of preload recruitable stroke volume is demonstrated. If the ventricle is on the steep part of the Starling curve **(A)**, then a given increase in preload will lead to a significant increase in stroke volume. By contrast, on the flatter part of the curve **(B)**, the stroke volume increases marginally if at all with the same increase in preload. Dynamic indices of preload-recruitable stroke volume are more accurate than static indices in identifying where on this curve the patient is at any point in time.

- **Afterload** – resistance against the ventricle contracting (**SVR**)
- **Contractility** – the force of contraction
- **Stroke volume** determined by LVEDV, contractility, and afterload
  - Stroke volume = LVEDV − LVESV

- **Ejection fraction** = stroke volume/LVEDV
- **EDV** (end-diastolic volume) – determined by preload and distensibility of the ventricle
- **ESV** (end-systolic volume) – determined by contractility and afterload
- Cardiac output increases with HR up to 120–150 beats/min, then starts to go down because of **decreased diastolic filling time.**
- **Atrial kick** – accounts for 20% of LVEDV
- **Anrep effect** – automatic increase in **contractility** secondary to ↑ **afterload**
- **Bowditch effect** – automatic increase in **contractility** secondary to ↑ **HR**
- **Arterial O$_2$ content** (CaO$_2$) = Hgb × 1.34 × O$_2$ saturation + (Po$_2$ × 0.003)
- **O$_2$ delivery** = CO × arterial O$_2$ content (CaO$_2$) × 10
- **O$_2$ consumption** (VO$_2$) = CO × (CaO$_2$ − CvO$_2$); CvO$_2$ = venous O$_2$ content
  - Normal O$_2$ delivery-to-consumption ratio is 4:1. CO increases to keep this ratio constant.
  - O$_2$ consumption is usually <u>supply independent</u> (consumption does not change until low levels of delivery are reached).
- Causes of **right shift** of **oxygen–Hgb dissociation curve** (increased O$_2$ unloading) – ↑ CO$_2$ (Bohr effect) ↑ temperature, ↑ ATP production, ↑ 2,3-DPG production, or ↓ pH
  - Opposite above causes left shift (increased O$_2$ binding)
  - Normal p50 (O$_2$ at which 50% of O$_2$ receptors are saturated) = 27 mm Hg
- ↑ **SvO$_2$** (saturation of venous blood, normally 75% ± 5%; used on some Swan–Ganz catheters) – occurs with ↑ shunting of blood or ↓ O$_2$ extraction (eg sepsis, cirrhosis, cyanide toxicity, hyperbaric O$_2$, hypothermia, paralysis, coma)
- ↓ **SvO$_2$** – occurs with ↑ O$_2$ extraction (eg malignant hyperthermia, fever, seizures) or ↓ O$_2$ delivery (eg ↓ O$_2$ saturation, ↓ CO, ↓ Hgb)
- **Wedge pressure** – may be thrown off by pulmonary hypertension, mitral stenosis, mitral regurgitation, high PEEP, poor LV compliance
- **Swan–Ganz catheter** – should be placed in **zone III** (lower lung; has less respiratory influence on wedge pressure)
  - **Hemoptysis after flushing Swan–Ganz catheter** – increase PEEP, which will tamponade the pulmonary artery bleed, mainstem intubate non-affected side; can try to place Fogarty balloon down mainstem on affected side
    - Definitive Tx: **angioembolization**; may need thoracotomy and lobectomy if that fails
  - Absolute contraindications – right-sided mechanical valve (rare)
  - **Relative contraindications** – previous pneumonectomy, left bundle branch block, recent pacemaker, right-sided endocarditis
  - Approximate **Swan–Ganz catheter distances to wedge** – R SCV 45 cm, R IJ 50 cm, L SCV 55 cm, L IJ 60 cm
  - **Pulmonary vascular resistance** (PVR) can be measured only by using a **Swan–Ganz catheter** (ECHO does not measure PVR).
  - **Wedge pressure** measurements should be taken at **end-expiration** (for both ventilated and nonventilated patients).
- ↑ **Ventricular wall tension** (#1) and **HR** are the primary determinants of myocardial O$_2$ consumption → can lead to myocardial ischemia
- **Unsaturated bronchial blood** – empties into pulmonary veins; thus, LV blood is 5 mm Hg (Po$_2$) lower than pulmonary capillaries
- **Alveolar–arterial gradient** – is 10–15 mm Hg in a normal nonventilated patient
- Blood with the **lowest** venous saturation → **coronary sinus blood** (30%)
- Blood with **highest** venous saturation → **renal veins** (80%)

SHOCK

- **Shock** = inadequate tissue perfusion/oxygenation (most basic definition)
  - **Tachypnea** and **mental status** changes occur with progressive shock.
  - Blood shunted to the **heart** and **brain**

- **Adrenal insufficiency**
  - MCC – withdrawal of exogenous steroids
  - **Acute** – cardiovascular collapse; characteristically **unresponsive to fluids and pressors**; nausea and vomiting, abdominal pain, fever, lethargy, ↓ glucose, ↑ K
  - Dx: random cortisol < 25 usually used
  - Tx: **hydrocortisone** (give empirically if adrenal insufficiency is suspected; does not interfere with test)
  - **Steroid potency**
    - 1× – cortisone, hydrocortisone
    - 5× – prednisone, prednisolone, methylprednisolone
    - 30× – dexamethasone
- **Neurogenic shock** (vasogenic shock) – loss of sympathetic tone (↓ SVR)
  - Causes – high spine or head injury; anaphylactic reactions (eg bee stings)
  - Usually have ↓ HR, ↓ BP, pink and warm skin
  - Tx: Give **volume 1st**, then **phenylephrine** after resuscitation.
- **Hemorrhagic shock** – initial alteration is ↑ <u>diastolic pressure and tachycardia</u> followed by a <u>drop in systolic pressure</u>
- **Cardiogenic shock** (eg massive MI, severe CHF exacerbation) – Tx: dobutamine, IABP
- **Cardiac tamponade** (causes a type of cardiogenic shock)
  - Mechanism of hypotension is **decreased ventricular filling** due to fluid in the pericardial sac around the heart.
  - Beck's triad – hypotension, jugular venous distention, and muffled heart sounds
  - Can present in **postcardiac surgery** patient as sudden **decreased chest tube output** followed by **hypotension** and **elevated wedge/CVP** or as **PEA**
    - If coding patient, open sternum in **ICU** (cut wires, chest spreader).
    - If patient still has BP and HR, return to OR for reentry.
  - Can also present after **penetrating chest trauma** (see Trauma chapter) or as **malignant pericardial effusion** (most common – lung CA)
  - Echocardiogram shows **impaired diastolic filling of right atrium initially** (1st sign of cardiac tamponade).
  - Pericardiocentesis blood does not form clot.
  - Tx: fluid resuscitation to temporize situation; need **pericardial window** or **pericardiocentesis**

Types of Shock

Shock	CVP and PCWP	CO	SVR
Hemorrhagic (hypovolemic)	↓	↓	↑
Septic (hyperdynamic)[a]	↓ (usually)	↑	↓
Cardiogenic (eg MI, cardiac tamponade)	↑	↓	↑
Neurogenic (eg head or spinal cord injury)	↓	↓	↓
Adrenal insufficiency	↓ (usually)	↓	↓

[a]Severe septic shock that leads to cardiac dysfunction can cause a hypodynamic state, leading to ↓ CO and ↑ SVRI.

- **Sepsis**
  - **Early sepsis triad** – hyperventilation, confusion, hypotension
  - **Early gram-negative sepsis** – ↓ insulin, ↑ **glucose** (impaired utilization)
  - **Late gram-negative sepsis** – ↑ insulin, ↑ **glucose** (secondary to insulin resistance)
  - **Hyperglycemia** – often occurs just before patient becomes clinically septic
  - **Pro-calcitonin** – elevated in patients with sepsis however not specific (higher sensitivity, lower specificity); good at ruling out sepsis; also good for discontinuing antibiotics when it normalizes
  - Use serial **lactic acids** to help guide **volume resuscitation** (want lactate < 2.0).
  - **Fungitell** (1,3 beta-D-glucan) – blood test for invasive **fungus**
  - **Mannan antigen/antibody** – blood test for invasive **candida**
  - Tx: **volume resuscitation** and **send cultures**; **antibiotics** after cultures sent
    - **Levophed** (primary) and **vasopressin** (secondary) for **septic shock**
    - Want **glucose < 180**

- **Neurohormonal response** to **hypovolemia**
  - **Rapid** – **epinephrine** and **norepinephrine** release (<u>adrenergic</u> release; results in vasoconstriction and increased cardiac activity)
  - **Sustained** – **renin** (from <u>kidney</u>; renin-angiotensin pathway activated resulting in vasoconstriction and water resorption), **ADH** (from <u>pituitary</u>; reabsorption of water), and **ACTH** release (from <u>pituitary</u>; increases cortisol)

EMBOLI

- **Fat emboli** – petechia, hypoxia, and confusion (can also present similar to pulmonary embolism [PE])
  - **Sudan red stain** may show fat in sputum and urine.
  - Most common with lower extremity (hip, femur) fractures/orthopedic procedures
  - Can turn into ARDS with hypoxemia and bilateral patchy infiltrates on CXR
  - Tx: supportive (mechanical ventilation)
- **Pulmonary emboli** (PE) – chest pain and dyspnea; ↓ Po_2 and Pco_2; respiratory alkalosis; ↑ HR and ↑ RR; anxiety and diaphoresis; hypotension and shock if massive
  - Intubated patients can present with **decreased ETCO$_2$** and **hypotension.**
  - MC EKG finding – **tachycardia**
  - Dx: **CT angio** *(best)*
  - **Echocardiogram** – shows RV strain and dilation
  - **D-Dimer** – high sensitivity, low specificity; if normal patient is very unlikely to have PE
  - Most PEs arise from **iliofemoral region.**
  - Tx: **heparin** bolus followed by drip (PTT 60–90), consider **tPA** or percutaneous (suction catheter) **embolectomy** if patient is in shock despite massive pressors and inotropes; ECMO if coding/coded patient; long-term Coumadin
- **Air emboli** – usually occurs when central vein is exposed to air (eg central line placement/removal, supraclavicular nodal biopsies)
  - **Tx** – CPR; place patient head down and roll to left (keeps air in RV and RA), then aspirate air out with central line or PA catheter to RA/RV
  - **Prevention** – use Trendelenburg when entering neck veins

INTRA-AORTIC BALLOON PUMP (IABP)

- <u>Inflates</u> on **T wave** (diastole); <u>deflates</u> on **P wave** (systole)
- Place tip of the catheter just distal to left subclavian (1–2 cm below the top of the arch).
- Used for **cardiogenic shock** (after CABG or MI), in patients with **refractory angina** awaiting revascularization, preop in high-risk patients, acute mitral regurgitation, and for ventricular septal ruptures
- **Decreases afterload** (deflation during ventricular systole)
- **Improves diastolic BP** (inflation during ventricular diastole), which **improves diastolic coronary perfusion**
- Absolute contraindications – aortic dissection, severe aortoiliac disease, aortic regurgitation
- Relative contraindications – vascular grafts, aortic aneurysms

RECEPTORS

- **Alpha-1** – vascular smooth muscle constriction
- **Alpha-2** – venous smooth muscle constriction
- **Beta-1** – myocardial contraction and rate
- **Beta-2** – relaxes bronchial smooth muscle, relaxes vascular smooth muscle; increases renin
- **Dopamine receptors** – relax renal and splanchnic smooth muscle

CARDIOVASCULAR DRUGS

- **Dopamine** (2–5 μg/kg/min initially)
  - 2–5 μg/kg/min – <u>dopamine receptors</u> (renal)
  - 6–10 μg/kg/min – <u>beta-adrenergic</u> (heart contractility and heart rate)
  - > 10 μg/kg/min – <u>alpha-adrenergic</u> (vasoconstriction and ↑ BP)
- **Dobutamine** (3 μg/kg/min initially)
  - <u>Beta-1</u> (↑ contractility mostly, tachycardia with higher doses)
- **Milrinone**
  - **Phosphodiesterase inhibitor** (↑ cAMP)
  - Results in ↑ Ca flux and ↑ myocardial contractility
  - Also causes vascular smooth muscle relaxation and **pulmonary vasodilation**; sometimes **systemic vasodilation** (hypotension)
  - Is <u>not</u> subject to receptor down-regulation (good for long-term Tx, eg chronic CHF)
- **Phenylephrine** (10 μg/min initially)
  - Alpha-1, vasoconstriction
- **Norepinephrine** (5 μg/min initially)
  - Alpha-1 and alpha-2; some beta-1
  - Potent splanchnic vasoconstrictor
- **Epinephrine** (1–2 μg/min initially)
  - <u>Low dose</u> – beta-1 and beta-2 (↑ contractility and vasodilation)
    - Can ↓ BP at low doses
  - <u>High dose</u> – alpha-1 and alpha-2 (vasoconstriction)
    - ↑ Cardiac ectopic pacer activity and myocardial O_2 demand
- **Isoproterenol** (1–2 μg/min initially)
  - Beta-1 and beta-2, ↑ HR and contractility, vasodilates
  - Side effects: extremely arrhythmogenic; ↑ heart metabolic demand (rarely used); may actually ↓ BP
- **Vasopressin**
  - V-1 receptors – arterial vasoconstriction
  - V-2 receptors (intrarenal) – water reabsorption at collecting ducts
  - V-2 receptors (extrarenal) – mediate release of factor VIII and von Willebrand factor (vWF)
- **Nipride** – arterial vasodilator
  - **Cyanide toxicity** at doses > 3 μg/kg/min for 72 hours; can check **thiocyanate levels** and signs of metabolic acidosis
  - **Tx for cyanide toxicity** – amyl nitrite, then sodium nitrite
- **Nitroglycerin** – predominately venodilation with ↓ myocardial wall tension from ↓ preload; moderate coronary vasodilator
- **Hydralazine** – α-blocker; lowers BP

PULMONARY SYSTEM

- **Compliance** – (change in volume)/(change in pressure)
  - <u>High pulmonary compliance</u> means lungs easy to ventilate (eg severe COPD).
  - Pulmonary compliance is *decreased* in patients with ARDS, fibrotic lung diseases, reperfusion injury, pulmonary edema, atelectasis.
- **Aging** – ↓ FEV_1 and vital capacity, ↑ functional residual capacity (FRC)
- **V/Q ratio** (ventilation/perfusion ratio) – highest in upper lobes, lowest in lower lobes
- **Ventilator**
  - ↑ <u>PEEP</u> to improve oxygenation (alveoli recruitment) → **improves FRC**
    - Can also ↑ <u>FiO_2</u> or ↑ <u>mean airway pressure</u> to improve oxygenation
  - ↑ <u>respiratory rate</u> (RR) or <u>tidal volume</u> (TV) to ↓ CO_2 (improved ventilation)
  - **Normal weaning parameters** – rapid shallow breathing index (RR/TV) < 100 (*best predictor of successful extubation*), negative inspiratory force (NIF; need expiratory pause

to measure) > 20, $FiO_2 \leq 40\%$, PEEP 5 (physiologic), pressure support 5, RR $<$ 24/min, HR < 120 beats/min, $Po_2 > 60$ mm Hg, $Pco_2 < 50$ mm Hg, pH 7.35–7.45, saturations $> 93\%$, off pressors, follows commands, can protect airway

- Usually need spontaneous awakening trial (**SAT**) and spontaneous breathing trial (**SBT**) at least once a day when on vent
- **Ventilator-induced lung injury** – caused by oxygen radicals (high FiO_2) and barotrauma (high pressure)
- Try to keep $FiO_2 \leq 60\%$ – prevents O_2 radical toxicity to lungs
- **Peak pressure** – indicates **large airway pressure** (normal < 40)
- **Plateau pressure** (need <u>inspiratory pause</u> to measure) – indicates **alveolar pressure** (normal < 20)
- **Airway obstruction** (eg bronchospasm, mucus plug) – <u>high</u> peak and <u>normal</u> plateau pressures (Tx: albuterol; remove any mechanical obstruction)
- **ARDS** (eg alveolar lung disease) – <u>high</u> peak and <u>high</u> plateau pressures
  - **Plateau pressure** better indicator of **potential barotrauma**
  - If plateau pressure $> 30 \rightarrow$ need to decrease TV; consider pressure control ventilation.
- **PEEP** – *improves FRC* and compliance by keeping alveoli open $\rightarrow$ best way to improve oxygenation
- **Excessive PEEP complications** – $\downarrow$ right atrial filling (main reason for $\downarrow$ed CO), $\downarrow$ BP, $\downarrow$ renal blood flow ($\uparrow$ed renin), $\downarrow$ urine output, $\uparrow$ wedge pressure, and $\uparrow$ pulmonary vascular resistance

- **Ventilator modes**
  - **AC** (assist control; continuous mechanical ventilation [CMV])
    - **RR** and **TV** are preset.
    - <u>Every breath</u> (either patient initiated or vent initiated) is supported by vent.
    - Can lead to **barotrauma** from preset TV (gives volume of air regardless of pressure)
    - Can lead to **hyperventilation** if patient RR is too high (every breath is supported)
  - **SIMV** (synchronous intermittent mechanical ventilation)
    - **RR** and **TV** are preset.
    - Vent attempts to synchronize with patient's own RR and deliver preset RR and TV.
    - Allows <u>unsupported</u> spontaneous breathing if above preset RR (<u>prevents</u> hyperventilation)
    - Can still get **barotrauma**
    - Often used when trying to **wean off vent** (more comfortable) although patients can tire out from the unsupported breaths (ie having to breathe on their own)
    - **Pressure support** often added to help with patient's spontaneous breaths (see below).
  - **PCV** (pressure control ventilation)
    - **RR** and **inspiratory pressure** (peak pressure) are preset (get variable TVs).
    - <u>Limits</u> barotrauma
    - Can lead to **hypoventilation** from low TV (eg patient coughing or fighting the vent can increase airway pressure, leading to a decrease in TV)
    - Used at times for **ARDS** and permissive **hypercapnia**
  - **Pressure support** (different from PCV above)
    - **Inspiratory pressure** (peak pressure) is preset (get variable TV's); <u>*no*</u> RR
    - Can be used in conjunction with **SIMV** (pressure support is added to the unsupported breaths) or as a separate vent mode (**PSV** [pressure support ventilation])
    - Decreases the work of breathing (Preset inspiratory pressure is held constant until minimum volume is achieved.)
    - Can result in **hypoventilation** if the patient is not taking enough breaths
  - **High-frequency ventilation** – used a lot in kids; tracheoesophageal fistula, bronchopleural fistula

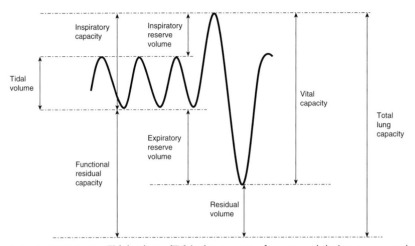

Lung measurements: Tidal volume (TV) is the amount of gas moved during one normal inspiration and expiration. Functional residual capacity (FRC) represents the volume of gas left in the lung following normal expiration. Inspiratory capacity is the maximum volume of air, which can be inspired following a normal expiration. Inspiratory reserve volume is the additional amount of air, which can be inspired following normal inspiration. Expiratory reserve volume is the additional amount of air, which can be expired following normal expiration. Residual volume is the minimum lung volume possible, which is the air that remains in the lung following maximum expiration. Vital capacity is the maximum amount of air, which can be moved, maximum inspiration following maximum expiration. Total lung capacity is the total amount of volume present in the lung.

- **Pulmonary function measurements**
  - **Total lung capacity** (TLC) – lung volume after maximal inspiration
    - TLC = FVC + RV
  - **Forced vital capacity** (FVC) – maximal exhalation after maximal inhalation
  - **Residual volume** (RV) – lung volume after maximal expiration (20% TLC)
  - **Tidal volume** (TV) – volume of air with normal inspiration and expiration
  - **Functional residual capacity** (FRC) – lung volume after normal exhalation
    - FRC = ERV + RV
    - Surgery (atelectasis), sepsis (ARDS), and trauma (contusion, atelectasis, ARDS) – all ↓ FRC
    - **PEEP** ↑s FRC
  - **Expiratory reserve volume** (ERV) – volume of air that can be forcefully expired after normal expiration
  - **Inspiratory capacity** – maximum air breathed in from FRC
  - **FEV_1** – forced expiratory volume in 1 second (after maximal inhalation)
  - **Minute ventilation** = TV × RR
  - **Restrictive lung disease** – ↓ TLC, ↓ RV, and ↓ FVC
    - FEV_1 can be normal or ↑.
  - **Obstructive lung disease** – ↑ TLC, ↑ RV, and ↓ FEV_1
    - FVC can be normal or ↓.
- **COPD** – ↑ work of breathing due to **prolonged expiratory phase**

- **Dead space**
  - Part of lung that is ventilated but <u>not</u> perfused
  - Normally, dead space is the airway to level of the bronchiole (comprises 150 mL; conductive airways).
    - **MCC of increased dead space** (high V/Q ratio) – **excessive PEEP** (due to capillary compression); others – ↓ed CO (capillary collapse), PE, pulmonary hypertension
  - *Increased* **dead space** leads to *increased* P_{CO_2}.
- **Shunt** (poor ventilation but good perfusion)
  - **MCC of increased shunt** (low V/Q ratio) – **atelectasis** *(alveolar hypoventilation)*; others – mucus plug, ARDS (alveoli filled with edema)
  - **Shunt** causes **hypoxia** *(decreased P_{O_2})*.
- **ARDS** – acute onset (< 1 week) inflammation of lung mediated primarily by PMNs
  - Get ↑ proteinaceous material, ↑ A-a gradient, ↑ pulmonary shunt
  - Most common cause is **pneumonia**; other causes – sepsis, multi-trauma, severe burns, pancreatitis, aspiration, DIC
  - Can result in SIRS, shock, and MSOF
  - **PaO_2/FiO_2 ratio**: 200–300 (mild), 100–200 (moderate), < 100 (severe)
  - Tx: Decrease barotrauma by allowing **permissive hypercapnia** (hypercarbia).
    - Use **low tidal volume** (4–6 cc/kg) to keep plateau pressures < 30; **PEEP** 10–15.
    - **Increase inspiratory time** to improve oxygenation.
    - Keep **pH > 7.20** (adjust vent, consider HCO_3^-).
    - **Paralytics** and **proning** patient useful; consider inhaled NO.
- Aspiration – pH < 2.5 and volume > 0.4 cc/kg is associated with ↑ degree of damage
  - **Mendelson's syndrome** – **chemical pneumonitis** from **aspiration of gastric secretions**
  - Most frequent site is **superior segment of the right lower lobe** (RLL).
- **Atelectasis** – collapse of alveoli resulting in reduced oxygenation; usually caused by poor inspiration postop
  - Most common cause of **fever** in first 48 hours after operation
  - Mediated by alveolar macrophages which release IL-1 (acts at the hypothalamus)

Acute Respiratory Distress Syndrome (ARDS) Criteria
Acute onset
Bilateral pulmonary infiltrates
$PaO_2/FiO_2 \leq 300$
Absence of heart failure (wedge < 18 mm Hg)

Characteristic chest radiograph **(A)** and CT scan **(B)** in a patient with severe ARDS following multiple trauma.

- MCC of hypoxia early postop
- Sx's – fever, tachycardia, hypoxia
- Increased in patients with COPD, upper abdominal surgery, obesity
- Tx: incentive spirometer, pain control, ambulation
- Lots of things can throw off a pulse oximeter → nail polish, dark skin, low-flow states, ambient light, anemia, vital dyes
- **Pulmonary vasodilation** – PGE_1, prostacyclin (PGI_2), inhaled nitric oxide, sildenafil
- **Pulmonary vasoconstriction** – **hypoxia** (#1), acidosis, histamine, serotonin, TXA_2
- **Alkalosis** – pulmonary vasodilator
- **Acidosis** – pulmonary vasoconstrictor
- **Pulmonary shunting** (causes hypoxia) – occurs with nitroprusside (Nipride), nitroglycerin, and nifedipine

RENAL SYSTEM

- MCC of poor urine output early postop – hypovolemia (Tx: give fluids)
- **Hypotension intraop** – the most common cause of postoperative renal failure
- 70% of nephrons need to be damaged before renal dysfunction occurs.
- Check serum and urine electrolytes; check urinary catheter for obstruction.
- **FeNa** (fractional excretion of sodium) = (urine Na/Cr)/(plasma Na/Cr) → **best test for azotemia**

Standard Measurements in the Diagnosis of Renal Failure

Test	Prerenal	Parenchymal
Urine osmolarity (mOsm)	> 500	250–350
U/P osmolality	> 1.5	< 1.1
BUN:creatinine ratio	> 20	< 10
Urine sodium	< 20	> 40
FE_{Na}	$< 1\%$	$> 3\%$

FE_{Na}, fraction of excreted sodium; U/P, urine-to-plasma ratio.

- **Oliguria**
  - 1st – make sure patient is volume loaded (CVP 11–15 mm Hg)
  - 2nd – try diuretic trial → furosemide (Lasix)
  - 3rd – dialysis if needed
- **Prerenal** oliguria/ARF – Tx: **fluid volume**
- **Renal** oliguria/ARF (eg acute tubular necrosis; ATN) – Tx: diuretic trial (try to make non-oliguric)
  - MCC of renal ATN – hypotension intraop
- **Post-renal** oliguria/ARF (obstructive uropathy; eg ureteral obstruction, severe BPH)
  - Dx: U/S (shows hydronephrosis)
  - Tx: Relieve obstruction.
- **Indications for dialysis** – fluid overload, ↑ K, metabolic acidosis, uremic encephalopathy, uremic coagulopathy, poisoning
- **Hemodialysis** – rapid, can cause large volume shifts; Hct increases by about 5 for each liter taken off
- **CVVH** – slower, good for ill patients who cannot tolerate the volume shifts (septic shock, etc.); Hct increases by 5–8 for each liter taken off with dialysis
- **Renin** (released from kidney)
  - Released in response to ↓ pressure sensed by **juxtaglomerular apparatus** in kidney
  - Also released in response to ↑ Na concentrations sensed by the **macula densa**
  - Beta-adrenergic stimulation and hyperkalemia also cause release.
  - Converts angiotensinogen (synthesized in the liver) to angiotensin I

- **Angiotensin-converting enzyme** (lung) – converts angiotensin I to angiotensin II
- **Adrenal cortex** – releases aldosterone in response to angiotensin II
- **Aldosterone** acts at the **distal convoluted tubule** to **reabsorb water** by up-regulating the **Na/K ATPase** on the membrane (Na reabsorbed, K secreted).
- **Angiotensin II** – also <u>vasoconstricts</u> as well as inhibits renin release
- Atrial natriuretic peptide (or factor)
  - Released from **atrial wall** with atrial distention (eg CHF)
  - **Inhibits Na and water resorption** in the collecting ducts
  - Also a **vasodilator**
- Antidiuretic hormone (ADH; vasopressin)
  - Released by **posterior pituitary gland** when osmolality is high
  - Acts on collecting ducts for **water resorption**
  - Also a **vasoconstrictor**
- **Efferent limb** of the kidney controls **GFR.**
- Renal toxic drugs
  - **NSAIDs** – cause renal damage by **inhibiting prostaglandin synthesis**, resulting in renal arteriole vasoconstriction
  - **Aminoglycosides** – direct tubular injury
  - **Myoglobin** – direct tubular injury; Tx: hydration (best), alkalinize urine
  - **Contrast dyes** – direct tubular injury; Tx: **prehydration** before contrast exposure best for patients with elevated creatinine; HCO_3^-, N-acetylcysteine

SYSTEMIC INFLAMMATORY RESPONSE SYNDROME (SIRS)

- Mediated by massive **IL-1** and **TNF-alpha release**
- **Causes** – shock, infection (MC – pneumonia), burns, multi-trauma, pancreatitis, ARDS
  - **Endotoxin** (lipopolysaccharide – **lipid A**) is the most potent stimulus for **SIRS.**
  - Lipid A is a very potent stimulator of **TNF release.**
- **Mechanism** – inflammatory response is activated systemically (**TNF-alpha** and IL-1 major components) and can lead to shock and eventually multi-organ dysfunction
  - Results in capillary leakage, microvascular thrombi, shock, and eventually end-organ dysfunction
- Need to Tx the underlying cause
- **Sepsis = SIRS + infection**
- **Septic shock = sepsis + hypotension**

Definitions of Systemic Inflammatory Response Syndrome (SIRS), Shock, and Multisystem Organ Dysfunction (MOD)		
SIRS →	Shock →	MOD
SIRS		
● Temperature $> 38°C$ or $< 36°C$		
● Heart rate > 90 beats/min		
● Respiratory rate > 20/min or $Paco_2 < 32$		
● White blood count $> 12,000/\mu L$ or $< 4,000/\mu L$		
Shock		
● Arterial hypotension despite adequate volume resuscitation (inadequate tissue oxygenation)		
MOD		
● Progressive but reversible dysfunction of 2 or more organs arising from an acute disruption of normal homeostasis		

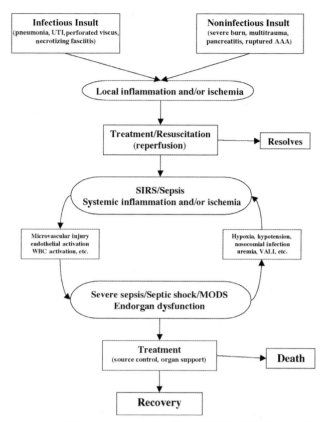

Pathophysiology of multisystem organ dysfunctions (MODS). AAA, abnormal aortic aneurysm; SIRS, systemic inflammatory response syndrome; UTI, urinary tract infection; VALI, ventilator-associated lung injury; WBC, white blood cell.

BRAIN DEATH

- **Precludes diagnosis** – temperature $< 32°C$, BP < 90 mm Hg, drugs (eg phenobarbital, pentobarbital, ETOH), metabolic derangements (hyperglycemia, uremia), desaturation with apnea test
- **Following must exist for 6–12 hours** → unresponsive to pain, absent cold caloric oculovestibular reflexes, absent oculocephalic reflex (patient doesn't track), no spontaneous respirations, no corneal reflex, no gag reflex, fixed and dilated pupils, positive apnea test
- **EEG** – shows electrical silence; **MRA** – will show no blood flow to brain
- **Apnea test** – the patient is pre-oxygenated, a catheter delivering O_2 at 8 L/min is placed at the carina through the ET tube and CO_2 should be normal before the start of the test. The patient is disconnected from ventilator for 10 minutes.
  - A $CO_2 > 60$ **mm Hg** or **increase in CO_2 by 20 mm Hg** at the end of the test is a <u>positive test for apnea</u> (meets brain death criteria).
  - If BP drops (< 90 mm Hg), the patient desaturates ($< 85\%$ on pulse oximeter), or spontaneous breathing occurs, the test is terminated (<u>negative test for apnea</u>) → place back on the ventilator (cannot declare brain death)

- **Organ donation** – UNOS should discuss donation with family, not the treating physician.
- *Can still have deep tendon reflexes with brain death*

OTHER CONDITIONS

- **Carbon monoxide**
  - Can **falsely** ↑ **oxygen saturation** reading on pulse oximeter
  - Binds hemoglobin directly (creates **carboxyhemoglobin** – HA, nausea, confusion, coma, death); CO has 250× more affinity for Hgb than oxygen
  - Causes a **left shift** on the oxygen–Hgb dissociation curve
  - Can usually correct with **100% oxygen on ventilator** (displaces carbon monoxide); rarely need hyperbaric O_2
  - Abnormal carboxyhemoglobin > 10%; in smokers > 20%
- **Methemoglobinemia** (from nitrites such as Hurricaine spray, fertilizers; nitrites bind Hgb) – **O_2 saturation reads 85%**
  - Tx: methylene blue
- **Cyanide toxicity** – disrupts the electron transport chain; can't utilize oxygen; get left to right shunt; **Tx** – amyl nitrite, then sodium nitrite; hydroxycobalamin
- **Critical illness polyneuropathy** – motor > sensory neuropathy; occurs with sepsis; can lead to failure to wean from ventilation
- **Xanthine oxidase** – in endothelial cells, forms toxic **oxygen radicals** with reperfusion, involved in **reperfusion injury**
  - Also involved in the metabolism of purines to **uric acid**
- Most important mediator of **reperfusion injury** – **PMNs**
- **DKA** – nausea and vomiting, thirst, polyuria, ↑ glucose, ↑ ketones, ↓ Na, ↑ K
  - Tx: **normal saline** and **insulin** initially
  - After treatment with insulin, hypokalemia can occur as K is driven back into cells along with glucose (Tx: potassium chloride).
- **ETOH withdrawal** – HTN, tachycardia, delirium, seizures after 48 hours
  - Tx: thiamine, folate, B_{12}, Mg, K, PRN lorazepam (Ativan)
- **ICU** (or hospital) **psychosis** – generally occurs after third postoperative day and is frequently preceded by lucid interval
  - Need to rule out metabolic (hypoglycemia, DKA, hypoxia, hypercarbia, electrolyte imbalances) and organic (MI, CVA) causes
- **Atrial fibrillation** – MCC of delayed discharge after cardiac surgery
- **Magnesium** – can be used to Tx ventricular fibrillation (torsades de pointes)

17 Burns

INTRODUCTION

Burn Classification	
Degree	**Description**
1st	Sunburn (epidermis)
2nd	
<u>Superficial</u> dermis (papillary)	Painful to touch; blebs and blisters; hair follicles intact; blanches (do <u>not</u> need skin grafts)
<u>Deep</u> dermis (reticular)	Decreased sensation; ***loss of hair*** follicles (need **skin grafts**)
3rd	Leathery (charred parchment); down to subcutaneous fat
4th	Down to bone; adjacent adipose or muscle tissue

- 1st- and superficial 2nd-degree burns heal by **epithelialization** (primarily from **hair follicles**).
- **Extremely deep burns**, **electrical burns**, or **compartment syndrome** can cause **rhabdomyolysis** with **myoglobinuria** (Tx: hydration, alkalinize urine).

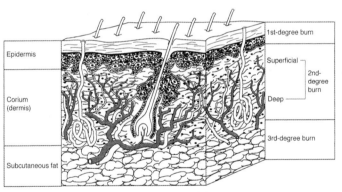

Schematic depiction of the skin.

ADMISSION CRITERIA[1]

- 2nd- and 3rd-degree burns > 10% BSA in patients aged < 10 or > 50 years
- 2nd- and 3rd-degree burns > 20% BSA in all other patients
- 2nd- and 3rd-degree burns to significant portions of hands, face, feet, genitalia, perineum, or skin overlying major joints
- 3rd-degree burns > 5% in any age group
- Electrical and chemical burns
- Concomitant inhalational injury, mechanical traumas, preexisting medical conditions
- Injuries in patients with special social, emotional, or long-term rehabilitation needs
- Suspected child abuse or neglect

[1]Modified from Feliciano DV, Moore EE, Mattox KL. *Trauma*. 3rd ed. Appleton & Lange; 1996:937.

BURN ASSESSMENT

- Deaths highest in children and elderly (trouble getting away)
- Scald burns – most common
- Flame burns – more likely to come to hospital and be admitted
- **Assessing percentage of body surface burned** (rule of 9s)
  - Head = 9, arms = 18, chest = 18, back = 18, legs = 36, perineum = 1
  - Can also use patient's palm to estimate injury (palm = 1%)
- **Parkland formula**
  - Use for **burns ≥ 20%** BSA (≥ 2nd degree; capped at 50% BSA) only – give 4 cc/kg × % burn in first 24 hours; give ½ the volume in the first 8 hours
- Use **lactated Ringer's** solution (LR) in first 24 hours.
  - **Urine output** best measure of resuscitation (> 0.5 cc/kg/h in adults, > 1 cc/kg/h in children, > 2 cc/kg/hr in infants < 6 months)
- Parkland formula can grossly underestimate volume requirements with inhalational injury, ETOH, electrical injury, post-escharotomy.
- Colloid (albumin) in 1st 24 hours causes ↑ pulmonary/respiratory complications → can use colloid after 24 hours

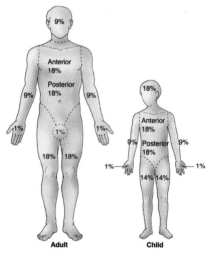

Estimating burn size accurately is essential for care of the burn patient. The rule of nines provides a simple algorithm for calculating the burned surface area.

- **Escharotomy indications** (perform within 4–6 hours):
  - Circumferential deep burns (can cut off blood supply to the extremity)
  - Low temperature, weak pulse, ↓ capillary refill, ↓ pain sensation, or ↓ neurologic function in extremity
  - Problems ventilating patient with significant chest torso burns
  - May need fasciotomy if compartment syndrome suspected after escharotomy
- **Risk factors for burn injuries** – alcohol or drug use, age (very young/very old), smoking, low socioeconomic status, violence, epilepsy

CHILD ABUSE

- Accounts for 15% of burn injuries in children
- History and exam findings that suggest abuse:
  - **History** – delayed presentation for care, conflicting histories, previous injuries
  - **Exam** – sharply demarcated margins, uniform depth, absence of splash marks, stocking or glove patterns, flexor sparing, dorsal location on hands, very deep localized contact injury; scalding burns

LUNG AND AIRWAY INJURY

- Caused primarily by inhalation of **carbonaceous materials** and **smoke**, not heat
- **Risk factors for injury** – ETOH, trauma, closed space, rapid combustion, extremes of age, delayed extrication
- **Signs and symptoms of possible injury** – facial burns, wheezing, carbonaceous sputum (soot)
- Dx: fiberoptic **bronchoscopy**
- **Indications for intubation** – upper airway stridor or obstruction, worsening hypoxemia, massive volume resuscitation (can worsen symptoms)
- **Pneumonia** – most common infection in patients with > 30% BSA burns; also most common cause of **death** after > 30% BSA burns; inhalational injury #1 RF for pneumonia in burn patients

UNUSUAL BURNS

- **Acid and alkali burns** – copious water irrigation as soon as possible
  - Alkalis (Liquid Plumr, Drano) produce deeper burns than acid due to liquefaction necrosis.
  - Acid burns (battery acid) produce coagulation necrosis.
- **Hydrofluoric acid burns** – spread **calcium** on wound
- **Powder burns** – wipe away before irrigation
- **Tar burns** – cool, then wipe away with a **lipophilic solvent** (glycerol; eg adhesive remover)
- **Electrical burns** – need cardiac monitoring; injury is always deeper and worse than skin findings
  - Can cause rhabdomyolysis and compartment syndrome
  - Other complications – polyneuritis (demyelinization), quadriplegia, transverse myelitis, cataracts, liver necrosis, intestinal perforation, gallbladder perforation, pancreatic necrosis, posterior shoulder dislocations, vertebral body fractures
- **Lightning** – cardiopulmonary arrest secondary to ventricular fibrillation

1ST WEEK – EARLY EXCISION OF BURNED AREAS AND START NUTRITION

- **Caloric need**: 25 kcal/kg/day + (30 kcal × % burn)
  - **Glucose** – best source of nonprotein calories in patients with burns
  - Burn wounds – use glucose in an obligatory fashion
  - Place **feeding tube** in patients with significant BSA burns.
- **Protein need**: 1 g/kg/day + (3 g × % burn)
  - Large burn wounds require a significant amount of **protein** for healing.
- **Excise burn wounds** in < 72 hours (but not until after appropriate fluid resuscitation).
  - Used for **deep 2nd-, 3rd-**, and some **4th-degree** burns
  - Viability is based on **punctate bleeding** (#1), color, and texture after removal (use dermatome).
  - **Early excision and grafting** (day 1 of burn) can be considered in stable patients with **limited burns** (< 20%) that are clearly **3rd degree** (saves costs; minimizes pain, suffering, and complications).
- Wounds to **face, palms, soles**, and **genitals** are **deferred** for the 1st week.

- **For each burn wound excision** – want < 1 L blood loss, < 20% of skin excised, and < 2 hours in OR
  - Patients can get extremely sick if too much time is spent in OR.
- **Skin grafts are contraindicated** if culture is positive for **beta-hemolytic strep** or **bacteria > 10^5**.
- **Autografts** (split-thickness [STSG] or full-thickness [FTSG]) – <u>best</u>
  - ↓ Infection, desiccation, protein loss, pain, water loss, heat loss, and RBC loss compared to dermal substitutes
  - Donor skin site is regenerated from **hair follicles** and **skin edges** on STSGs.
  - **Imbibition** (osmotic) – blood supply to skin graft for days 0–3
  - **Neovascularization** – starts around day 3
  - Poorly vascularized beds are unlikely to support skin grafting → includes tendon, bone without periosteum, XRT areas
  - **Split-thickness grafts** are 0.12–0.15 mm (includes epidermis and part of dermis).
- **Homografts** (allografts; cadaveric skin) – not as good as autografts
  - Can be a good temporizing material; last 4 weeks
  - Allografts vascularize and are eventually rejected at which time they must be replaced.
- **Xenografts** (porcine) – not as good as homografts; last 2 weeks; these do not vascularize
- **Dermal substitutes** – not as good as homografts or xenografts
- **Meshed grafts** – use for back, flank, trunk, arms, and legs
  - **Reasons to delay autografting** – infection, not enough skin donor sites, patient septic or unstable, do not want to create any more donor sites with concomitant blood loss
  - **Most common reason for skin graft loss** – seroma or hematoma formation under graft (prevents attachment)
    - Need to apply pressure dressing (cotton balls) to the skin graft to prevent seroma and hematoma buildup underneath the graft
  - **STSGs** are more likely to survive – graft not as thick so easier for **imbibition** and subsequent revascularization to occur
  - **FTSGs** have less wound contraction – good for areas such as the palms and back of hands
- **Burn scar hypopigmentation** and **irregularities** can be improved with dermabrasion thin split-thickness grafts.

2ND TO 5TH WEEKS – SPECIALIZED AREAS ADDRESSED, ALLOGRAFT REPLACED WITH AUTOGRAFT

- **Face** – topical antibiotics for 1st week, **FTSG** for unhealed areas (nonmeshed)
- **Hands**
  - **Superficial** – ROM exercises; splint in extension if too much edema
  - **Deep** – immobilize in extension for 7 days after skin graft (need **FTSG**), then physical therapy. May need wire fixation of joints if unstable or open
- **Palms** – try to preserve specialized palmar aponeurosis. Splint hand in extension for 7 days after **FTSG**.
- **Genitals** – can use **STSG** (meshed)

BURN WOUND INFECTIONS

- The larger the burn, the greater the risk.
- <u>No</u> role for prophylactic IV antibiotics
- **Pseudomonas** is most common organism in burn wound infection (some texts say staph but *Pseudomonas* is the classic answer), followed by *Staphylococcus*, *E. coli*, and *Enterobacter*.
- More common in burns > **30% BSA**
- Topical agents have decreased incidence of burn wound bacterial infections.

- *Candida* infections have increased incidence secondary to topical antimicrobials.
- Granulocyte chemotaxis and cell-mediated immunity are impaired in burn patients.
- **Silvadene** (silver sulfadiazine) – can cause **neutropenia** and **thrombocytopenia**
  - Standard topical agent used for burns
  - Do not use in patients with sulfa allergy.
  - Limited eschar penetration; can inhibit epithelialization
  - Ineffective against some *Pseudomonas*; effective for *Candida*
- **Silver nitrate** – can cause **electrolyte imbalances** (hyponatremia, hypochloremia, hypocalcemia, and hypokalemia)
  - Discoloration
  - Limited eschar penetration
  - Ineffective against some *Pseudomonas* species and GPCs
  - Can cause **methemoglobinemia** – contraindicated in patients with G6PD deficiency (causes hemolysis)
- **Sulfamylon** (mafenide sodium) – <u>painful</u> application
  - Can cause **metabolic acidosis** due to carbonic anhydrase inhibition ($\downarrow$ renal conversion of $H_2CO_3 \rightarrow H_2O + CO_2$)
  - Good **eschar penetration** (good for deep burns); good for burns overlying **cartilage**
  - Broadest spectrum against *Pseudomonas* and GNRs
- **Triple antibiotic ointment** – good for burns near the eyes (Silvadene is irritating)
- **Mupirocin** – good for MRSA; very expensive
- **Signs of burn wound infection** – peripheral edema, 2nd- to 3rd-degree burn conversion, hemorrhage into scar, erythema gangrenosum, green fat, black skin around wound, rapid eschar separation, focal discoloration
- **Burn wound sepsis** – usually due to *Pseudomonas*
- **HSV** – most common viral infection in burn wounds
- **< 10^5 organisms** – <u>not</u> a burn wound infection
- Best way to detect burn wound infection (and differentiate from colonization) – **biopsy of burn wound**
- Tx of burn wound infection:
  - Burn wound excision with allograft placement (<u>not</u> autograft)
  - Systemic antibiotics
  - If just cellulitis around the wound, no excision and just give IV antibiotics

COMPLICATIONS AFTER BURNS

- **Tetanus prophylaxis** – required in patients with burn wounds
- **Seizures** – usually iatrogenic and related to **Na concentration**
- **Peripheral neuropathy** – secondary to small vessel injury and demyelination
- **Ectopia** – from contraction of burned adnexa. Tx: eyelid release
- **Eyes** – fluorescein staining to find injury. Tx: topical fluoroquinolone or gentamicin
- **Corneal abrasion** – Tx: topical antibiotics
- **Symblepharon** – eyelid stuck to conjunctiva. Tx: release with glass rod
- **Heterotopic ossification of tendons** – Tx: physical therapy; may need surgery
- **Fractures** – Tx: often need external fixation to allow for treatment of burns
- **Curling's ulcer** – gastric ulcer that occurs with burns
- **Marjolin's ulcer** – highly malignant **squamous cell CA** that arises in chronic (many years) nonhealing burn wounds or unstable scars
- **Hypertrophic scar**
  - Usually occurs 3–4 months after injury secondary to $\uparrow$ **neovascularity**
  - More likely to be deep thermal injuries that take > 3 weeks to heal, heal by contraction and epithelial spread, or heal across flexor surfaces
  - Tx: **steroid injection into lesion** (best), silicone, compression; wait 1–2 years before scar modification surgery

RENAL ISSUES WITH SEVERE BURNS
- **Hyperkalemia** – from dead tissue and myonecrosis; avoid succinylcholine
- **Myoglobinuria** – from dead muscle; Tx: fluids; alkalinize urine
- **Renal failure** – from volume loss and myoglobinuria

FROSTBITE
- Tx: rapid re-warming in 40°C circulating water
- Tetanus shot, Silvadene; avoid early amputations

ERYTHEMA MULTIFORME AND VARIANTS
- **Erythema multiforme** – least severe form (self-limited, target lesions)
- **Stevens–Johnson syndrome** (more serious) – 10%–30% BSA
- **Toxic epidermal necrolysis** (TEN) – most severe form (> 30% BSA)
- **Staph scalded skin syndrome** (caused by *Staphylococcus aureus*)
- Skin <u>epidermal–dermal separation</u> seen in all
- Caused by a variety of drugs (penicillin [#1], Dilantin, Bactrim) and viruses
- Tx: fluid resuscitation and supportive; need to prevent wound desiccation with Telfa wraps; topical antibiotics; IV antibiotics if due to *Staphylococcus*; may need future skin grafts
- **No steroids**

18 Plastics, Skin, and Soft Tissues

SKIN

- **Epidermis** – primarily cellular
  - **Keratinocytes** – main cell type in epidermis; originate from basal layer; provide mechanical barrier
  - **Melanocytes** – neuroectodermal origin (neural crest cells); in basal layer of epidermis
    - Have dendritic processes that transfer melanin to neighboring keratinocytes via melanosomes
    - Density of melanocytes is the same among races; difference is in melanin production.
- **Dermis** – primarily structural proteins (collagen) for the epidermis
- **Langerhans cells** (dendritic cells)
  - Act as antigen-presenting cells (MHC class II)
  - Originate from bone marrow
  - Have a role in contact hypersensitivity reactions (type IV)
- **Sensory nerves**
  - **Pacinian corpuscles** – pressure
  - **Ruffini's endings** – warmth
  - **Krause's end-bulbs** – cold
  - **Meissner's corpuscles** – tactile sense
- **Eccrine sweat glands** – aqueous sweat (thermal regulation, usually hypotonic)
- **Apocrine sweat glands** – milky sweat
  - Highest concentration of glands in palms and soles; most sweat is the result of sympathetic nervous system via acetylcholine.
- **Lipid-soluble drugs** – ↑ skin absorption
- **Type I collagen** – predominant type in skin; 70% of dermis; gives tensile strength
- **Tension** – resistance to stretching (collagen)
- **Elasticity** – ability to regain shape (branching proteins that can stretch to 2× normal length)
- **Cushing's striae** – decreased collagen results in loss of tensile strength and elasticity in the dermis; blood vessel dilation and neovascularization occur.

FLAPS

- MCC of **pedicled** or **anastomosed free flap necrosis** – **venous thrombosis**
- **Tissue expansion** occurs by local recruitment, thinning of the dermis and epidermis, mitosis.
- **DIEP Flap**
  - Used more commonly than TRAM flap
  - Transfers **deep inferior epigastric perforators** (DIEP) along with overlying fat and skin to breast area (*no muscle is transferred*)
  - **Inferior epigastric artery / vein** are sewn to **internal mammary artery / vein** respectively (thoracodorsal vessels are alternative)
  - Less hernias and muscle weakness long term compared to TRAM
- **TRAM flaps**
  - Transfers portion of **rectus muscle** with flap (unlike above)
  - Complications – flap necrosis, ventral hernia, infection, abdominal wall weakness
  - Pedicled TRAM – relies on **superior** epigastric vessels
  - Free TRAM – relies on **inferior** epigastric vessels
  - **Periumbilical muscle perforators** most important determinant of **TRAM flap viability**

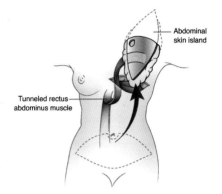

Transverse rectus abdominis myocutaneous (TRAM) flap reconstruction.

Pressure Sores		
Stage	**Description**	**Treatment**
I	**Erythema** and pain, no skin loss (epidermis)	Keep pressure off
II	**Partial** skin loss with yellow debris (into the dermis)	Local treatment, keep pressure off
III	Full-thickness skin loss (**subcutaneous fat exposure**)	Sharp debridement; likely need myocutaneous flap
IV	Involves **bony cortex**, **muscle**, **adipose tissue**, **tendon**	Myocutaneous flaps (eg gluteal flap)

UV RADIATION

- Damages DNA and repair mechanisms
- Both a promoter and initiator
- **Melanin** single best factor for protecting skin from UV radiation
- **UV-B** – responsible for chronic sun damage
- Blistering sunburns in childhood place patient at higher risk for skin CA in later years.

MELANOMA

- Most lethal skin CA – represents only 15% of skin CA but accounts for 65% of the deaths
- **Risk factors** for melanoma:
  - Dysplastic, atypical, or large **congenital nevi** – 10% lifetime risk for melanoma
  - Familial **BK mole syndrome** – almost 100% risk of melanoma
  - **Xeroderma pigmentosum**
  - Fair complexion, easy sunburn, intermittent sunburns, previous skin CA, previous XRT
  - 10% of melanomas familial
- **Most common melanoma site on skin** – back in men, legs in women
- **Prognosis worse** for men, ulcerated lesions, ocular and mucosal lesions
- **Signs of melanoma** (ABCDE) – <u>a</u>symmetry (angulations, indentation, notching, ulceration, bleeding), <u>b</u>orders that are irregular, <u>c</u>olor change (darkening), <u>d</u>iameter increase, <u>e</u>levation or evolving over time
- Originates from **neural crest cells** (melanocytes) in **basal layer** epidermis

- **Blue** color → most ominous
- **Lung** – most common location for distant melanoma metastases
- Most common metastasis to <u>small bowel</u> – **melanoma**
- **Dx:**
  - < **2 cm lesion** – <u>excisional</u> biopsy (Tru-Cut core needle biopsy) unless cosmetically sensitive area – need resection with margins if pathology comes back as melanoma
  - > **2 cm lesions** or **cosmetically sensitive area** – <u>incisional</u> biopsy (or punch biopsy), will need to resect with margins if pathology shows melanoma
  - Changes in a **nevus** – get biopsy
  - Stains for S-100 and HMB-45 proteins
- **Types:**
  - **Melanoma in situ** or **thin lentigo maligna** (ie Hutchinson's freckle) – just in the **epidermis**; <u>0.5-cm margins</u> are appropriate here
  - **Lentigo maligna melanoma** – least aggressive, minimal invasion, radial growth 1st; presents as an elevated nodule
  - **Superficial spreading** (MC type) – intermediate malignancy; originates from nevus or sun-exposed areas
  - **Acral lentiginous** – very aggressive; palms/soles of African Americans; **subungual** (below fingernail)
  - **Nodular** – *most aggressive type*; most likely to have metastasized at time of Dx; deepest growth at time of Dx; vertical growth 1st; bluish-black with smooth borders; occurs *anywhere* on the body
- **Staging** – chest/abd/pelvic CT, LFTs, and LDH for all melanoma ≥ 1 mm; examine all possible draining lymph nodes
- **Tx for all stages** → 1) resection of primary tumor with appropriate margins (get down to muscle fascia) and; 2) management of lymph nodes

Recommended Surgical Margins for Melanoma Excision	
Melanoma Thickness (mm)	Clinical Excision Margin (cm)
In situ	0.5
Thin (≤ 1.0)	1.0
Intermediate (1.1–2.0)	1.0–2.0
Thick (> 2.0)	2.0

Margins may need to be modified based on anatomic considerations but still require histologic confirmation of tumor-free margins. For clinically ill-defined lentigo maligna melanoma, wider margins may be required for histologic confirmation of tumor-free margins.

- **Nodes**
  - Always need formal lymphadenectomy for **clinically positive nodes** or if **sentinel lymph node biopsy** (SLNB) is **positive**
  - You are trying to clear the tumor here, not stage
  - Perform **SLNB** if nodes clinically negative and tumor > 1 mm deep
  - Consider **SLNB** for tumor 0.8 – 1.0 mm deep with ulceration, high mitotic index, or lymphovascular invasion
  - **Involved nodes** usually nontender, round, hard, 1–2 cm
  - Need to include **superficial parotidectomy** for all **scalp and face melanomas anterior to the ear (tragus)** and **above the lower lip** ≥ 1 mm deep including melanomas on the **ear** (20% metastasis rate to parotid)

- **Axillary node melanoma with no other primary** – Tx: complete axillary node dissection (remove level I, II, and III nodes – unlike breast CA); primary lesion may have regressed or the melanoma primary is unpigmented
- **Resection of metastases** has provided some patients with long disease-free interval and is the best chance for cure.
- **Isolated metastases** (ie lung or liver) that can be resected with a low-risk procedure should probably undergo resection.
- **Head and neck melanoma**
  - **Margins** can be **modified** if abutting **critical structures** (eg carotid artery), although margin should still be tumor free.
  - Preserve facial nerve unless already clinically involved (ie is non-functional).
  - Head and neck melanomas anterior to the ear and above the lower lip metastasize to **parotid**; melanomas posterior to the ear go to **posterior neck**.
- Dacarbazine first-line chemo for metastatic melanoma
- Interferon-alpha, immunotherapy, and tumor vaccines can be used for systemic disease.
- XRT can help regional control (*no survival benefit*).
- No Mohs surgery for melanoma

BASAL CELL CARCINOMA

- **Most common malignancy in United States**; 4× more common than squamous cell skin CA
- 80% on head and neck
- Originates from **epidermis** – basal epithelial cells and hair follicles
- **Pearly** appearance, **rolled borders**, slow and indolent growth
- Pathology – **peripheral palisading of nuclei** and **stromal retraction**
- Rare metastases or nodal disease
- **Regional adenectomy** for rare **clinically positive nodes**
- **Morpheaform type** – most aggressive; has **collagenase** production
- Tx: **0.3–0.5-cm** margins (or Mohs surgery)
  - XRT and chemotherapy – may be of limited benefit for inoperable disease, metastases or neuro/lymphatic/vessel invasion

SQUAMOUS CELL CARCINOMA

- Overlying erythema, papulonodular with crust and ulceration; usually red-brown
- May have surrounding induration and satellite nodules
- Metastasizes more frequently than basal cell CA but less common than melanoma
- Can develop in post-XRT areas or in old burn scars
- **Risk factors** – actinic keratoses, xeroderma pigmentosum, Bowen's disease, atrophic epidermis, arsenics, hydrocarbons (coal tar), chlorophenols, HPV, immunosuppression, sun exposure, fair skin, previous XRT, previous skin CA
- Risk factors for metastasis – poorly differentiated, greater depth, recurrent lesions, immunosuppression
- Tx: **0.5–1.0-cm** margins usual (2-cm margins for Marjolin's ulcers and penile/vulvar areas)
  - Can treat high risk with **Mohs surgery** (margin mapping using conservative slices; not used for melanoma) when trying to minimize area of resection (ie lesions on face)
  - **Regional adenectomy** for **clinically positive nodes**
  - XRT and chemotherapy – may be of limited benefit for inoperable disease, metastases or neuro/lymphatic/vessel invasion

SOFT TISSUE SARCOMA

- **Most common soft tissue sarcomas** – #1 malignant fibrous histiosarcoma, #2 liposarcoma
- 50% arise from extremities; 50% in children (arise from embryonic mesoderm)

- Most sarcomas are large, grow rapidly, and are painless.
- Symptoms: asymptomatic mass (most common presentation), GI bleeding, bowel obstruction, neurologic deficit
- CXR – to R/O lung mets
- **MRI** *before* **biopsy** to R/O vascular, neuro, or bone invasion
- **Core needle biopsy** (best, 95% accurate); if that fails →
  - **Excisional biopsy** if mass < 4 cm
  - **Longitudinal incisional biopsy** for masses > 4 cm
  - Need to eventually resect biopsy skin site if biopsy shows sarcoma
  - Biopsy along the long axis plane of future incision for resection
- **Hematogenous spread**, not to lymphatics → <u>metastasis to nodes is rare</u>
  - **Lung** – most common site for metastasis
- **Staging** based on **grade**, not size
- **Tumor grade** is the most important prognostic factor (undifferentiated worse).
- Tx: Want **1–3 cm margins** (varies based tumor grade) and if possible **1 uninvolved fascial plane** → try to perform limb-sparing operation
  - **Place clips** to mark site of likely recurrence → will XRT these later
  - **Postop XRT** – for high-grade tumors, close margins, or tumors > 5 cm
  - Chemotherapy is **doxorubicin** (Adriamycin) based.
  - Tumors > 10 cm may benefit from preop chemo-XRT → may allow limb-sparing resection; 90% do not require an amputation

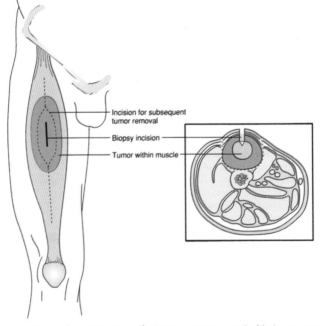

Technique for biopsy of an extremity soft-tissue mass suspected of being a sarcoma. The incision should be oriented along the long axis of the extremity, at the point where the lesion is closest to the surface, and situated so that it can be readily excised along with the tumor if a diagnosis of sarcoma is made. There should be no raising of flaps or disturbance of tissue planes superficial to the tumor. The mass should not be enucleated within the pseudocapsule; rather, incisional biopsy leaving the bulk of the lesion undisturbed should be carried out. Before wound closure, hemostasis should be achieved to avoid a hematoma, which could disseminate tumor cells through normal tissue planes. Drains are not used routinely.

- **Isolated sarcoma metastases** without other evidence of systemic disease can be **resected** and are the best chance for survival; otherwise can palliate with XRT
- Midline incision favored for pelvic and retroperitoneal sarcomas
- With resection, try to preserve motor nerves and retain or reconstruct vessels.
- **Poor prognosis overall**
  - Delay in diagnosis
  - Difficulty with total resection
  - Difficulty getting XRT to pelvic tumors
  - Chemo and XRT have not changed survival.
  - 40% 5-year survival rate with complete resection
- **Head** and **neck sarcomas** – usually in the pediatric population (usually rhabdomyosarcoma)
  - Hard to get margins because of proximity to vital structures
  - Postop XRT for positive or close margins as negative margins may be impossible to obtain
- **Retroperitoneal sarcomas** – most commonly are leiomyosarcomas and liposarcomas
  - Especially poor prognosis due to delayed diagnosis and incomplete resection; also trouble getting XRT to the tumor due to proximity of vital structures
  - Ability to completely remove the tumor the most important prognostic factor
  - Need to rule out **lymphoma** in this location (MC retroperitoneal tumor overall)
- **Risk factors**
  - **Asbestos** – mesothelioma
  - **PVC** and **arsenic** – angiosarcoma
  - **Chronic lymphedema** – lymphangiosarcoma
- **Kaposi's sarcoma** (KS) – vascular sarcoma
  - Oral and pharyngeal mucosa are the most common sites; bleeding, dysphagia
  - Associated with immunocompromised state; most common malignancy in AIDS
  - Rarely a cause of death in AIDS (very slow growing)
    - Tx: Primary goal is **palliation**.
    - **AIDS Tx** (HAART) shrinks AIDS-related KS – *best Tx*
    - Consider XRT or intra-lesional vinblastine for local disease.
    - Interferon-alpha for disseminated disease
    - Surgery for severe intestinal hemorrhage
- **Childhood rhabdomyosarcoma**
  - #1 soft tissue sarcoma in **kids**
  - Head/neck, genitourinary, extremities, and trunk (poorest prognosis)
  - **Embryonal** subtype – most common
  - **Alveolar** subtype – worst prognosis
  - Rhabdomyosarcoma contains **desmin**.
  - **Botryoides** tumor – vaginal rhabdomyosarcoma
  - Tx: surgery; **doxorubicin**-based chemotherapy
- **Bone sarcomas**
  - Most are metastatic at the time of diagnosis.
  - **Osteosarcoma**
    - Increased incidence around the knee
    - Originates from **metaphyseal cells**
    - Usually in children
- **Genetic syndromes for soft tissue tumors**
  - Neurofibromatosis – CNS tumors, peripheral sheath tumors, pheochromocytoma
  - Li–Fraumeni syndrome – childhood rhabdomyosarcoma, many others
  - Hereditary retinoblastoma – also includes other sarcomas
  - Tuberous sclerosis – angiomyolipoma
  - Gardner's syndrome – familial adenomatous polyposis and intra-abdominal desmoids tumors

OTHER CONDITIONS

- **Lip lacerations** – important to line up vermillion border
- **Xanthoma** (cholesterol-rich) – yellow, contains histiocytes; benign
- **Warts** (verruca vulgaris) – viral origin, contagious, autoinoculable, can be painful
  - Tx: salicylic acid; liquid nitrogen
- **Lipomas** – common but rarely malignant; back, neck, between shoulders
  - Most common mesenchymal tumor
- **Neuromas** – can be associated with neurofibromatosis and von Recklinghausen's disease (café-au-lait spots, axillary freckling; peripheral nerve and CNS tumors)
- **Keratoses**
  - **Actinic keratosis** – premalignant in sun-damaged areas; need excisional biopsy if suspicious; Tx: diclofenac sodium; liquid nitrogen
  - **Seborrheic keratosis** – <u>not</u> premalignant; trunk on elderly; can be dark
  - **Arsenical keratosis** – associated with squamous cell carcinoma
- **Merkel cell carcinoma** – are **neuroendocrine**
  - Very aggressive malignant tumor with early regional and systemic spread
  - Red to purple papulonodule or indurated plaque
  - Have **neuron-specific enolase** (NSE), **cytokeratin**, and **neurofilament protein**
  - All patients get **SLNBx** or **formal lymph node dissection**.
  - Need **2–3-cm margins**
- **Glomus cell tumor**
  - Painful tumor composed of **blood vessels** and **nerves**
  - **Benign**; most common in the **terminal aspect of the digit**
  - Tx: tumor excision
- **Desmoid tumors** – benign but locally very invasive
  - **Anterior abdominal wall** (most common location) desmoids can occur during or following pregnancy; can also occur after trauma or surgery; occur in fascial planes
  - **Intra-abdominal desmoids** associated with Gardner's syndrome and retroperitoneal fibrosis; often **encases bowel**, making it hard to get en bloc resection
  - High risk of local recurrences; no distant spread
  - Tx: surgery if possible; chemotherapy (**sulindac, tamoxifen**) if vital structure involved or too much bowel would be taken (high risk of short bowel syndrome with surgery)
- **Bowen's disease** – SCCA in situ; 10% turn into invasive SCCA; associated with **HPV**
  - Tx: **imiquimod**, cautery ablation, topical 5FU, **_avoid wide local excision_** if possible (high recurrence rate w/ HPV); regular biopsies to R/O CA
- **Keratoacanthoma**
  - Rapid growth, rolled edges, crater filled with **keratin**
  - Is <u>not</u> malignant but can be confused with SCCA
  - Involutes spontaneously over months
  - Always biopsy these to be sure.
  - If small, excise; if large, biopsy and observe.
- **Hyperhidrosis** – ↑ sweating, especially noticeable in the palms. Tx: **thoracic sympathectomy** if refractory to variety of antiperspirants
- **Hidradenitis** – infection of the apocrine sweat glands, usually in axilla and groin regions
  - Staph/strep most common organisms; avoid antiperspirants.
  - Tx: antibiotics, improved hygiene 1st; may need surgery to remove skin and associated sweat glands (excise from skin to fascia)
- **Benign cysts**
  - **Epidermal inclusion cyst** – most common; have completely mature epidermis with creamy **keratin** material
  - **Trichilemmal cyst** – in scalp, no epidermis; contain keratin from hair follicles

- **Ganglion cyst** – over joints, usually the wrist; filled with **synovial fluid**
  - Aspiration cures 50%
  - Need to remove the **one-way check valve** that leads back to the joint with resection to prevent recurrence
- **Dermoid cyst** – midline intra-abdominal and sacral lesions usual; need resection due to malignancy risk
- **Pilonidal cyst** – congenital coccygeal sinus (at sacrococcygeal junction) with ingrown hair; gets infected and needs to be excised

ANATOMY AND PHYSIOLOGY

- **Anterior neck triangle** – neck midline (and sternal notch), sternocleidomastoid muscle (SCM), and the inferior border mandible; contains the **carotid sheath**
- **Posterior neck triangle** – posterior border of the SCM, trapezius muscle, and the clavicle; contains the **accessory nerve** (innervates SCM, trapezius, and platysma) and the **brachial plexus**
- **Parotid glands** – secrete mostly serous fluid
- **Sublingual glands** – secrete mostly mucin
- **Submandibular glands** – 50/50 serous/mucin
- In larynx, the false vocal cords are superior to the true vocal cords.
- Trachea has U-shaped cartilage and a posterior portion that is membranous.

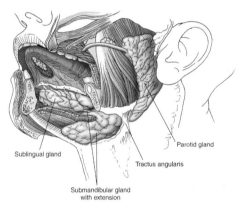

Sublingual gland

Parotid gland

Tractus angularis

Submandibular gland with extension

Major salivary glands. The lateral view, illustrating the tractus angularis and submandibular gland with extension under the mylohyoid muscle and the sublingual gland.

- **Vagus nerve** – runs between internal jugular (IJ) vein and carotid artery
- **Phrenic nerve** – runs on top of anterior scalene muscle (*runs lateral to medial as it enters chest*)
- **Long thoracic nerve** – runs posterior to the middle scalene muscle
- **Trigeminal nerve** – ophthalmic, maxillary, and mandibular branches
  - Gives **sensation** to most of face; mastication muscles
  - Marginal mandibular nerve comes off trigeminal nerve – gives fibers to the corner of the mouth
- **Facial nerve** – temporal, zygomatic, buccal, marginal mandibular, and cervical branches
  - **Motor** function to face
- **Glossopharyngeal nerve** – taste to posterior ⅓ tongue
  - Motor to stylopharyngeus
  - Injury affects **swallowing**.
- **Hypoglossal nerve** – motor to all of tongue except palatoglossus
  - Tongue deviates to the **same side** of a hypoglossal nerve injury.
- **Recurrent laryngeal nerve** – innervates all of larynx except cricothyroid muscle

- **Superior laryngeal nerve** – innervates the cricothyroid muscle
- **Frey's syndrome** – occurs after parotidectomy; injury of **auriculotemporal nerve** that then cross-innervates with **sympathetic fibers** to sweat glands of skin
  - Symptom: **gustatory sweating** (sweating while eating or tasting)
- **Thyrocervical trunk** – "STAT": **s**uprascapular artery, **t**ransverse cervical artery, **a**scending cervical artery, inferior **t**hyroid artery
- **External carotid artery** – 1st branch is superior thyroid artery
- **Trapezius flap** – based on transverse cervical artery
- **Pectoralis major flap** – based on either the thoracoacromial artery or the internal mammary artery
- **Torus palatini** – congenital bony mass on upper palate of mouth. Tx: nothing
- **Torus mandibular** – similar to above but on lingual surface of mandible. Tx: nothing
- **Modified radical neck dissection** (MRND) – takes omohyoid, submandibular gland, sensory nerves C2–C5, cervical branch of facial nerve, and ipsilateral thyroid
  - No mortality difference compared with RND
- **Radical neck dissection** (RND) – same as MRND *plus* accessory nerve (CN XII), sternocleidomastoid, and internal jugular resection (rarely done anymore)
  - Most morbidity occurs from accessory nerve resection
- ENT chemotherapy – **5FU** and **cisplatin** usual
- ENT tumors often present as an enlarged lymph node in the neck.

ORAL CAVITY CANCER

- **Most common cancer of the oral cavity, pharynx**, and **larynx** – squamous cell CA
  - **Biggest risk factors** – tobacco and ETOH
  - **Erythroplakia** – considered more premalignant than leukoplakia
- **Oral cavity includes** mouth floor, anterior ⅓ tongue, gingiva, hard palate, anterior tonsillar pillars, and lips
- **Lower lip** – most common site for oral cavity CA (due to sun exposure)
- **Survival rate lowest** for **hard palate tumors** – hard to resect
- **Oral cavity CA** increased in patients with **Plummer–Vinson syndrome** (glossitis, cervical dysphagia from esophageal web, spoon fingers, iron-deficiency anemia).
- **Treatment**
  - **Wide resection** (1 cm margins)
  - **MRND** for tumors > 4 cm, clinically positive nodes, or bone invasion
  - **Postop XRT** for advanced lesions (> 4 cm, positive margins, or nodal/bone involvement)
- **Lip CA** – may need **flaps** if more than ⅓ of the lip is removed
  - Lesions along the **commissure** are **most aggressive**.
- **Tongue CA** – can still operate with jaw invasion (commando procedure)
- **Verrucous ulcer** – a well-differentiated SCCA; often found on the cheek; oral tobacco
  - Not aggressive, rare metastasis
  - Tx: full cheek resection ± flap; *__no lymph node dissection__*
- **Cancer of maxillary sinus** – Tx: maxillectomy
- **Tonsillar CA** – ETOH, tobacco, males; SCCA most common; asymptomatic until large; 80% have lymph node metastases at time of diagnosis
  - Tx: **tonsillectomy** best way to biopsy; wide resection with margins after that

PHARYNGEAL CANCER

- **Nasopharyngeal SCCA** – EBV; Chinese; presents with nose bleeding or obstruction
  - Goes to **posterior cervical neck nodes**
  - Tx: *__XRT primary therapy__* (*very sensitive*; give chemo-XRT for advanced disease – *no surgery*)
  - **Children** – lymphoma #1 tumor of nasopharynx. Tx: chemotherapy
  - **Papilloma** – most common benign neoplasm of nose/paranasal sinuses

- **Oropharyngeal SCCA** – neck mass, sore throat
  - Goes to **posterior cervical neck nodes**
  - Tx: **XRT** for tumors **< 4 cm** and no nodal or bone invasion
  - Combined surgery, MRND, and XRT for advanced tumors (> 4 cm, bone invasion or nodal invasion)
- **Hypopharyngeal SCCA** – hoarseness; <u>early metastases</u>
  - Goes to **anterior cervical nodes**
  - Tx: **XRT** for tumors **< 4 cm** and no nodal or bone invasion
  - Combined **surgery**, **MRND**, and **XRT** for **advanced tumors** (> 4 cm, bone invasion or nodal invasion)
- **Nasopharyngeal angiofibroma** – benign tumor
  - Presents in males < 20 years (obstruction or epistaxis)
  - Extremely **vascular**
  - Tx: angiography and **embolization** (usually internal maxillary artery), followed by **resection**

LARYNGEAL CANCER

- Hoarseness, aspiration, dyspnea, dysphagia
- Try to **preserve larynx**
- Tx: **XRT** (if vocal cord only) or **chemo-XRT** (if beyond vocal cord)
  - Spread XRT to ipsilateral neck nodes; bilateral neck nodes if the tumor crosses the midline
  - Surgery is <u>not</u> the primary Tx; try to **preserve larynx**.
  - MRND needed if nodes clinically positive
  - Take **ipsilateral thyroid lobe** with MRND.
- Papilloma – most common benign lesion of larynx

SALIVARY GLAND CANCERS

- Parotid, submandibular, sublingual, and minor salivary glands (*listed by size, large to small*)
- Submandibular or sublingual tumors – can present as a neck mass or swelling in the floor of the mouth
- **Mass in <u>large</u> salivary gland** → more likely mass is <u>benign</u>
- **Mass in <u>small</u> salivary gland** → more likely mass is <u>malignant</u>, although the parotid gland is the most frequent site for malignant tumor
- **Pre-auricular masses** are **parotid tumors** until proven otherwise.
  - Dx: **superficial parotidectomy** (do <u>not</u> shell out; <u>no</u> enucleation)
  - <u>No</u> FNA unless in the deep parotid gland, is felt to be a metastasis from another site, or if the patient is a poor surgical risk
- **Malignant tumors**
  - Often present as a painful mass but can also present with facial nerve paralysis or lymphadenopathy (pain or facial nerve paralysis from a parotid mass is highly suggestive of malignancy)
  - Lymphatic drainage is to the intra-parotid and anterior cervical chain nodes.
  - Most commonly metastasizes to the **lung**
  - **Mucoepidermoid CA** – #1 malignant tumor of the salivary glands
    - Wide range of aggressiveness
  - **Adenoid cystic CA** – #2 malignant tumor of the salivary glands
    - Slow, long, indolent course; propensity to invade **nerve roots**
    - Very sensitive to **XRT**
    - Consider XRT as sole (definitive) therapy if resection would result in high morbidity or the patient is a poor surgical candidate
  - Tx for both: **resection of salivary gland** (eg total parotidectomy), **prophylactic MRND**, and **postop XRT**
    - If in parotid, need to take **whole lobe**; try to **preserve facial nerve**.

- **Benign tumors**
  - Often present as a painless mass
  - **Pleomorphic adenoma** (mixed tumor) – #1 tumor overall of the salivary glands
    - **Malignant degeneration** in 5%
    - Tx: superficial parotidectomy
    - If malignant degeneration, need total parotidectomy
  - **Warthin's tumor** – #2 benign tumor of the salivary glands
    - Males, bilateral in 10%
    - Tx: superficial parotidectomy
- Most common injured nerve with **parotid** surgery – **greater auricular nerve** (numbness over lower portion of ear)
- Most common injured nerve with **submandibular gland** resection – **marginal mandibular nerve** (branch of the facial nerve; get droop at the corner of the mouth)
- Most common salivary gland tumor in children – **hemangiomas**

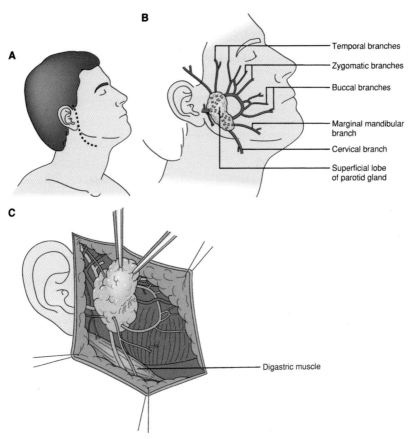

Superficial parotidectomy. **(A)** The standard Blair incision or the cosmetically superior facelift incision can be used. **(B)** Branches of the facial nerve course between the superficial and deep lobes of the parotid. **(C)** The main trunk of the facial nerve is identified 8 mm deep to the tympanomastoid suture line and at the same level as the digastric muscle.

EAR

- **Pinna lacerations** – need suture through involved cartilage
- **Outer ear infections** – early antibiotics to avoid cartilage necrosis
- **Cauliflower ear** – undrained hematomas that organize and calcify; need to be drained to avoid this
- **Cholesteatoma** – epidermal inclusion cyst of ear; slow growing but erode as they grow; present with conductive hearing loss and clear drainage from ear. Tx: surgical excision; can involve mastoid with possible need for mastoidectomy
- **Chemodectomas** – vascular tumor of middle ear (paraganglionoma). Tx: surgery ± XRT
- **Acoustic neuroma** – CN VIII (vestibulocochlear nerve) tinnitus, hearing loss, unsteadiness; can grow into cerebellar/pontine angle. Dx: MRI; Tx: craniotomy and resection; XRT is alternative to surgery.
- **Ear SCCA** – 20% metastasize to parotid gland. Tx: resection and parotidectomy, MRND for positive nodes or large tumors
- **Rhabdomyosarcoma** – most common childhood aural malignancy (although rare) of the middle or external ear

NOSE

- **Nasal fractures** – set after swelling decreases
- **Septal hematoma** – need to drain to avoid infection and necrosis of septum
- **CSF rhinorrhea** – usually a cribriform plate fracture (CSF has **tau protein**)
  - Repair of facial fractures may help leak; may need contrast study to help find leak
  - Tx: conservative 2–3 weeks; try epidural catheter drainage of CSF; may need transethmoidal repair
- **Epistaxis** – 90% are <u>anterior</u> and can be controlled with packing; consider **internal maxillary artery** or **ethmoid artery embolization** for persistent <u>posterior</u> bleeding despite packing/balloon; can be life-threatening in elderly patients with HTN

NECK AND JAW

- **Radicular cyst** – inflammatory cyst at the root of teeth; can cause bone erosion; lucent on X-ray; Tx: local excision or curettage
- **Ameloblastoma** – slow-growing malignancy of odontogenic epithelium (outside portion of teeth); soap bubble appearance on X-ray. Tx: wide local excision
- **Osteogenic sarcoma** – poor prognosis. Tx: multimodality approach that includes surgery
- **Maxillary jaw fractures** – most treated with wire fixation
- **TMJ dislocations** – treated with closed reduction
- **Lower lip numbness** – inferior alveolar nerve damage (branch of mandibular nerve)
- **Stensen's duct laceration** – repair over catheter stent
  - Ligation can cause painful parotid atrophy and facial asymmetry.
- **Suppurative parotitis** – usually in elderly patients; occurs with **dehydration**; **staph** most common organism
  - Fever, pain, and swelling near angle of jaw
  - Tx: fluid hydration, salivation, antibiotics; drainage if abscess develops or patient not improving; may need to remove salivary calculi if present
  - Can be life-threatening
- **Sialoadenitis** – acute inflammation of a salivary gland related to a stone in the duct; most calculi near orifice
  - 80% of the time affects the submandibular or sublingual glands
  - Recurrent sialoadenitis is due to ascending infection from the oral cavity.
  - Tx: Incise duct and remove stone.
  - Gland excision may eventually be necessary for recurrent disease.

ABSCESSES

- **Peritonsillar abscess** – older kids (> 10 years)
  - Symptoms: trismus, odynophagia; usually does not obstruct airway
  - Tx: needle aspiration 1st, then drainage through tonsillar bed if no relief in 24 hours (may need to intubate to drain; will self-drain with swallowing once opened)
- **Retropharyngeal abscess** – younger kids (< 10 years)
  - Symptoms: fever, odynophagia, drool; is an **airway emergency**
  - Can occur in elderly with Pott's disease
  - Tx: intubate the patient in a calm setting; drainage through posterior pharyngeal wall; will self-drain with swallowing once opened
- **Parapharyngeal abscess** – all age groups; occurs with **dental infections**, tonsillitis, pharyngitis
  - Morbidity comes from vascular invasion and **mediastinal spread** via prevertebral and retropharyngeal spaces.
  - Tx: drain through lateral neck to avoid damaging internal carotid and internal jugular veins; need to leave drain in
- **Ludwig's angina** – acute infection of the floor of the mouth, involves **mylohyoid muscle**
  - Most common cause is **dental infection** of the mandibular teeth.
  - May rapidly spread to deeper structures, causing **airway obstruction** and **mediastinitis**
  - Tx: airway control, surgical drainage (intra- or extra-oral), antibiotics; may needs VATS drainage if mediastinitis present

ASYMPTOMATIC HEAD AND NECK MASSES (UNKNOWN PRIMARY HEAD AND NECK MASS)

- **Neck mass workup**
  - 1st – H and P, larynx and nasopharynx fiberoscopy, and **FNA (best test for Dx)**; can consider antibiotics for 2 weeks with re-evaluation if thought to be inflammatory
  - 2nd – if above nondiagnostic → panendoscopy (direct laryngoscopy, upper endoscopy, and bronchoscopy) with multiple random biopsies (looking for primary); head, neck, and chest CT
  - 3rd – still cannot figure it out → perform excisional biopsy; need to be prepared for MRND
  - Adenocarcinoma in lymph node suggests breast, GI, or lung primary.
  - Squamous cell CA in lymph node suggests lung or head/neck primary.
- **Posterior neck masses** – if no obvious malignant epithelial tumor, considered to have **lymphoma** (Sx's – fever, night sweats; Tx – chemotherapy) until proved otherwise. Need FNA (core needle biopsy may be better if lymphoma suspected) or open biopsy
- Most common distant metastases for primary head and neck tumors → **lung**
- **Epidermoid CA** (SCCA variant) found in **cervical node without known primary** →
  - 1st – panendoscopy to look for primary; get random biopsies
  - 2nd – CT head/neck/chest
  - 3rd – still cannot find primary → ipsilateral MRND, ipsilateral tonsillectomy (most common location for occult head/neck tumor), bilateral XRT (nodal region and potential primary sites)

OTHER CONDITIONS

- **Esophageal foreign body** – dysphagia; most just below the cricopharyngeus (95%)
  - Dx and Tx: **rigid EGD** under anesthesia
  - Perforation risk increases with length of time in the esophagus.
- **Fever and pain** after EGD for foreign body → Gastrografin followed by barium swallow to rule out perforation

- **Laryngeal foreign body** – coughing; emergent cricothyroidotomy as a last resort may be needed to secure airway
- **Sleep apnea** – associated with MIs, arrhythmias, and death
  - More common in obese and those with micrognathia/retrognathia → have snoring and excessive daytime somnolence; can get cor pulmonale (right heart failure)
  - Tx: CPAP, **uvulopalatopharyngoplasty** (best surgical solution), or permanent trach
- **Prolonged intubation** – can lead to subglottic stenosis, Tx: tracheal resection and reconstruction
- **Tracheostomy** – consider in patients who will require intubation for > 7–14 days
  - Decreases secretions, provides easier ventilation, decreases pneumonia risk
- **Median rhomboid glossitis** – failure of tongue fusion. Tx: none necessary
- **Cleft lip** (primary palate) – involves lip, alveolus, or both
  - Repair at 10 weeks, 10 lb, Hgb 10. Repair nasal deformities at same time.
  - May be associated with poor feeding
- **Cleft palate** (secondary palate) – involves hard and soft palates; may affect speech and swallowing if not closed soon enough; may affect maxillofacial growth if closed too early → repair at 12 months
- **Hemangioma** – most common benign head and neck tumor in adults
- **Mastoiditis** – infection of the mastoid cells; can destroy bone
  - Rare; results as a complication of untreated **acute supportive otitis media**
  - Ear is pushed forward.
  - Tx: antibiotics, tympanostomy tube; may need emergency **mastoidectomy**
- **Epiglottitis**
  - Rare since immunization against *H. influenzae* type B
  - Mainly in children aged 3–5
  - Symptoms: stridor, drooling, leaning forward position, high fever, throat pain, thumbprint sign on lateral neck film
  - Can cause airway obstruction
  - Tx: early control of the airway; antibiotics

20 Pituitary

ANATOMY AND PHYSIOLOGY

- **Hypothalamus** – releases TRH, CRH, GnRH, GHRH, and dopamine into median eminence; passes through neurohypophysis on way to adenohypophysis
- **Dopamine** – inhibits prolactin secretion
- **Posterior pituitary** (neurohypophysis)
  - **ADH** – supraoptic nuclei, regulated by osmolar receptors in hypothalamus
  - **Oxytocin** – paraventricular nuclei in hypothalamus
  - Neurohypophysis does not contain cell bodies.
- **Anterior pituitary** (80% of gland, adenohypophysis)
  - Releases ACTH, TSH, GH, LH, FSH, and prolactin
  - Does not have its own direct blood supply; passes through neurohypophysis 1st (portal venous system)
- **Bi-temporal hemianopia** – pituitary mass compressing optic nerve (CN II) at chiasm
- **Nonfunctional tumors** – almost always macroadenomas; present with mass effect and decreased ACTH, TSH, GH, LH, FSH. Tx: transsphenoidal resection
- **Contraindications to transsphenoidal approaches** – suprasellar extension, massive lateral extension, dumbbell-shaped tumor
- Most pituitary tumors respond to **bromocriptine** (dopamine agonist).

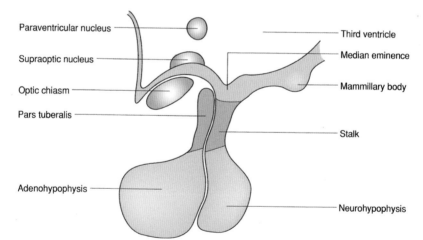

Paraventricular nucleus

Supraoptic nucleus

Optic chiasm

Pars tuberalis

Adenohypophysis

Third ventricle

Median eminence

Mammillary body

Stalk

Neurohypophysis

Schematic diagram of the pituitary and floor of the third ventricle as seen in a midline sagittal view. Anterior is to the left.

PROLACTINOMA

- **Most common pituitary adenoma**
- Mostly **microadenomas**
- Most patients do not need surgery. Prolactin is usually > 150 for symptoms to occur.
- Symptoms: galactorrhea, irregular menses, ↓ libido, infertility

- If asymptomatic and a microadenoma (< 10 mm) – just follow with MRI
- If symptomatic or is a macroadenoma, need Tx.
  - **Bromocriptine** (safe in pregnancy) or **cabergoline** (both are dopamine agonists)
  - Transsphenoidal resection for failure of medical management
  - Macroadenomas – transsphenoidal resection with hemorrhage, visual loss, wants pregnancy, CSF leak

ACROMEGALY (GROWTH HORMONE)

- Symptoms: HTN, DM, gigantism; can be life-threatening secondary to **cardiac symptoms** (valve dysfunction, cardiomyopathy)
- Usually macroadenomas
- Dx: **elevated IGF-1** (*best test*) growth hormone > 10 in 90%; MRI
- Tx: **transsphenoidal resection** (first-line therapy); XRT, bromocriptine, octreotide, and pegvisomant (GH receptor antagonist) can be used as secondary therapies.

OTHER CONDITIONS

- **Sheehan's syndrome**
  - Postpartum **trouble lactating** – usually **1st sign**
  - Can also have amenorrhea, adrenal insufficiency, and hypothyroidism
  - Due to **anterior pituitary ischemia** following hemorrhage and hypotensive episode during childbirth
  - Tx: **corticosteroids** and **hormone replacement**
- **Pituitary apoplexy**
  - Bleeding into a pituitary tumor with subsequent destruction of the gland
  - May have history of chronic headache, visual loss, or endocrine problems
  - Acute bleeding Sx's – severe headache, vision loss, stupor, hypotension
  - Tx: emergent corticosteroids; hormone replacement
- **Craniopharyngioma** – benign calcified cyst, remnants of Rathke's pouch; grows along pituitary stalk to suprasellar location (anterior pituitary)
  - Symptoms: most frequently presents with endocrine abnormalities, visual disturbances (bitemporal hemianopsia), headache, hydrocephalus
  - Tx: surgery to resect cyst
  - **Diabetes insipidus** – frequent complication postoperatively
- **Bilateral pituitary masses** – check pituitary axis hormones; if OK, probably metastases
- **Nelson's syndrome**
  - Occurs after **bilateral adrenalectomy**; ↑ CRH causes <u>pituitary enlargement</u>, resulting in **amenorrhea** and **visual problems** (bi-temporal hemianopia)
  - Also get **hyperpigmentation** from beta-MSH (melanocyte-stimulating hormone), a peptide byproduct of ACTH
  - Tx: **steroids** (prednisone)
- **Waterhouse–Friderichsen syndrome** – adrenal gland hemorrhage that occurs after meningococcal sepsis infection; can lead to adrenal insufficiency

21 Adrenal

INTRODUCTION

- **Vascular supply**
  - **Superior adrenal** – inferior phrenic artery
  - **Middle adrenal** – aorta
  - **Inferior adrenal** – renal artery
  - **Left adrenal vein** goes to **left renal vein**.
  - **Right adrenal vein** goes to **inferior vena cava**.
- Made up of adrenal cortex and adrenal medulla
- No innervation to the cortex
- Medulla receives innervation from the sympathetic splanchnic nerves.
- Lymphatics drain to subdiaphragmatic and renal lymph nodes.

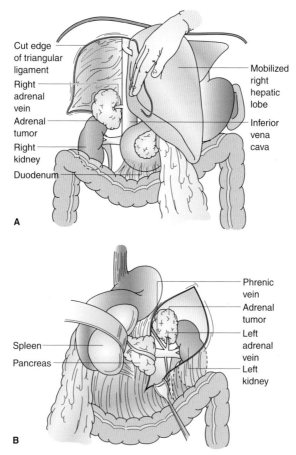

Anterior approach to right **(A)** and left **(B)** adrenalectomy. Note position of phrenic vein in relationship to the left adrenal vein and tumor.

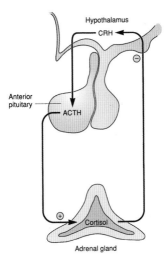

Schematic of hypothalamic–pituitary–adrenal axis for cortisol. Regulatory feedback relationships are designated with arrows.

ASYMPTOMATIC ADRENAL MASS

- 1%-2% of abdominal CT scans show incidentaloma (5% are metastases).
- Benign adenomas are common.
- Adrenals are also common sites for metastases.
- Dx: **always** check for **functioning tumor** _before_ biopsy or surgery – urine metanephrines/VMA/catecholamines, urinary hydroxycorticosteroids, serum K with plasma renin and aldosterone levels
  - Consider CXR, colonoscopy, and mammogram to check for a primary tumor.
- Surgery is indicated if mass has **ominous CT scan characteristics** (non-homogenous), is > **4–6 cm**, is **functioning**, is > **10 HU** (Hounsfield Units), or is **enlarging**.
- If going to follow an incidentaloma, need repeat imaging every 3 months for 1 year, then yearly
- Anterior approach for adrenal CA resection
- **Common metastases to adrenal** – lung CA (#1), breast CA, melanoma, renal CA
- Cancer history with asymptomatic adrenal mass – **need biopsy**
- Some **isolated metastases** to the adrenal gland can be resected with adrenalectomy.

ADRENAL CORTEX

- From **mesoderm**; **cortical cells**; remember GFR = salt, sugar, sex steroids
  - **Zona glomerulosa** – aldosterone; **fasciculata** – glucocorticoids; **reticularis** – androgens/estrogens
- Cholesterol → progesterone → androgens/cortisol/aldosterone
- All zones have **21-** and **11-beta hydroxylase**.
- **Corticotropin-releasing hormone** (CRH) is released from the hypothalamus and goes to anterior pituitary gland.
- **ACTH** is released from the anterior pituitary gland and causes the release of **cortisol**.
- Cortisol has a diurnal peak at 4–6 a.m.
- **Cortisol** – inotropic, chronotropic, and increases vascular resistance; proteolysis and gluconeogenesis; decreases inflammation, glycogenolysis

- **Aldosterone** stimulates renal sodium resorption and secretion of potassium and hydrogen ion.
  - Aldosterone secretion is stimulated by **angiotensin II** and **hyperkalemia**, and to some extent ACTH.
- **Excess estrogens** and **androgens** by adrenals – almost always cancer
- **Congenital adrenal hyperplasia** (enzyme defect in cortisol synthesis)
  - **21-Hydroxylase deficiency** (90%) – most common; precocious puberty in males, virilization in females
    - ↑ 17-OH progesterone leads to ↑ **testosterone**
    - Is **salt wasting** (↓ sodium and ↑ potassium) and causes **hypotension** (↓ **aldosterone**)
    - Tx: cortisol
  - **11-Hydroxylase deficiency** – precocious puberty in males, virilization in females
    - ↑ **11-Deoxycortisone** leads to ↑ **testosterone**
    - Is **salt saving** (11-deoxycortisone is a **mineralocorticoid**) and causes **hypertension**
    - Tx: cortisol
  - **17-hydoxylase deficiency** – lack of sexual characteristics
    - Results in ↑ **pregnenolone** (is a **mineralocorticoid**; is **salt saving**, **hypertension**) and ↓ **testosterone**
- **Hyperaldosteronism** (Conn's syndrome)
  - **Symptoms: HTN** secondary to sodium retention without edema and **hypokalemia**; also have weakness, polydipsia, and polyuria
  - **Primary disease** (renin is low) – bilateral idiopathic adrenal hyperplasia (65%) → #1 cause of primary hyperaldosteronism; adenoma (15%), ovarian tumors (rare), CA (rare)
  - **Secondary disease** (renin is high) – more common than primary disease; CHF, renal artery stenosis, liver failure, diuretics, Bartter's syndrome (renin-secreting tumor)
  - Dx for **primary hyperaldosteronism** (1 and 2 below, best)
    1. **Salt-load suppression test** (best, **urine aldosterone** will <u>stay high</u>)
    2. **Aldosterone:renin ratio > 25**
    - Labs – ↓ serum K, ↑ serum Na, ↑ urine K, metabolic alkalosis
    - Plasma renin activity will be low.
  - **Localizing studies** – CT scan initially; consider MRI, NP-59 scintigraphy (shows hyperfunctioning adrenal tissue; differentiates adenoma from hyperplasia; 90% accurate); adrenal venous sampling if others nondiagnostic
  - Preop need **control of HTN** and **K replacement**
  - **Adenoma Tx** – adrenalectomy
  - **Hyperplasia Tx** – ↑ morbidity with bilateral resection
    - Try **medical therapy** first (treats majority) for hyperplasia using <u>spironolactone</u> (inhibits aldosterone), <u>calcium channel blockers</u> (nifedipine), and <u>potassium</u>
    - If **bilateral resection** is performed (usually done for **refractory hypokalemia**), patient will need **fludrocortisone** postoperatively.
- **Hypocortisolism** (adrenal insufficiency, Addison's disease)
  - #1 cause – **withdrawal of exogenous steroids**
  - #1 primary disease – **autoimmune disease**
  - Also caused by pituitary disease, adrenal infection/hemorrhage/metastasis/resection
  - Causes ↓ **cortisol** (ACTH will be high) and ↓ **aldosterone**
  - Dx: **cosyntropin test** (ACTH given, cortisol measured) – cortisol will remain low
  - **Acute adrenal insufficiency** – hypotension (refractory to fluids and pressors), fever, lethargy, abdominal pain, nausea and vomiting, ↓ glucose, ↑ K
    - Tx: **dexamethasone**, fluids, and give **cosyntropin test** (dexamethasone does **not** interfere with test)
  - **Chronic adrenal insufficiency** – hyperpigmentation, weakness, weight loss, GI symptoms, ↑ K, ↓ Na; Tx: **corticosteroids**

- **Hypercortisolism** (Cushing's syndrome)
  - Most commonly **iatrogenic** (exogenous steroids)
  - **Sx's** - moon face, acne, weight gain, buffalo hump, abdominal stria, DM, HTN, mental status changes
  - 1st – measure **24-hour urine cortisol** (most sensitive test) and **ACTH**
    - If **ACTH is low** (and cortisol is high), patient has a cortisol secreting lesion (eg **adrenal adenoma, adrenal hyperplasia**).
    - If **ACTH is high** (and cortisol is high), patient has a pituitary adenoma or an ectopic source of ACTH (eg small cell lung CA) → go to 2nd below.
  - 2nd – if **ACTH is high**, give **high-dose dexamethasone suppression test**
    - If urine cortisol is suppressed → **pituitary adenoma**
    - If urine cortisol is not suppressed → **ectopic producer of ACTH** (eg small cell lung CA)
  - NP-59 scintigraphy can help localize tumors and differentiate adrenal adenomas from hyperplasia.
  - **Pituitary adenoma** (Cushing's disease)
    - **#1 non-iatrogenic cause of Cushing's syndrome** → 80% of cases
    - Cortisol should be suppressed with either low- or high-dose dexamethasone suppression test.
    - Mostly **microadenomas**
    - Dx: brain MRI
    - Tx: most tumors removed with transsphenoidal approach; unresectable or residual tumors treated with XRT
  - **Ectopic ACTH**
    - **#2 non-iatrogenic** cause of Cushing's syndrome
    - Most commonly from **small cell lung CA**
    - Cortisol is <u>not</u> suppressed with either low- or high-dose dexamethasone suppression test.
    - Dx: Chest/abdominal/pelvic CT can help localize.
    - Tx: resection of primary if possible; medical suppression for inoperable lesions
  - **Adrenal adenoma**
    - **#3 non-iatrogenic** cause of Cushing's syndrome
    - ↓ ACTH, unregulated steroid production
    - Dx: CT scan
    - Tx: adrenalectomy
  - **Adrenal hyperplasia** (macro or micro)
    - Tx: **metyrapone** (blocks cortisol synthesis) and **aminoglutethimide**; (inhibits steroid production); bilateral adrenalectomy if medical Tx fails
  - **Adrenocortical carcinoma** - rare cause of Cushing's syndrome (see below)
  - **Bilateral adrenalectomy** - consider in patients with ectopic ACTH from tumor that is unresectable (would need to be a slow growing tumor – rare) or ACTH from pituitary adenoma that cannot be found
  - Give **steroids postop** when operating for Cushing's syndrome (and mineralocorticoid [fludrocortisone] if bilateral adrenalectomy).
- **Adrenocortical carcinoma**
  - Bimodal distribution (before age 5 and in the 5th decade); more common in females
  - **50% are functioning tumors** - cortisol, aldosterone, sex steroids
  - Children display virilization 90% of the time (precocious puberty in boys, virilization in females); feminization in men; masculinization in women and/or Cushing's syndrome can occur.
  - Symptoms: abdominal pain, weight loss, weakness
  - Very aggressive - 80% have **advanced disease** at the time of diagnosis
  - Dx: CT scan findings usually suggests diagnosis.
  - Tx: **radical adrenalectomy** (take kidney); <u>debulking</u> helps symptoms, prolongs survival
    - **Mitotane** (adrenal-lytic) for residual, recurrent, or metastatic disease
  - 5-year survival rate - 20%

ADRENAL MEDULLA

- From **ectoderm**; **neural crest cells** (neuroendocrine, chromaffin cells)
- Catecholamine production: **tyrosine** → **dopa** → **dopamine** → **norepinephrine** → **epinephrine**
- **Tyrosine hydroxylase** – rate-limiting step (tyrosine to dopa)
- **PNMT** (phenylethanolamine *N*-methyltransferase) – enzyme converts norepinephrine → epinephrine
  - Enzyme is found only in the **adrenal medulla** (exclusive producers of epinephrine).
  - Extra-adrenal tumors do *not* produce epinephrine.
- Only **adrenal pheochromocytomas** will produce **epinephrine**.
- **MAO** (monoamine oxidase) – breaks down catecholamines; converts norepinephrine to normetanephrine, epinephrine to metanephrine; **VMA** (vanillylmandelic acid) produced from these
- **Extra-adrenal rests of neural crest tissue** can exist, usually in the retroperitoneum, most notably in the organ of Zuckerkandl at the aortic bifurcation.
- **Pheochromocytoma** (chromaffin cells)
  - Rare; usually slow growing; arise from sympathetic ganglia or ectopic neural crest cells
  - MC location – **adrenal gland**
  - **10% rule** – malignant, bilateral, in children, familial, extra-adrenal
  - Can be associated with MEN IIa, MEN IIb, von Recklinghausen's disease, tuberous sclerosis, Sturge–Weber disease
  - **Right-sided** predominance
  - **Extra-adrenal tumors** are more likely **malignant**.
    - Extra-adrenal pheochromocytomas also called **paragangliomas**
  - Symptoms: HTN (frequently **episodic**), headache, diaphoresis, palpitations
  - Dx: **urine metanephrines** (24-hour urine; *best test*) and VMA
    - **MIBG scan** (norepinephrine analogue) – can help identify location if having trouble finding tumor with CT scan/MRI (best test for localization)
    - **Clonidine suppression test** – tumor doses not respond, keeps catecholamines ↑
    - **No venography** → can cause hypertensive crisis
  - <u>Preoperatively</u>: **volume replacement** and **α-blocker first** (phenoxybenzamine, prazosin → avoids hypertensive crisis); then β-blocker if patient has tachycardia or arrhythmias
    - Need to be careful with β-blocker and give after α-blocker → can precipitate **hypertensive crisis** (unopposed alpha stimulation, can lead to **stroke**), **heart failure**, and **MI**
  - Tx: **adrenalectomy** – ligate adrenal veins first to avoid spilling catecholamines during tumor manipulation
    - Debulking helps symptoms in patients with unresectable disease.
    - **Metyrosine** – inhibits tyrosine hydroxylase causing ↓ synthesis of catecholamines (given preop or for unresectable disease)
    - Should have Nipride, Neo-Synephrine, and antiarrhythmic agents (eg amiodarone) ready during the time of surgery
  - **Postop conditions** – persistent hypertension, hypotension, hypoglycemia, bronchospasm, arrhythmias, intracerebral hemorrhage, CHF, MI
  - **Other sites of pheochromocytomas** (paraganglionomas) – aortic bifurcation (#1), vertebral bodies, opposite adrenal gland, bladder
    - Most common extramedullary tissue site – **organ of Zuckerkandl** (inferior aorta near bifurcation)
  - **Falsely elevated VMA** – coffee, tea, fruits, vanilla, iodine contrast, labetalol, α- and β-blockers
  - **Extramedullary tissue** – responsible for **medullary CA of thyroid** and **extra-adrenal pheochromocytoma**
- **Ganglioneuroma** – rare, benign, asymptomatic tumor of neural crest origin in the adrenal medulla or sympathetic chain; Tx: resection

22 Thyroid

ANATOMY AND PHYSIOLOGY

- From the 1st and 2nd pharyngeal <u>arches</u> (not from pouches)
- **Thyrotropin-releasing factor** (TRF) – released from the hypothalamus; acts on the anterior pituitary gland and causes release of TSH
- **Thyroid-stimulating hormone** (TSH) – released from the anterior pituitary gland; acts on the thyroid gland to release T3 and T4 (through a mechanism that involves ↑ cAMP)
- TRF and TSH release are controlled by T3 and T4 through a negative feedback loop.
- **Superior thyroid artery** – 1st branch off external carotid artery
  - Ligate close to superior pole of thyroid to avoid injury to superior laryngeal nerve with thyroidectomy.
- **Inferior thyroid artery** – off thyrocervical trunk; supplies <u>*both*</u> the **inferior** and **superior parathyroids**
  - Ligate close to thyroid to avoid injury to parathyroid glands with thyroidectomy.
- **Ima artery** – occurs in 1%, arises from the innominate or aorta and goes to the isthmus
- **Superior** and **middle thyroid veins** – drain into internal jugular vein
- **Inferior thyroid vein** – drains into innominate vein
- **Superior laryngeal nerve**
  - Motor to cricothyroid muscle
  - Runs lateral to thyroid lobes
  - Tracks close to superior thyroid artery but is variable
  - MC injured nerve following thyroidectomy
  - Injury results in **loss of projection** and **easy voice fatigability** (opera singers).
- **Recurrent laryngeal nerves** (RLNs; branch off vagus nerve)
  - Motor to all of larynx except cricothyroid muscle
  - Controls **vocal cords**
  - Run posterior to thyroid lobes in the tracheoesophageal groove
  - Can track with inferior thyroid artery but are variable
  - **Left** RLN loops around **aorta**; **right** RLN loops around **innominate artery** (*RLNs loop anterior to posterior around these structures*).

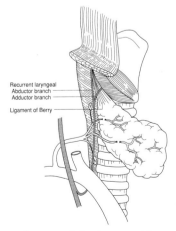

The ligament of Berry and distal recurrent laryngeal nerves.

127

- Injury results in **hoarseness**; bilateral injury can **obstruct airway** → need emergency tracheostomy
- **Non-recurrent laryngeal nerve** – in 2%; more common on the right
- **Risk of injury** is higher for a non-recurrent laryngeal nerve during thyroid surgery.
- **Ligament of Berry** – posterior medial suspensory ligament close to RLNs; need careful dissection
- **Follicular cells** – produce T3 and T4
- **Thyroglobulin** – stores T3 and T4 in colloid
  - Plasma T4:T3 ratio is 15:1; **T3** is the more active form (is tyrosine + iodine).
  - Most T3 is produced in periphery from T4 to T3 conversion by **deiodinases**.
- **Peroxidases** link iodine and tyrosine together.
- **Deiodinases** separate iodine from tyrosine.
- **Thyroxine-binding globulin** – thyroid hormone transport; binds the majority of T3 and T4 in circulation
- **TSH** – most sensitive indicator of gland function
- **Tubercles of Zuckerkandl** – most lateral, posterior extension of thyroid tissue
  - Rotate medially to find RLNs.
  - This portion is left behind with subtotal thyroidectomy because of proximity to RLNs.
- **Parafollicular C cells** – produce **calcitonin** (lowers Ca)
- **Thyroxine treatment** – TSH levels should fall 50%; osteoporosis long-term side effect
- **Post-thyroidectomy stridor** – open neck and remove hematoma emergently → can result in airway compromise; can also be due to bilateral RLN injury → would need emergent tracheostomy

THYROID STORM

- Symptoms: ↑ HR, fever, numbness, irritability, vomiting, diarrhea, high-output cardiac failure (most common cause of death)
- Most common after surgery in patient with undiagnosed **Graves' disease**
- Can be precipitated by anxiety, excessive gland palpation, adrenergic stimulants
- Tx: **β-blockers** (*first drug to give*), Lugol's solution (KI, most effective but takes while to work), cooling blankets, oxygen, glucose
  - Emergent thyroidectomy rarely indicated
- **Wolff–Chaikoff effect** – very effective for thyroid storm; patient given high doses of iodine (Lugol's solution, potassium iodide), which inhibits TSH action on thyroid and inhibits organic coupling of iodide, resulting in less T3 and T4 release

ASYMPTOMATIC THYROID NODULE

- 90% of thyroid nodules are benign; female predominance
- Get U/S-guided **FNA** (*best initial test*) and **thyroid function tests**.
  - Needs to be ≥ **5 mm** to warrant FNA
  - FNA determinant in 80% → follow appropriate treatment
  - FNA results and Tx:
    - **Indeterminant** → repeat FNA
    - **Benign** (**1% CA** risk) → repeat U/S in 6–12 months (repeat FNA if it enlarges)
    - **AUS/FLUS** (atypia of undetermined significant/follicular lesion of undetermined significance; **10% CA** risk) → repeat FNA
      - If same on repeat FNA → <u>lobectomy</u> (*preferred*) versus <u>careful U/S-FNA follow-up</u> (3 months)
      - **Molecular testing** increasingly used here – determines specific CA risk and guides Tx
    - **Follicular neoplasm** → lobectomy (**25% CA** risk; see Thyroid CA section)
    - **Suspicious for malignancy** → lobectomy (**70% CA** risk)
    - **Thyroid CA** → total thyroidectomy usual and appropriate F/U treatment (see Thyroid CA section for lobectomy criteria)

- **Cyst fluid** → drain fluid (send for cytology)
  - If it recurs or is bloody → lobectomy
- **Colloid tissue** → most likely colloid goiter; low chance of malignancy ($< 1\%$)
  - Tx: **thyroxine**; lobectomy if it enlarges
- **Normal thyroid tissue** and **TFTs are elevated** → likely solitary toxic nodule
  - Tx: if asymptomatic can just monitor; **methimazole** and ^{131}I if symptomatic
- **Cold nodule** more likely to be malignant than hot nodule

- **Goiter**
  - Any abnormal enlargement
  - Most identifiable cause is iodine deficiency; Tx: iodine replacement
  - MCC in U.S. – low-grade stimulation of the thyroid gland
  - Diffuse enlargement without evidence of functional abnormality = nontoxic colloid goiter
    - Unusual to have to operate unless goiter is causing **airway compression** or there is a **suspicious nodule**
    - Tx: **thyroxine**; need **subtotal** or **total thyroidectomy** for failure of medical Tx or if a suspicious nodule appears; subtotal has decreased risk of RLN injury
    - If the goiter is hyperfunctioning (toxic goiter) – do <u>not</u> use thyroxine
- **Substernal goiter**
  - Usually secondary (vessels originate from superior and inferior thyroid arteries)
  - Primary substernal goiter – rare (vessels originate from innominate artery)
- **Mediastinal thyroid tissue** – most likely from acquired disease with inferior extensions of a normally placed gland (eg substernal goiter)

ABNORMALITIES OF THYROID DESCENT

- **Pyramidal lobe** – occurs in 10%, extends **superiorly** from the thyroid isthmus
- **Lingual thyroid**
  - Thyroid tissue that persists in foramen cecum at **base of the tongue**
  - Symptoms: dysphagia, dyspnea, dysphonia
  - 2% malignancy risk
  - Tx: thyroxine suppression; abolish with ^{131}I
    - Resection if worried about CA or if it does not shrink after medical therapy
  - Is the only thyroid tissue in 70% of patients who have it
- **Thyroglossal duct cyst** (develops in pyramidal lobe)
  - Midline cervical mass between the hyoid bone and the thyroid isthmus
  - May be all the thyroid tissue the patient has
  - Classically moves upward with swallowing
  - Susceptible to **infection** and may be **premalignant**; dysphonia
  - Tx: resection → need to take midportion or all of **hyoid bone** along with the **thyroglossal duct cyst** (Sistrunk procedure; lateral neck incision)

HYPERTHYROIDISM TREATMENT

- **Thioamides** – propylthiouracil (PTU) and **methimazole**
- **Methimazole** – *1st-line drug*
  - <u>Not</u> used in pregnancy
  - **Inhibits peroxidases** and prevents iodine–tyrosine coupling
  - Side effects: **cretinism** in newborns (crosses placenta), **aplastic anemia**, **agranulocytosis** (rare)
- **PTU** (thioamides) – not used 1st line anymore due to hepatotoxicity (especially in children)
  - Safe with pregnancy
  - **Inhibits peroxidases** and prevents iodine–tyrosine coupling
  - Side effects: **aplastic anemia**, **agranulocytosis** (rare)

- **Radioactive iodine** (^{131}I)
  - For patients who are poor surgical risks or unresponsive to methimazole
  - ^{131}I should <u>not</u> be used in <u>children</u> or during <u>pregnancy</u> → can traverse placenta
- **Thyroidectomy**
  - Good for cold nodules, toxic adenomas, Graves' disease not responsive to medical therapy, pregnant patients not controlled with PTU, multinodular goiters with compressive symptoms of suspicious nodule, and toxic multinodular goiters (^{131}I doesn't work well)
  - Best time to operate during pregnancy is **2nd trimester** (↓ risk of teratogenic events and premature labor).
  - Subtotal thyroidectomy can leave patient euthyroid.

CAUSES OF HYPERTHYROIDISM

- **Graves' disease** (toxic diffuse goiter)
  - MCC of hyperthyroidism
  - Women; exophthalmos, pretibial edema, atrial fibrillation, heat intolerance, thirst, ↑ appetite, weight loss, sweating, palpitations
  - Sx's found only in Graves' – exophthalmos, pretibial edema
  - Most common cause of hyperthyroidism (80%)
  - Caused by **IgG antibodies** to **TSH receptor** (long-acting thyroid stimulator [LATS], thyroid-stimulating immunoglobulin [TSI])
  - Dx: low TSH, high T3 and T4; LATS level; diffuse ^{123}I uptake (thyroid scan) in thyrotoxic patient with goiter
  - Medical therapy usually manages hyperthyroidism (95% success rate).
  - Tx: **thioamides** (50% recurrence), ^{131}I (5% recurrence), or **thyroidectomy** if medical therapy fails; beta-blockers help symptoms only
    - *Avoid* radioactive iodide in patients with active/severe ophthalmopathy (can worsen symptoms).
  - **Unusual to have to operate** on these patients (suspicious nodule most common reason)
    - **Preop preparation**: <u>methimazole</u> until euthyroid, β-blocker, <u>Lugol's solution</u> for 14 days to decrease friability and vascularity (start only after euthyroid)
    - **Operation**: bilateral subtotal (5% recurrence) or total thyroidectomy (need lifetime thyroxine replacement)
    - **Indications for surgery**: noncompliant patient, recurrence after medical therapy, children, pregnant women not controlled with PTU, or concomitant suspicious thyroid nodule (most common indication)
- **Toxic multinodular goiter**
  - Women; age > 50 years, usually nontoxic 1st
  - Symptoms: tachycardia, weight loss, insomnia, airway compromise; symptoms can be precipitated by contrast dyes.
  - Caused by hyperplasia secondary to chronic low-grade TSH stimulation
  - Pathology shows **colloid**.
  - Tx: Most consider *surgery (subtotal or total thyroidectomy)* the ***preferred initial Tx*** for toxic multinodular goiter, but a **trial of** ^{131}I should be considered, especially in the elderly and frail (generally doesn't work well due to non-homogenous uptake).
    - If compression or a suspicious nodule is present, need to go with surgery
- **Single toxic nodule**
  - Women; younger; usually > 3 cm to be symptomatic; function autonomously
  - Dx: **thyroid scan** (hot nodule) – 20% of hot nodules eventually cause symptoms
  - Tx: **thioamides** and ^{131}I (95% effective); lobectomy if medical Tx ineffective
- **Rare causes of hyperthyroidism** – trophoblastic tumors, TSH-secreting pituitary tumors

CAUSES OF THYROIDITIS

- **Hashimoto's disease**
  - Most common cause of **hypothyroidism** in adults
  - **Enlarged gland**, painless, chronic thyroiditis
  - Women; history of childhood XRT
  - Can cause thyrotoxicosis in the acute early stage
  - Caused by both **humeral** and **cell-mediated autoimmune disease** (microsomal and thyroglobulin **antibodies**)
  - Goiter secondary to **lack of organification of trapped iodide inside gland**
  - Pathology shows a **lymphocytic infiltrate.**
  - Tx: **thyroxine** (*first line*); **partial thyroidectomy** if continues to grow despite thyroxine, if nodules appear, or if compression symptoms occur
  - Frequently, no surgery is necessary for Hashimoto's disease.
- **Bacterial thyroiditis** (rare)
  - Usually secondary to **contiguous spread**
  - **Bacterial upper respiratory tract infection** (URI) usual precursor (staph/strep)
  - Normal thyroid function tests, fever, dysphagia, tenderness
  - Tx: **antibiotics**
    - May need **lobectomy** to rule out cancer in patients with unilateral swelling and tenderness
    - May need total thyroidectomy for persistent inflammation
- **De Quervain's thyroiditis** (subacute granulomatous thyroiditis)
  - Can be associated with hyperthyroidism initially
  - **Viral URI** precursor; tender thyroid, sore throat, mass, weakness, fatigue; women
  - Elevated **ESR**
  - Tx: **steroids** and **NSAIDs**
    - May need **lobectomy** to rule out cancer in patients with unilateral swelling and tenderness
    - May need total thyroidectomy for persistent inflammation
- **Riedel's fibrous struma** (rare)
  - <u>Woody, fibrous component</u> that can involve adjacent strap muscles and carotid sheath
  - Can resemble thyroid CA or lymphoma (need biopsy)
  - Disease frequently results in **hypothyroidism** and **compression symptoms**.
  - Associated with sclerosing cholangitis, fibrotic diseases, methysergide Tx, and retroperitoneal fibrosis
  - Tx: **steroids** and **thyroxine**
    - May need **isthmectomy** or **tracheostomy** for airway symptoms
    - If resection needed, watch for RLNs.

THYROID CANCER

- Most common endocrine malignancy in the United States
- Thyroid CA generally does not affect thyroid function.
- FNA shows just **follicular cells** – can be hard to differentiate between FLUS, hyperplasia, adenoma, and CA; often end up performing lobectomy for diagnosis/therapy
- **Worrisome for malignancy** – solid, solitary, cold, slow growing, hard; male, age > 50, previous neck XRT, MEN IIa or IIb
- **Sudden growth** – could be hemorrhage into previously undetected nodule or malignancy
- Patients can also present with **voice changes** or **dysphagia**.
- **Follicular adenomas** – colloid, embryonal, fetal → no increase in cancer risk
  - Still need **lobectomy** to prove it is an adenoma
- **Papillary thyroid carcinoma**
  - Most common (85%) thyroid CA
  - Least aggressive, slow growing, has the best prognosis; women, children

- Risk factors: **childhood XRT** (very ↑ risk) → most common tumor following neck XRT
- Older age (> 40–50 years) predicts a worse prognosis.
- **Lymphatic spread 1st** but is not prognostic → prognosis based on **local invasion**
- <u>Rare</u> metastases (**lung**)
- **Children** are more likely to be **node positive** (80%) than are adults (20%).
- Large, firm nodules in children are worrisome.
- Many are **multicentric**.
- Pathology – **psammoma bodies** (calcium) and **Orphan Annie nuclei**
- 95% 5-year survival rate; death secondary to local disease
- **Follicular thyroid carcinoma**
  - **Hematogenous** spread (**bone** most common) → 50% have metastatic disease at the time of presentation
  - More aggressive than thyroid papillary cell CA; older adults (50–60s), women
  - If FNA shows just **follicular cells** – have 10% chance of malignancy, need lobectomy
  - 70% 5-year survival rate; prognosis based on stage
- **Surgery** for **papillary** and **follicular** thyroid CA → start with lobectomy
  - Indications for **total** thyroidectomy:
    - Tumor > **1 cm**
    - **Extrathyroidal disease** (beyond thyroid capsule, clinically positive nodes, metastases)
    - **Multi-centric** or **bilateral** lesions
    - **Previous XRT**
    - *Vast majority of patients in U.S. get total thyroidectomy.*
  - Indications for **MRND**:
    - **Extrathyroidal disease**
  - Indications for **postop ^{131}I** (6 weeks after surgery, want TSH high for maximum uptake):
    - Tumor > **1 cm**
    - **Extrathyroidal disease**
    - *Need <u>total thyroidectomy for</u> ^{131}I to be effective*
  - Enlarged lateral neck lymph node that shows **thyroid tissue** (**lateral aberrant thyroid tissue**; ie papillary thyroid CA with lymphatic spread) → Tx: **total thyroidectomy, MRND, and ^{131}I**
  - Risk factors for thyroid CA <u>recurrence</u> or <u>metastases</u>: **X-GAMES** – previous XRT, high grade, age (< 20 or > 50), males, extrathyroidal disease, and size (> 1 cm)
- **Medullary thyroid carcinoma**
  - 20% associated with **MEN IIa** or **IIb** (RET proto-oncogene)
  - 80% are sporadic.
  - Usually the **1st manifestation** of MEN IIa and IIb (**diarrhea**)
  - Tumor arises from **parafollicular C cells** (which secrete calcitonin).
  - **C-cell hyperplasia** considered premalignant
  - **Pathology** – shows **amyloid** deposition
  - **Calcitonin** – can cause **diarrhea** (most common symptom) and **flushing**
  - Need to screen for **hyperparathyroidism** and **pheochromocytoma**
  - **Lymphatic spread** – most have involved nodes at time of diagnosis
  - **Early metastases** to lung, liver, and bone
  - **Worse prognosis** – IIb and sporadic types
  - Tx: **total thyroidectomy** with **central neck node dissection**
    - **MRND** if patient has a palpable thyroid mass or clinically positive lymph nodes
    - **Bilateral MRND** if both lobes have tumor or if extrathyroidal disease present
    - Liver and bone metastases prevent attempt at cure.
    - XRT may be useful for unresectable local and distant metastatic disease.
  - May be useful to **monitor calcitonin levels** for disease recurrence

- More aggressive than follicular and papillary CA
- 5-year survival – 50% (prognosis based on presence of regional and distant metastases)
- Age for **prophylactic thyroidectomy** and **central node dissection** is determined by specific RET proto-oncogene codon mutation risk:
  - Level **A** codon – before **age 10** or earlier if lacks low-risk criteria
  - Level **B** codon – before **age 5** or later if low-risk criteria
  - Level **C** codon – before **age 5**
  - Level **D** codon – **first year of life**
  - *Low-risk criteria – normal calcitonin level, normal neck U/S, less aggressive MTC family history*
- **Hürthle cell carcinoma**
  - Most are **benign** (80%; Hürthle cell adenoma); presents in older patients
  - Metastases go to bone and lung if malignant.
  - Pathology shows Ashkenazi cells.
  - Can <u>not</u> make the diagnosis of benign vs malignant on biopsy alone – need lobectomy
  - Tx: lobectomy; total thyroidectomy if malignant; MRND for clinically positive nodes
- **Anaplastic thyroid cancer**
  - Elderly patients with long-standing goiters
  - **Most aggressive thyroid CA**
  - Pathology shows vesicular appearance of nuclei.
  - Rapidly lethal (0% 5-year survival rate); usually beyond surgical management at diagnosis
  - Tx: total thyroidectomy for the rare lesion that can be resected
  - Can perform palliative thyroidectomy for compressive symptoms (or tracheostomy) or give palliative chemo-XRT
- **XRT effective** for papillary, follicular, medullary, and Hürthle cell thyroid CA
- ^{131}**I effective** for papillary and follicular thyroid CA *only* (not MTC, anaplastic, or Hürthle)
  - <u>Not</u> used in **children** (CA risk), **pregnancy** (cretinism), or in **lactating mothers** (cretinism)
  - Can cure bone and lung metastases
  - Given 4–6 weeks after surgery when TSH levels are highest
  - Do not give thyroid replacement until <u>after</u> treatment with ^{131}I → would suppress TSH and uptake of ^{131}I
  - **Indications** (used only for papillary and follicular thyroid CA)
    - **Recurrent CA**
    - **Primary inoperable tumors** due to **local invasion**
    - **Tumors that are** > 1 **cm** or have **extrathyroidal disease** (extracapsular invasion, nodal spread, or metastases)
  - Patients with papillary or follicular cell CA and metastases → need to perform total thyroidectomy to facilitate uptake of ^{131}I to the metastatic lesions (otherwise all gets absorbed by the thyroid gland)
  - ^{131}**I Side effects** (rare): sialoadenitis, GI symptoms, infertility, bone marrow suppression, parathyroid dysfunction, leukemia
- **Thyroglobulin** level used to detect **recurrence** of papillary and follicular cell thyroid CA after thyroidectomy (must have had a total thyroidectomy for this to work)
- **Thyroxine** – can help suppress TSH and slow metastatic disease; administered only after ^{131}I therapy has finished

23 Parathyroid

ANATOMY AND PHYSIOLOGY

- **Superior parathyroids** – 4th pharyngeal <u>pouch</u>; associated with **thyroid complex**
  - Found lateral to recurrent laryngeal nerves (RLNs), posterior surface of superior portion of gland, above inferior thyroid artery
- **Inferior parathyroids** – 3rd pharyngeal <u>pouch</u>; associated with **thymus**
  - Found medial to RLNs, more anterior, below inferior thyroid artery
  - Inferior parathyroids have more **variable location** and are more likely to be **ectopic**.
  - Occasionally are found in the **tail of the thymus** (most common ectopic site) and can migrate to the anterior mediastinum
  - Other ectopic sites – intra-thyroid, mediastinal, near tracheoesophageal groove
- 90% have all 4 glands.
- **Inferior thyroid artery** – blood supply to <u>both</u> **superior** and **inferior parathyroid glands**
  - Artery approaches glands from a medial direction under thyroid.

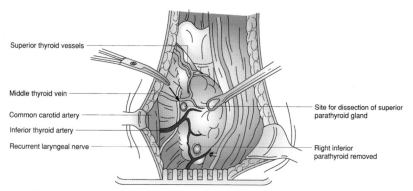

Superior thyroid vessels

Middle thyroid vein

Common carotid artery

Inferior thyroid artery

Recurrent laryngeal nerve

Site for dissection of superior parathyroid gland

Right inferior parathyroid removed

Lateral view of the right side of the neck after rotation of the thyroid lobe. The important anatomic landmarks are emphasized.

- **PTH** – *increases* <u>serum Ca</u>
  - Released by **chief cells** in the <u>parathyroid</u> in response to <u>low</u> calcium
  - ↑ kidney Ca reabsorption in distal convoluted tubule, ↓ kidney PO_4 and HCO_3^- absorption
  - ↑ bone osteoclasts to release Ca (and PO_4^-; resorption)
  - ↑ vitamin D production in kidney (↑ 1-OH hydroxylation by 1-alpha hydroxylase) → ↑ Ca-binding protein in intestine → ↑ intestinal Ca reabsorption
- **Vitamin D** – ↑ intestinal Ca and PO_4 absorption by increasing **calcium-binding protein**
- **Calcitonin** – *decreases* <u>serum Ca</u>
  - Released by **parafollicular C cells** in the <u>thyroid</u> gland in response to <u>high</u> calcium
  - ↓ bone Ca resorption (osteoclast inhibition)
  - ↓ kidney Ca and PO_4 reabsorption (renal tubules)
- **Normal Ca level**: 8.5–10.5 (ionized 1.0–1.5)
- **Normal PTH level**: 10–60 pg/mL

- **Normal PO₄ level**: 2.5–5.0
- **Normal Cl⁻ level**: 98–107
- Most common cause of hypoparathyroidism is **previous thyroid surgery**.

PRIMARY HYPERPARATHYROIDISM

- Women, older age
- Due to **autonomously high PTH**
- Dx: ↑ PTH and ↑ Ca; ↓ PO₄⁻; Cl⁻ to PO₄⁻ ratio > 33; ↑ renal cAMP; high urinary Ca (24-hour urine collection)
  - HCO₃⁻ secreted in urine
  - PO₄⁻ may _not_ be low in patients with renal failure.
- Can get **hyperchloremic metabolic acidosis**
- **Osteitis fibrosa cystica** (brown tumors) – bone lesions from Ca resorption; characteristic of hyperparathyroidism
- Most patients **have no symptoms** – ↑ Ca found on routine lab work for some other problem or on checkup
- Symptoms: muscle weakness, myalgia, nephrolithiasis, pancreatitis, ulcers, depression, bone pain, pathologic fractures, mental status changes, constipation, anorexia
- Hypertension can result from renal impairment.
- **Normocalcemic hyperparathyroidism variant** – elevated PTH with normal Ca level; indications for surgery same as primary hyperparathyroidism

Diagnostic Workup for Primary Hyperparathyroidism

Take careful history, including records or medications, symptoms, prior head and neck radiotherapy, and other endocrinopathies in the patient and the patient's family.

Establish elevated calcium through 2 or 3 determinations.

Order a chest radiograph and search for bony metastases, sarcoidosis, and pulmonary tumors (ie looking for PTHrP source).

Order an excretory urogram and search for nephrolithiasis and, rarely, renal tumors.

Order a serum protein electrophoresis to rule out multiple myeloma.

Order a 24-hour urinary calcium determination (ie benign familial hypocalciuric hypercalcemia – would show low urine Ca).

Rule out multiple endocrine neoplasia (usually multiple endocrine neoplasia type I).

Check the absolute or relative elevation of the parathyroid hormone level.

Indications for surgery
  - Symptomatic disease
  - Asymptomatic disease with: elevated Ca (> 1 mg/dL above normal), decreased Cr clearance (< 60 mL/min), kidney stones, substantially ↓ bone mass (densitometry T score < −2.5), age < 50, poor access to follow-up
- **Single adenoma** – occurs in 80% of patients
- **Multiple adenomas** – occur in 4% of patients
- **Diffuse hyperplasia** – occurs in 15%; patients with MEN I or IIa have 4-gland hyperplasia
- **Parathyroid adenocarcinoma** – very rare; can get very high Ca levels
- **Treatment**
  - **Adenoma** – resection; inspect other glands to rule out hyperplasia or multiple adenomas
  - **Parathyroid hyperplasia**
    - Do not biopsy all glands → risks hemorrhage and hypoparathyroidism
    - Tx: Resect 3½ glands or total parathyroidectomy and autoimplantation (forearm brachioradialis or neck strap muscle).

- **Parathyroid CA** → need radical parathyroidectomy (need to take **ipsilateral thyroid lobe**)
- **Pregnancy** – surgery in 2nd trimester; ↑ risk of stillbirth if not resected
- **Intraop frozen section** → can confirm that the tissue taken was indeed parathyroid
- **Intraop PTH levels** → can help determine if the causative gland is removed (PTH should go to < ½ of the preop value in 10 minutes)
- **Find 4 normal glands** at surgery (likely ectopic adenoma) – resect tail of thymus, if not there check missing gland locations below
- **Missing gland** – check inferiorly in thymus tissue (most common ectopic location, can remove tail of the thymus and see if PTH drops), near carotids, near vertebral bodies, superior to pharynx, intra-thyroid
- **Still cannot find gland** – close and follow PTH; if PTH still ↑, get **sestamibi scan** to localize
- **At reoperation for a missing gland,** the most common location for the gland is **normal anatomic position**.
- **Hypocalcemia postop** – from bone hunger or failure of parathyroid remnant/graft
  - **Bone hunger** – normal PTH, decreased HCO_3^-, ↑ urine cAMP
  - **Aparathyroidism** – decreased PTH, normal HCO_3^-, normal urine cAMP
  - Remember to give Ca postop.
- **Persistent hyperparathyroidism** (1%) – most commonly due to missed adenoma remaining in the neck
- **Recurrent hyperparathyroidism** – occurs after a period of hypocalcemia or normocalcemia
  - Can be due to new adenoma formation
  - Can be due to tumor implants at the original operation that have now grown
  - Need to consider recurrent parathyroid CA
- **Reoperation** associated with ↑ risk of RLN injury, permanent hypoparathyroidism
- **Sestamibi scan**
  - Will have preferential uptake by the overactive parathyroid gland
  - Good for picking up adenomas but not 4-gland hyperplasia
  - Best for trying to pick up missing / ectopic glands and for reops
  - If still having trouble locating a missing gland, can use angiography with select venous sampling for PTH

SECONDARY HYPERPARATHYROIDISM

- Seen in patients with **renal failure**
- ↑ **PTH** in response to **low Ca** (lose Ca with dialysis)
- Most do <u>not</u> need surgery (95%).
- Osteoporosis can occur.
- Tx: **Ca supplement**, vitamin D, control diet PO_4, PO_4-binding gel (sevelamer chloride)
  - **Cinacalcet** – mimics Ca, inhibits PTH from the parathyroid glands
  - Surgery for **bone pain** (most common indication), fractures, or pruritus (80% get relief) despite medical Tx
  - Surgery involves total parathyroidectomy with autotransplantation or subtotal parathyroidectomy.

TERTIARY HYPERPARATHYROIDISM

- Renal disease now corrected with transplant but still overproduces PTH.
- Has similar lab values as primary hyperparathyroidism (hyperplasia)
- Tx: subtotal (3½ glands) or total parathyroidectomy with autoimplantation

FAMILIAL HYPERCALCEMIC HYPOCALCIURIA

- Patients have ↑ serum Ca and ↓ urine Ca (should be ↑ if hyperparathyroidism).
- Caused by defect in PTH receptor in distal convoluted tubule of the kidney that causes ↑ resorption of Ca
- Dx: Ca 9-11, have normal PTH, ↓ urine Ca
- Tx: nothing (Ca generally not that high in these patients); **no parathyroidectomy**

PSEUDOHYPOPARATHYROIDISM

- Because of defect in PTH receptor in the kidney, does not respond to PTH

PARATHYROID CANCER

- Rare cause of hypercalcemia; can have a palpable mass
- ↑ Ca, PTH, and alkaline phosphatase (can have extremely high Ca levels)
- **Lung** most common location for metastases
- Tx: wide en bloc excision (parathyroidectomy, ipsilateral thyroidectomy, and central node dissection)
- 50% 5-year survival rate
- Mortality is due to **hypercalcemia**.
- Recurrence in 50%
- Chemo-XRT not really effective
- Palliation – consider palliative surgery (debulking to lower calcium)
  - Meds – cinacalcet, bisphosphonates (Alendronate), Fosamax

MULTIPLE ENDOCRINE NEOPLASIA SYNDROMES

- Derived from APUD cells
- Neoplasms can develop synchronously or metachronously.
- Autosomal dominant, 100% penetrance
- **MEN I**
  - **Parathyroid hyperplasia**
    - Usually the 1st part to become symptomatic; urinary symptoms
    - Tx: 4-gland resection with autotransplantation
  - **Pancreatic neuro-endocrine tumors** (PNET)
    - Gastrinoma #1 – 50% multiple, 50% malignant; major morbidity of syndrome
  - **Pituitary adenoma**
    - Prolactinoma #1
  - Need to correct hyperparathyroidism 1st if simultaneous tumors
- **MEN IIa**
  - **Parathyroid hyperplasia**
  - **Medullary CA of thyroid**
    - Nearly all patients; diarrhea most common symptom; often bilateral
    - #1 cause of death in these patients
    - Usually 1st part to be symptomatic (diarrhea)
  - **Pheochromocytoma**
    - Often bilateral, nearly always benign
  - Need to correct pheochromocytoma 1st if simultaneous tumors
- **MEN IIb**
  - **Medullary CA of thyroid**
    - Nearly all patients; diarrhea most common symptoms; often bilateral
    - #1 cause of death in these patients
    - Usually 1st part to be symptomatic (diarrhea)
  - **Pheochromocytoma**
    - Often bilateral, nearly always benign

- **Mucosal neuromas**
- **Marfan's habitus, musculoskeletal abnormalities**
- Need to correct pheochromocytoma 1st if simultaneous tumors
- **MEN I** – MENIN gene
- **MEN IIa and IIb** – RET proto-oncogene

Disease Phenotypes Related to Mutation of the RET Proto-Oncogene

Phenotype	Genetic Defect	Clinical Features	Prevalence (%)
MEN 2A (60%)	Germline mutations in cysteine codons of extracellular and transmembrane domains of RET	Medullary thyroid carcinoma Pheochromocytoma Hyperparathyroidism	100 10–60 5–20
MEN 2B (5%)	Germline activating mutation in tyrosine kinase domain of RET	Medullary thyroid carcinoma Pheochromocytoma Marfanoid habitus Mucosal neuromas (gut) and ganglioneuromatosis	100 50 100 100
FMTC (35%)	Germline mutations in cysteine codons of extracellular or transmembrane domains of RET	Medullary thyroid carcinoma	100

FMTC, familial medullary thyroid carcinoma; MEN, multiple endocrine neoplasia.

HYPERCALCEMIA

- Causes (90% from hyperparathyroidism or CA):
  - Malignancy (MCC of inpatient hypercalcemia)
    - **PTHrP** (75%) – cancers that release PTHrP (eg squamous cell lung CA, breast CA); MCC of malignant hypercalcemia (_not_ lytic bone destruction)
    - **Bone destruction** by CA (25%) – lytic bone lesions (eg multiple myeloma)
  - Hyperparathyroidism (MCC of outpatient hypercalcemia)
  - Hyperthyroidism
  - Familial hypercalcemic hypocalciuria
  - Immobilization
  - Granulomatous disease (sarcoidosis or tuberculosis)
  - Excess vitamin D
  - Milk–alkali syndrome (excessive intake of milk and calcium supplements)
  - Thiazide diuretics
- **Mithramycin** – inhibits osteoclasts (used with malignancies or failure of conventional treatment); has hematologic, liver, and renal side effects
- **Hypercalcemic crisis** – usually secondary to another surgery in patients with preexisting hyperparathyroidism (see Fluid and Electrolytes chapter)
- **Breast CA** – releases **PTHrP** (rP = related peptide); can cause **hypercalcemia**
  - Squamous cell lung CA and other nonhematologic cancers can do this as well → this is _not_ due to bone destruction
  - Associated with ↑ urinary cAMP (from action of **PTHrP on kidney PTH receptors**)
- **Hematologic malignancies** – these can cause bone destruction with ↑ Ca (urinary cAMP will be low)

24 Breast

ANATOMY AND PHYSIOLOGY

- **Breast development**
  - Breast formed from ectoderm milk streak.
  - **Estrogen** – duct development (double layer of columnar cells)
  - **Progesterone** – lobular development
  - **Prolactin** – synergizes estrogen and progesterone
- **Cyclic changes**
  - **Estrogen** – ↑ breast swelling, growth of glandular tissue
  - **Progesterone** – ↑ maturation of glandular tissue; withdrawal causes menses
  - **FSH, LH surge** – cause ovum release
  - After menopause, lack of estrogen and progesterone results in atrophy of breast tissue.
- **Nerves near axilla**
  - **Long thoracic nerve** – innervates **serratus anterior**; injury results in winged scapula
    - **Lateral thoracic artery** supplies serratus anterior.
  - **Thoracodorsal nerve** – innervates **latissimus dorsi**; injury results in weak arm pull-ups and adduction
    - **Thoracodorsal artery** supplies latissimus dorsi.
  - **Medial pectoral nerve** – innervates pectoralis major and pectoralis minor
  - **Lateral pectoral nerve** – pectoralis major only
  - **Intercostobrachial nerve** – lateral cutaneous branch of the 2nd intercostal nerve; provides sensation to medial arm and axilla; encountered just below axillary vein when performing axillary dissection
    - Can transect without serious consequences
    - Most common injured nerve with MRM or ALND
- Branches of **internal thoracic (mammary) artery**, **intercostal arteries**, **thoracoacromial artery**, and **lateral thoracic artery** supply breast.

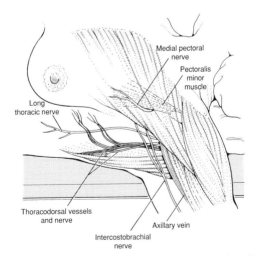

Major neurovascular structures to be preserved in an axillary dissection.

- **Batson's plexus** – valveless vein plexus that allows direct hematogenous metastasis of breast CA to spine
- **Lymphatic drainage**
  - 97% is to the axillary nodes.
  - 2% is to the internal mammary nodes.
  - Any quadrant can drain to the internal mammary nodes.
  - Supraclavicular nodes – considered **N3 disease**
  - Primary axillary adenopathy – ≤**1 is lymphoma**
- **Cooper's ligaments** – suspensory ligaments; divide breast into segments
  - Breast CA involving these strands can dimple the skin.

BENIGN BREAST DISEASE

- **Infectious mastitis** – most commonly associated with **breastfeeding**
  - **S. aureus** most common; strep; RF – smoking
  - **Lactational** – from blockage of lactiferous ducts; Tx: **antibiotics alone** (continue breastfeeding) for 2 weeks
  - **Nonlactational** – can be due to chronic inflammatory diseases (eg actinomyces) or autoimmune disease (eg SLE) → **antibiotics** for 2 weeks
  - **Failure to resolve** after 2 weeks or **recurs** – need **excisional biopsy** including skin to rule out necrotic breast CA
- **Breast abscess** – sequala from **infectious mastitis** or **periductal mastitis**
  - **Lactational** Tx: **percutaneous drainage**, **antibiotics**, continue breastfeeding.
    - Incision and drainage if it does not resolve promptly (complication – milk fistula)
  - **Nonlactational** breast abscess is **breast CA** until proven otherwise (need **incision/drainage** and **antibiotics**; send **skin** and **abscess cavity** biopsies for pathology and **fluid** for cytology).
  - **Failure to resolve** after 2 weeks or **recurs** – need **excisional biopsy** including skin to rule out necrotic breast CA
- **Periductal mastitis** (mammary duct ectasia or plasma cell mastitis)
  - Symptoms: **noncyclical mastodynia**, **erythema**, nipple retraction, creamy discharge from nipple; can have sterile or infected <u>subareolar abscess</u>
  - Risk factors – smoking, nipple piercings
  - Usually in peri- or postmenopausal women
  - Biopsy – **dilated subareolar mammary ducts**, inspissated secretions, periductal inflammation
  - Tx: if typical creamy discharge is present that is not bloody and not associated with nipple retraction, give **antibiotics** and **reassure**; if not or if it recurs (or if it persists > 2 weeks) → need to rule out inflammatory CA (incisional biopsy including the skin)
- **Galactocele** – breast cysts filled with milk; occurs with breastfeeding
  - Tx: ranges from aspiration to incision and drainage
- **Galactorrhea** – can be caused by ↑ prolactin (pituitary prolactinoma), OCPs, TCAs, phenothiazines, metoclopramide, alpha-methyl dopa, reserpine
  - Is often associated with amenorrhea
- **Gynecomastia** – 2-cm pinch; can be associated with cimetidine, spironolactone, marijuana; idiopathic in most
  - Tx: vast majority will regress; family reassurance and follow-up
- **Neonatal breast enlargement** – due to circulating maternal estrogens; will regress
- **Accessory breast tissue** (polymastia) – can present in axilla (most common location)
- **Accessory nipples** (polythelia) – can be found from axilla to groin (most common breast anomaly)
- **Breast asymmetry** – common
- **Breast reduction** – ability to lactate frequently compromised

- **Poland's syndrome** – hypoplasia of chest wall, amastia, hypoplastic shoulder, no pectoralis muscle
- **Mastodynia** – breast pain; very common; rarely represents breast CA
  - Dx: history and breast exam; bilateral mammogram
  - Tx: reassurance; OCPs, NSAIDs, evening primrose oil, bromocriptine, vitamin E
    - 2nd-line Tx: danazol, tamoxifen
  - Discontinue caffeine, nicotine, methylxanthines (eg theophylline).
  - **Cyclic mastodynia** – pain before menstrual period; most commonly from fibrocystic disease
  - **Continuous mastodynia** – continuous pain, many represents acute or subacute infection; continuous mastodynia is **more refractory** to treatment than cyclic mastodynia.
- **Mondor's disease** – superficial vein thrombophlebitis of breast (usually **lateral thoracic vein** or a branch); feels cordlike, can be painful; rarely represents CA
  - Associated with trauma and strenuous exercise
  - Usually occurs in lower outer quadrant
  - Tx: NSAIDs
- **Fibrocystic disease**
  - Lots of types: fibromatosis, sclerosing adenosis, apocrine metaplasia, duct adenosis, epithelial hyperplasia, ductal hyperplasia, and lobular hyperplasia
  - **Sclerosing adenosis** – has microcalcifications that can be confused with breast CA (no CA risk unless atypia)
  - Most common in **perimenopausal** women (40–50s); rare after menopause
  - **Symptoms**: breast pain, nipple discharge (usually yellow to brown), lumpy breast tissue that varies with hormonal cycle
  - Dx: mammogram, U/S, breast exam, and core needle biopsy
  - Only **cancer risk** is <u>atypical</u> ductal or **lobular hyperplasia** – ***need to resect these lesions*** (excisional biopsy)
    - Do <u>not</u> need to get negative margins with atypical hyperplasia; just remove all suspicious areas (ie calcifications) that appear on mammogram.
    - **Atypical lobular hyperplasia** (ALH) – is <u>not</u> premalignant although is a **marker** for increased risk of breast CA (4–5×; both breasts at risk); resected to avoid discordant findings (ie CA next to ALH)
    - **Atypical ductal hyperplasia** (ADH) – considered **premalignant**; 4–5× increased risk of breast CA; **pathology upgrade** after excision – 15% upgraded to DCIS, 3% upgraded to invasive CA
- **Intraductal papilloma**
  - Most common cause of **bloody nipple discharge**
  - Are usually small, nonpalpable, and close to the nipple
  - These lesions are <u>not</u> premalignant → get **contrast ductogram** to find papilloma, then needle localization
  - Tx: subareolar resection of the involved duct and papilloma

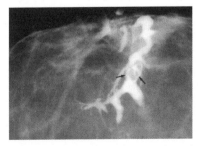

Ductogram. A large defect (*arrow*) represents an intraductal papilloma.

- **Fibroadenoma**
  - Most common breast lesion in adolescents and young women; 10% multiple
  - Usually painless, slow growing, well circumscribed, firm, and rubbery mass
  - Often grows to several cm in size and then stops
  - Can change in size with menstrual cycle and can enlarge in pregnancy
  - Generally considered benign
  - Giant fibroadenomas can be > 5 cm (treatment is the same)
  - Prominent **fibrous tissue compressing epithelial cells** on pathology
  - Can have large, coarse calcifications (popcorn lesions) on mammography from degeneration
  - **In patients ≤ 35 years old**:
    1. Mass needs to feel clinically benign (firm, rubbery, rolls, not fixed)
    2. Ultrasound or mammogram needs to be consistent with fibroadenoma
    3. Need core needle biopsy to show fibroadenoma (*safest answer*)
    - **Need all 3** of the above to be able to observe (with biannual U/S), otherwise need excisional biopsy
    - If the fibroadenoma continues to **enlarge** or is **symptomatic** – need **excisional biopsy**
    - Avoid resection of breast tissue in teenagers and younger children → can affect breast development
  - **In patients > 35 years old** → excisional biopsy to ensure diagnosis (core needle biopsy if you are trying for 1-step surgery)
  - **Complex fibroadenoma** – have slightly increased risk of CA
    - Is **complex** if any of the following: epithelial calcification, apocrine hyperplasia/metaplasia, sclerosing adenosis, or cysts > 3 cm
    - Tx: excisional biopsy
  - **Tubular fibroadenoma** – has tightly packed epithelial component with sparse connective tissues; are benign
- **Radial scar** (complex sclerosing lesions)
  - Stellate, irregular, spiculated mass that resembles breast CA
  - Has central **fibroelastic core** with ducts and lobules radiating outward (_not_ really a scar)
  - 2× increased risk of breast CA
  - Can _not_ make Dx on core biopsy alone – all need **excisional biopsy**

NIPPLE DISCHARGE

- Most nipple discharge is **benign**; CA risk increases with age.
- All need a history, breast exam, bilateral mammogram, and U/S.
- Try to find the trigger point or mass on exam; can send fluid for cytology.
- **Green/yellow/brown discharge** – usually due to fibrocystic disease; should have lumpy breast tissue consistent with fibrocystic disease
  - Tx: If cyclical and nonspontaneous, **reassure patient**.
- Worrisome for **CA** – persistent, unilateral, bloody, serous, or spontaneous
- **Bloody discharge** – most commonly intraductal papilloma; occasionally ductal CA
  - Tx: need **ductogram** and **subareolar excision** of involved ductal area and papilloma (wire-guided)
- **Serous discharge** – worrisome for cancer, especially if coming from only 1 duct or spontaneous
  - Tx: subareolar excisional biopsy of that ductal area
- **Spontaneous discharge** – no matter what the color or consistency is, this is worrisome for CA → all these patients need excisional biopsy of duct area causing the discharge
- **Nonspontaneous discharge** (occurs only with pressure, tight garments, exercise, etc.) – not as worrisome but may still need excisional biopsy (eg if bloody)
- May have to do a complete subareolar resection if the duct area cannot be properly identified (eg no trigger point or mass felt, no mass identified on imaging)

DUCTAL CARCINOMA IN SITU (DCIS)

- **Malignant cells of the ductal epithelium *without* invasion of basement membrane**
- 50% get cancer if not resected (ipsilateral breast).
- 5% get cancer in contralateral breast.
- Considered a **premalignant lesion**
- Usually not palpable and presents as a cluster of calcifications on mammography
- Can have solid, cribriform, papillary, and comedo patterns
  - **Comedo pattern** – most aggressive subtype; has necrotic areas
    - High risk for multicentricity, microinvasion, and recurrence
    - Tx: simple mastectomy
- ↑ **recurrence risk** with **comedo type** and **lesions > 2.5 cm**
- Tx: **lumpectomy** and adjuvant **whole breast XRT**; need ≥ **2 mm** margins
  - **No *ALND* or *SLNB***
  - XRT reduces recurrence 50% (*no* change in survival).
  - Postop **tamoxifen** (premenopausal) or **anastrazole** (aromatase inhibitor; postmenopausal)
  - **Simple mastectomy needed** if high grade (eg comedo type, multicentric, multifocal), if large tumor not amenable to lumpectomy, or if not able to get good margins; ***also need SLNB*** (last chance to sample the nodes if it turns out to be breast CA on final pathology [20% upgrade rate to invasive ductal CA])

LOBULAR CARCINOMA IN SITU (LCIS)

- Does not have basement membrane invasion
- 40% get cancer (either breast).
- Considered a marker for the development of breast CA, **not premalignant itself**
- Has *no* calcifications; is *not* palpable
- Primarily found in **premenopausal** women (genetic predisposition)
- Patients who develop breast CA are more likely to develop a **ductal CA** (70%).
- Usually an incidental finding; multifocal and bilateral disease is common.
- Majority are ER+/PR+/HER−.
- 5% risk of having a synchronous breast CA at time of LCIS diagnosis (most likely ductal CA)
- Tx: wire-guided excisional biopsy of the suspicious area (do *not* need negative margins)
  - Postop **tamoxifen** (premenopausal) or **raloxifene** (postmenopausal)
  - Consider bilateral subcutaneous mastectomy (*no* ALND).
- **Pleomorphic LCIS** – aggressive subtype with greater risk of breast CA; should be treated like **DCIS**

Indications for Excisional Biopsy After Core Biopsy

Atypical ductal hyperplasia
Atypical lobular hyperplasia
Radial scar
Lobular carcinoma in situ
Columnar cell hyperplasia with atypia
Papillary lesions
Phyllodes tumor
Lack of concordance between appearance of mammographic lesion and histologic diagnosis
Nondiagnostic specimen (including absence of calcifications on specimen radiograph when biopsy is performed for calcifications)

BREAST CANCER

- Breast CA decreased in economically poor areas.
- Japan has lowest rate of breast CA worldwide.
- U.S. breast CA risk – **1 in 8 women (12%)**; 5% in women with no risk factors
- **Gail model** (calculates 5 year and lifetime risk of breast CA) – uses age, race, ethnicity, age at first menses, age at birth of first child, number of first-degree relatives with breast CA, number of past biopsies, number of atypical hyperplasia biopsies
    - Does _not_ account for BRCA, at risk hereditary syndromes, or personal history LCIS, DCIS, or breast CA (underestimates risk; should _not_ use Gail in these scenarios)
- Breast CA in **younger women** (< 40) tends to be more aggressive.
- **Screening** decreases mortality by 25%.
- Untreated breast cancer – median survival 2–3 years
- 10% of breast CAs have negative mammogram and negative ultrasound.
- **Clinical features of breast CA** – distortion of normal architecture; skin/nipple distortion or retraction; hard, tethered, indistinct borders
- **Symptomatic breast mass workup**
    - **< 40 years old** – need **U/S** and **core needle Bx** (CNBx)
        - Need mammogram in patients < 40 if clinical exam or U/S is indeterminate or suspicious for CA although in general want to avoid excess radiation in this group
    - **> 40 years old** – need **bilateral mammograms**, **U/S**, and **CNBx**
    - If **CNBx** is **indeterminate**, **nondiagnostic**, or **nonconcordant** with exam findings/imaging studies → will need **excisional biopsy**
    - Clinically **indeterminate** or **suspect solid masses** will eventually need **excisional biopsy** unless CA diagnosis is made prior to that.
    - **Cyst fluid** (send fluid for cytology) – if **bloody**, need cyst excisional biopsy; if **clear and recurs**, need cyst excisional biopsy; if **complex cyst**, need cyst excisional biopsy; if **unresolved** after aspiration, need cyst excisional biopsy; if clear, does not recur, and cytology is negative (ie is a simple cyst) – no further therapy
    - **CNBx** – gives architecture (histology)
    - **FNA** – gives just cytology (just the cells)
    - CNBx and FNA can be performed with mammography or U/S guidance.

Management of Breast Masses Based on CNBx

Diagnosis	Treatment
Malignant	Definitive therapy
Suspicious	Surgical biopsy
Atypia	Surgical biopsy
Nondiagnostic	Repeated CNBx or surgical biopsy
Benign	Possible observation – exam and imaging studies need to concordant with benign disease, otherwise need excisional biopsy (if age > 40, lean toward excisional biopsy)

- **Mammography**
    - Has 90% sensitivity/specificity
    - Sensitivity increases with age as the dense parenchymal tissue is replaced with fat.
    - Mass needs to be ≥ 5 mm to be detected.
    - **Suggestive of CA** – irregular borders; spiculated; multiple clustered, small, thin, linear, crushed-like and/or branching calcifications; ductal asymmetry, distortion of architecture

BI-RADS Classification of Mammographic Abnormalities

Category	Assessment	Recommendation
0	Incomplete	Need further imaging
1	Negative	Routine screening
2	Benign finding	Routine screening
3	Probably benign finding	Short-interval follow-up mammogram (3-6 months)
4	Suspicious abnormality (eg indeterminate calcifications or architecture)	Definite probability of CA (**4a** – 15%, **4b** – 35%, **4c** – 80%); get **CNBx**
5	Highly suggestive of CA (suspicious calcifications or architecture)	High probability of CA (95%); get **CNBx**
6	Biopsy confirmed cancer	Excision

BI-RADS, breast imaging, reporting, and data system.

- **BI-RADS 4** lesion CNBx shows:
  - **Malignancy** → follow appropriate Tx
  - **Nondiagnostic**, **indeterminate**, or **benign and nonconcordant** with mammogram → need needle localization excisional biopsy
  - **Benign and concordant** with mammogram → 6-month follow-up
- **BI-RADS 5** lesion CNBx shows:
  - **Malignancy** → follow appropriate Tx
  - *Any other finding* (nondiagnostic, indeterminate, or benign) → all need needle localization excisional biopsy
- CNBx *without* excisional biopsy allows **appropriate staging with SLNB** (mass is still present) and **one-step surgery** (avoids 2 surgeries) for patients diagnosed with breast CA.
- Screening
  - **Average risk** – **annual mammogram** starting at **age 40**
  - **High-risk** – **annual mammogram** and **MRI** starting **age 25-40** (starting age depends on gene mutation and youngest age of breast CA in the family); also need **clinical breast exam** every 6-12 months once screening starts
  - Clinical breast exam *not* recommended for average risk women
  - **No** mammography in patients < **40** unless high risk → hard to interpret because of dense parenchyma
  - Want to **decrease radiation dose** in young patients
  - Mammograms are not performed in patients < 20 (breast is too dense)
- Node levels
  - **I** – lateral to pectoralis minor muscle
  - **II** – beneath pectoralis minor muscle
  - **III** – medial to pectoralis minor muscle (extends to thoracic inlet)
  - **Rotter's nodes** – between the pectoralis major and pectoralis minor muscles
  - **ALND** – need to take **level I** and **II nodes** (take level III nodes only if grossly involved)
  - **Nodes** are the most important **prognostic staging factor**. Other factors include tumor size, tumor grade, progesterone, and estrogen receptor status.
    - Survival is directly related to the number of positive nodes.
      - 0 nodes positive   75% 5-year survival
      - 1-3 nodes positive   60% 5-year survival
      - 4-10 nodes positive   40% 5-year survival
- **Bone** – most common site for distant metastasis (can also go to lung, liver, brain)
- Takes approximately 5-7 years to go from single malignant cell to 1-cm tumor
- **Central** and **subareolar tumors** have increased risk of multicentricity.
- **Breast cancer risk**
  - **High risk** (lifetime risk of breast CA > 20%)
    - BRCA gene with family history of breast CA

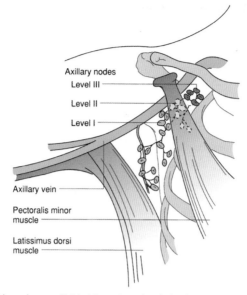

The axillary lymph nodes are divided into three levels by the pectoralis minor muscle. The level I nodes are inferior and lateral to the pectoralis minor, the level II nodes are below the axillary vein and behind the pectoralis minor, and the level III nodes are medial to the muscle against the chest wall.

- > 20% lifetime risk based on family history (eg ≥ 2 primary relatives with bilateral or premenopausal breast CA)
- DCIS (ipsilateral breast at risk) and LCIS (both breasts have same high risk)
- Atypical hyperplasia
- Prior breast CA
- Chest XRT between ages of 10–30
- Li-Fraumeni, Cowden/*PTEN* or Bannayan-Riley-Ruvalcaba syndrome
- *ATM, BARD1, BRIP1, CDH1, CHEK2, NBN, NF1, PALB2, PTEN, RAD51C, RAD51D, STK11* or *TP53* gene mutations
- **Moderately increased risk** – first-degree relative with breast cancer, age > 35 first birth
- **Lower increased risk** – early menarche, late menopause, nulliparity, proliferative benign disease, obesity, alcohol use, hormone replacement therapy
- **BRCA I and II** (+ family history of breast CA) and **CA risk**:
  - **BRCA I**:
    - Female breast CA   **60%** lifetime risk
    - Ovarian CA   **40%** lifetime risk
    - Male breast CA   **1%** lifetime risk
  - **BRCA II**:
    - Female breast CA   **60%** lifetime risk
    - Ovarian CA   **20%** lifetime risk
    - Male breast CA   **10%** lifetime risk
  - BRCA is the strongest RF for breast CA.
  - Women with BRCA breast CA have the same prognosis stage for stage as non-BRCA breast CA.
- **BRCA screening** – yearly mammogram and breast MRI starting at age 25
  - Yearly pelvic exam + U/S and CA-125 starting at age 25

- Consider **total abdominal hysterectomy** (TAH) and **bilateral salpingo-oophorectomy** (BSO) in BRCA families with history of breast CA.

TNM Definitions

Tx	Primary tumor cannot be assessed.
T0	No evidence of primary tumor
Tis	Carcinoma in situ, ductal, or lobular or Paget's disease of the nipple with no tumor
T1	Tumor 2 cm or less in greatest dimension
T2	Tumor more than 2 cm but not more than 5 cm in greatest dimension
T3	Tumor more than 5 cm in greatest dimension
T4	Tumor of any size with direct extension to the chest wall (not including pectoralis muscle), skin edema, skin ulceration, satellite skin nodules, or inflammatory carcinoma

REGIONAL LYMPH NODES (PATHOLOGIC)

Nx	Nodes cannot be assessed.
N0	No regional node metastases histologically, no additional examination for isolated tumor cells (ITCs)
N1	Metastasis to one to three axillary nodes or in internal mammary (IM) nodes with microscopic disease detected by sentinel node biopsy, which is not clinically apparent
N2	Metastases in four to nine axillary nodes or in clinically apparent IM nodes in the absence of axillary node metastasis
N3	Metastases in 10 or more axillary nodes, or in infraclavicular nodes, or in IM nodes in the presence of one or more positive axillary nodes; or in more than three axillary nodes with IM metastases, or in supraclavicular nodes

DISTANT METASTASES

Mx	Distant metastasis cannot be assessed.
M0	No distant metastasis
M1	Distant metastasis

STAGE GROUPING

Stage	T	N	M
Stage 0	Tis	N0	M0
Stage I	T1	N0	M0
Stage IIA	T0	N1	M0
	T1	N1	M0
	T2	N0	M0
Stage IIB	T2	N1	M0
	T3	N0	M0
Stage IIIA	T0	N2	M0
	T1	N2	M0
	T2	N2	M0
	T3	N1	M0
	T3	N2	M0
Stage IIIB	T4	N0	M0
	T4	N1	M0
	T4	N2	M0
Stage IIIC	Any T	N3	M0
Stage IV	Any T	Any N	M1

- **Considerations for prophylactic mastectomy** (vs careful follow-up +/− tamoxifen/raloxifene)
  - Family history + BRCA gene *or*
  - LCIS
  - **Also need one of the following**: high patient anxiety, poor patient access for follow-up exams and mammograms, difficult lesion to follow on exam or with mammograms, or patient preference for mastectomy

- **Hormone receptors** (estrogen/progesterone)
  - **Positive receptors** – better response to hormones, chemotherapy, surgery, and better overall prognosis
  - Receptor-positive tumors are more common in **postmenopausal women.**
  - **Progesterone receptor–positive tumors** have better prognosis than estrogen receptor–positive tumors.
  - Tumors that are both progesterone receptor and estrogen receptor positive have the best prognosis.
  - 10% of breast CA is negative for both receptors.
- **HER2/neu receptor** – worse prognosis stage for stage
  - Is a receptor tyrosine kinase
  - Trastuzumab (Herceptin) antibody blocks this receptor.
- **Male breast cancer**
  - < 1% of all breast CAs; usually **ductal**: RF – **BRCA2** (15% of breast CA in males)
  - **Poorer prognosis** compared to women because of late presentation (same prognosis stage for stage)
  - Have ↑ pectoral muscle involvement
  - Associated with steroid use, previous XRT, family history, Klinefelter's syndrome
  - Tx: BCT with post-op XRT _or_ modified radical mastectomy (MRM)
- **Ductal CA**
  - 85% of all breast CA (most common type of breast CA)
  - Various subtypes
    - **Medullary** – smooth borders, ↑ **lymphocytes**, bizarre cells, more favorable prognosis
    - **Tubular** – small **tubule** formations, more favorable prognosis
    - **Mucinous** (colloid) – produces an abundance of **mucin**, more favorable prognosis
    - **Cirrhotic** – worse prognosis
  - Tx: **MRM or BCT with postop XRT**
- **Lobular cancer**
  - 10% of all breast CAs
  - Does not form calcifications; extensively infiltrative; ↑ bilateral, multifocal, and multicentric disease
  - **Signet ring cells** confer worse prognosis.
  - Tx: **MRM or BCT with postop XRT**
- **Inflammatory cancer**
  - Considered T4 disease
  - Very aggressive → median survival of 36 months
  - Has **dermal lymphatic invasion**, which causes <u>peau d'orange lymphedema</u> appearance on breast skin (T4d); erythematous and warm
  - Dx: full-thickness incisional breast biopsy including the skin
  - Tx: **neoadjuvant chemo**, then **MRM**, then **adjuvant chemo-XRT** (most common method); BCT contraindicated here
- **Surgical options** (usually surgery first, followed by adjuvant Tx)
  - **Subcutaneous mastectomy** (simple mastectomy)
    - Leaves 1%–2% of breast tissue, preserves the nipple-areolar complex
    - <u>Not</u> indicated for breast CA treatment
    - Used for DCIS and LCIS
  - **Breast-conserving therapy** (BCT = lumpectomy, quadrantectomy, etc. plus ALND or SLNB); combined with **postop whole breast XRT**; need **"no ink on tumor"** margins
  - **Modified radical mastectomy**
    - Removes all breast tissue, including the nipple areolar complex
    - Includes axillary node dissection (**level I and II** nodes)

Contraindications to Breast-Conserving Therapy in Invasive Carcinoma

Absolute Contraindications to BCT
- Two or more primary tumors in separate quadrants of the breast
- Persistent positive margins after reasonable surgical attempts
- Pregnancy is an absolute contraindication to the use of breast irradiation. When cancer is diagnosed in the 3rd trimester; it may be possible to perform breast-conserving surgery and treat the patient with irradiation after delivery.
- A history of prior therapeutic irradiation to the breast region that would result in retreatment to an excessively high radiation dose
- Diffuse malignant-appearing microcalcifications

Relative Contraindications to BCT
- A history of scleroderma or active systemic lupus erythematosus
- Large tumor in a small breast that would result in cosmesis unacceptable to the patient

---

- **SLNB**
  - Fewer complications than ALND
  - Indicated for **early stage T1-2** breast CA (tumors ≤ **5 cm**)
  - <u>Not</u> indicated for clinically positive nodes (confirmed on FNA or CNBx) – need ALND
  - Not indicated for patients with distant metastases
  - Accuracy best when primary tumor is present (finds the right lymphatic channels)
  - Well suited for small tumors with low risk of axillary metastases
  - Lymphazurin blue dye or radiotracer is injected directly into tumor area.
  - **Type I hypersensitivity reactions** have been reported with Lymphazurin blue dye.
  - Usually find 1–3 nodes; 95% of the time, the sentinel node is found.
  - **Tumor deposits** need to be ≥ **2 mm** to be considered **positive**.
  - During **SLNB** – if no radiotracer or dye is found, need to do a formal ALND
  - If **tumor found** on SLNB, usually need **formal ALND**; <u>exception</u>:
    - Women > 18 with early stage tumors (**T1/T2,M0**) and **< 3 positive nodes** on SLNB who are receiving BCT (lumpectomy and whole breast XRT) do not need formal ALND.
  - **Contraindications to SLNB** – multicentric disease, neoadjuvant therapy, clinically positive nodes, prior axillary surgery, inflammatory or locally advanced disease
- **ALND** – take **level I and II nodes**
- **Complications of MRM** – infection, flap necrosis, seromas
- **Complications of ALND**
  - Infection, lymphedema, lymphangiosarcoma
  - **Axillary vein thrombosis** – sudden, early, postop swelling
  - **Lymphatic fibrosis** – slow swelling over 18 months
  - **Intercostal brachiocutaneous nerve injury** – hyperesthesia of inner arm and lateral chest wall; most commonly injured nerve after mastectomy; no significant sequelae
  - **Drains** – leave in until drainage < 40 cc/day
- **Radiotherapy**
  - **5,000 rad** for **BCT** and **XRT** (whole breast XRT with boost to tumor bed)
  - XRT decreases local recurrence and improves survival.
  - XRT given after chemo
  - **Complications of XRT** – edema, erythema, rib fractures, pneumonitis, ulceration, sarcoma, contralateral breast CA
  - **Contraindications to XRT** – pregnancy, scleroderma (results in severe fibrosis and necrosis), previous XRT and would exceed recommended dose, SLE (relative), active rheumatoid arthritis (relative)

- **Indications for XRT after <u>mastectomy</u>:**
  - **Advanced nodal disease** – > 4 nodes, extracapsular nodal invasion, fixed axillary nodes (N2), or internal mammary nodes (N3)
  - **Skin** or **chest wall** involvement
  - **Positive margins**
  - **T3** (> 5 cm) or **T4** (eg inflammatory CA) tumor
- **Indications for XRT to <u>regional nodes</u>:**
  - **> 4 positive** lymph nodes – XRT for supraclavicular, infraclavicular, axillary nodes
  - Tumors near **inner area of breast** – XRT for internal mammary nodes
- **BCT with XRT**
  - Need to have **no ink on tumor** margins following BCT before starting XRT
  - 10% chance of local recurrence, usually within 2 years of 1st operation, need to re-stage with recurrence
  - Need **salvage MRM** for local recurrence
- **Lumpectomy *without* XRT** – only indication is women **aged > 70** with early stage breast CA (T1,N0,M0, ER+, with negative margin lumpectomy) who are undergoing **hormonal therapy** (If <u>not</u> getting XRT, surgical margins should be 1 cm.)
- Chemotherapy
  - **TAC** (taxanes, Adriamycin, and cyclophosphamide) for 6-12 weeks
  - **Positive nodes** – everyone gets chemo *except* <u>postmenopausal women</u> with <u>positive hormonal receptors</u> → they can get hormonal therapy only with **aromatase inhibitor** (anastrozole)
  - **> 1 cm** and **negative nodes** – everyone gets chemo *except* patients with <u>positive hormonal receptors</u> → they can get hormonal therapy only with **tamoxifen** if they are <u>premenopausal</u> or **aromatase inhibitor** (anastrozole) if they are <u>postmenopausal</u>
  - **Triple receptor negative** – everyone gets chemo
  - **< 1 cm** *and* **negative nodes** *and* has **some receptor(s)** – no chemo; hormonal therapy as above or Herceptin
  - **After chemo**, patients who are **ER+** and/or **PR+** should receive **appropriate hormonal therapy**.
  - Both **chemotherapy** and **hormonal therapy** have been shown **to decrease recurrence** and **improve survival**.
  - **Neoadjuvant chemo** considered for:
    - **T4** – locally advanced or inflammatory breast CA to **shrink tumor** and **improve resectability** (obtain negative margins)
    - **T3** – to shrink tumor for patients desiring **BCT** who would otherwise require mastectomy due to large tumor relative to breast size
    - **Pregnancy** and breast CA
  - **Taxanes** – docetaxel, paclitaxel
  - **Tamoxifen** (Tx for 5 years) – decreases risk of breast CA recurrence by 50%
    - Blocks estrogen and progesterone hormonal receptors
    - Side effects – 1% risk of thromboembolism; 0.1% risk of endometrial CA
    - Decreases risk of osteoporosis and fractures
  - **Aromatase inhibitors** (Tx for 5 years) – decreases risk of breast CA recurrence by 50%
    - Block conversion of testosterone to estrogen in the periphery
    - Side effects – fractures
    - Decreased risk of thromboembolic events and endometrial CA compared to tamoxifen
  - **Trastuzumab** (Herceptin; Tx for 1 year) – decreases risk of breast CA recurrence 50%
    - Should be given for **HER2/neu receptor–positive** tumors either **> 1 cm** or if **nodes are positive**
    - Side effects – cardiac disease (heart failure)

- **Almost all women with recurrence die of disease.**
- Increased recurrences and metastases occur with **positive nodes**, **large tumors**, **negative receptors, unfavorable subtype**.
- **Metastatic flare** – pain, swelling, erythema in metastatic areas; XRT can help.
  - XRT is good for bone or brain metastases.
- **Occult breast CA** – breast CA that presents as axillary metastases with unknown primary; Tx: **MRM** (70% are found to have breast CA)
- **Paget's disease**
  - **Scaly** (eczematous, ulcerated) skin lesion on nipple
  - Biopsy shows Paget's cells (clear cytoplasm and large nucleoli).
  - Patients have underlying DCIS or ductal CA in breast.
  - Dx: full-thickness incisional breast biopsy including the skin
  - Tx: need **MRM** if cancer present; otherwise simple mastectomy with SLNB if DCIS is present (need to include the **nipple-areolar complex** with Paget's)
- **Phyllodes tumor**
  - Benign, borderline, and malignant subclasses
  - 10% **malignant** (cystosarcoma phyllodes; based on > 5–10 mitoses per high-power field)
  - **No nodal metastases**, hematogenous spread if any (rare)
  - Resembles giant fibroadenoma; has stromal and epithelial elements (mesenchymal tissue)
  - Can often be large tumors
  - Tx: WLE with negative margins (1 cm); **no ALND**
- **Stewart–Treves syndrome**
  - **Lymphangiosarcoma** from **chronic lymphedema** following axillary dissection
  - Patients present with dark purple nodule or lesion on arm 5–10 years after surgery.
- **Pregnancy with mass**
  - Tends to present late, leading to worse prognosis
  - Mammography and ultrasound do not work as well during pregnancy.
  - Try to use ultrasound to avoid radiation.
  - If **cyst**, drain it and send FNA for cytology.
  - If **solid**, perform core needle biopsy.
  - If core needle equivocal, need to go to excisional biopsy
  - **Breast CA** in pregnancy
    - No hormonal or radiation therapy at any time during the pregnancy
    - Chemotherapy can be used after the 1st trimester.
  - **1st trimester** breast CA – need MRM
  - **Late 2nd/3rd trimester** breast CA – lumpectomy with low-dose SLNB (BCT), then chemo during pregnancy, then postdelivery XRT

25 Thoracic

ANATOMY AND PHYSIOLOGY

- **Azygous vein** runs along the right side and dumps into superior vena cava.
- **Thoracic duct** starts at **cisterna chyli** in abdomen (L2), then runs along the right side of the chest (between azygous vein and esophagus), crosses midline at T4–5, and then dumps into left subclavian vein at junction with internal jugular vein.
- **Phrenic nerve** – runs anterior to hilum
- **Vagus nerve** – runs posterior to hilum
- Right lung volume 55% (3 lobes: RUL, RML, and RLL)
- Left lung volume 45% (2 lobes: LUL and LLL; also has lingula)
- Quiet inspiration – diaphragm 80%, intercostals 20%
- Greatest change in dimension **superior/inferior**
- Accessory muscles – sternocleidomastoid muscle (SCM), levators, serratus posterior, scalenes
- **Type I pneumocytes** – gas exchange
- **Type II pneumocytes** – surfactant production (mainly phosphatidylcholine – keeps alveoli open
- **Pores of Kahn** – direct air exchange between alveoli

LUNG CANCER SCREENING

- Annual low-dose CT scan
- Indicated for patients **50–80 years old** with **> 20 pack-year** smoking history and are **currently smoking** or who have **quit within last 15 years**
- Screening stops when the patient has not smoked for 15 years or if becomes ineligible for surgery due to comorbidities or patient preference.

SOLITARY PULMONARY NODULE (COIN LESION)

- Malignancy related to **age**: **< 50** – 5%; **> 50** – 50%
- Malignancy related to **size**:
  - **< 5 mm – 1%**
  - **5–10 mm – 10%**
  - **11–20 mm – 50%**
  - **21–30 mm – 70%**
  - **> 30 mm** considered mass
- MC lesion – **granuloma**
- MC tumor – **hamartoma**
- MC CA – **lung adenocarcinoma**
- Noncalcified lesions – more likely CA
- **Benign disease** (no growth in 2 years, smooth contour, and popcorn calcification suggests benign disease) – no further workup needed
- **Low-risk lesions** – serial chest CT (frequency based on clinical suspicion – start at 3 months if worried; if it grows need biopsy)
- **Intermediate-/high-risk lesions:**
  - Biopsy indicated for suspicious lesions **> 10 mm** (**growth** over 2 years worrisome)
  - **Bronchoscopy** guided for **central** lesions, **CT** guided for **peripheral** lesions
  - **VATS wedge resection** if those fail (need full CA workup _before_ VATS – will proceed with formal lung resection at that time if frozen section shows CA)

PULMONARY FUNCTION TESTS

- Need predicted postop **FEV$_1$ > 0.8** (or > 40% of the predicted postop value)
  - If it is close → get qualitative V/Q scan to see contribution of **diseased lung** to overall FEV$_1$ → if low, may still be able to resect
  - FEV$_1$ is the best predictor of **pulmonary complications** and being able to wean off the ventilator.
- Need predicted postop **DLCO > 10** mL/min/mm Hg (or > 40% of the predicted postop value)
  - Measures **carbon monoxide diffusion** and represents **oxygen exchange capacity**
  - This value depends on pulmonary capillary surface area, hemoglobin content, and alveolar architecture.
- No resection if preop **pCO$_2$ > 50** or **pO$_2$ < 60** at rest
- No resection if preop VO$_2$ max **< 10–12 mL/min/kg** (maximum oxygen consumption)
- **Persistent air leak** – most common after segmentectomy/wedge
- **Atelectasis** – most common after lobectomy
  - MC complication following lung resection
  - Tx: incentive spirometer
- **Arrhythmias** – most common after pneumonectomy

LUNG CANCER

- Symptoms: can be asymptomatic with finding on routine CXR; cough, hemoptysis, atelectasis, PNA, pain, weight loss
- **Most common cause of cancer-related death in the United States**
- **Nodal involvement** has strongest influence on survival.
  - Hilar nodal involvement does not preclude resection (N1).
- **Brain** – single most common site of metastasis
  - Can also go to supraclavicular nodes, other lung, bone, liver, and adrenals
- **Recurrence** usually appears as disseminated metastasis.
  - 80% of recurrences are within the 1st 3 years.
- **Non–small cell carcinoma**
  - **80%** of lung CA
  - **Squamous cell carcinoma** usually more central
  - **Adenocarcinoma** usually more peripheral
  - **Adenocarcinoma** is the most common lung CA (not squamous).
- **Small cell carcinoma**
  - **20%** of lung CA; **neuroendocrine** in origin; usually **central**
  - Usually unresectable at time of diagnosis (< 5% candidates for surgery)
  - Overall 5-year survival rate < 5% (very poor prognosis)
  - Stage T1,N0,M0 5-year survival rate – 50%
  - Most get just chemo-XRT.
- **Paraneoplastic syndromes**
  - **Squamous cell CA** – PTH-related peptide
  - **Small cell CA** – ACTH and ADH
  - Small cell **ACTH** – most common paraneoplastic syndrome
- **Bronchoalveolar CA** – can look like pneumonia; grows along alveolar walls; multifocal
- **Chest and abdominal CT scan** – single best test for clinical assessment of **T** and **N status** (*best test overall for resectability*)
- **PET scan** – best test for **M status**
- **Brain MRI** – indicated for neuro symptoms, stage III/IV, small cell, and Pancoast tumors
- **Mediastinoscopy**
  - Use for **centrally located tumors** and patients with **suspicious adenopathy** (> 0.8 cm or subcarinal > 1.0 cm) on chest CT.
  - Does not assess aorto-pulmonary (AP) window nodes (left lung drainage)

- Assesses **ipsilateral** (N2) and **contralateral** (N3) **mediastinal nodes**
- If **mediastinal nodes** are **positive**, tumor is ***unresectable***.
- Looking into **middle mediastinum** with mediastinoscopy
  - Left-side structures – RLN, esophagus, aorta, main pulmonary artery (PA)
  - Right-side structures – azygous and SVC
  - Anterior structures – innominate vein, innominate artery, right PA
- **Chamberlain procedure** (anterior thoracotomy or parasternal mediastinotomy) – assesses enlarged **AP window nodes**; go through left 2nd rib cartilage
- **Bronchoscopy** – needed for centrally located tumors to check for airway invasion

---

TNM STAGING SYSTEM FOR LUNG CANCER

- **T1**: ≤ 3 cm. **T2**: 3.1–5.0 cm but > 2 cm away from carina. **T3**: 5.1–7.0 cm _or_ invasion of chest wall, pericardium, or diaphragm, _or_ < 2 cm from carina. **T4**: ≥ 7.1 cm (still possibly resectable) _or_ invasion of mediastinum, esophagus, trachea, vertebra, heart, great vessels, or malignant effusion (usually all indicate unresectability)
- **N1**: ipsilateral hilum nodes
- **N2**: ipsilateral mediastinal, subcarinal, or aortopulmonary window (unresectable)
- **N3**: contralateral mediastinal or supraclavicular (unresectable)
- **M1**: distant metastasis

Stage	TNM Status
I	T1–2,N0,M0
IIa	T1,N1,M0
IIb	T2,N1,M0 or T3,N0,M0
IIIa	T1–3,N2,M0 or T3,N1,M0
IIIb	Any T4
IIIc	Any N3
IV	M1

- For **lung CA**, patients need to 1) be **operable** (eg have appropriate FEV_1 and DLCO values) and 2) be **resectable** (ie can't have N2, N3, or M disease).
  - **Lobectomy** or **pneumonectomy** most common procedure (need formal lung resection for lung CA); sample suspicious nodes
  - **VATS resection** – consider for **stage I peripheral tumors** (no nodal or local invasion)
- **Treatment**
  - **Stage I** and **II** – resection (definitive XRT if not surgical candidate)
    - **Stage II** – need postop chemo
  - **Stage IIIa** – T3,N1,M0 usually resectable (neoadjuvant chemo-XRT, re-stage, resection)
    - Any N2 disease is _not_ resectable (definitive chemo-XRT).
  - **Stage IIIb** – generally _not_ resectable (definitive chemo-XRT)
    - Some T4,N0–1,M0 tumors can be resected after neoadjuvant chemo-XRT.
  - **Stage IIIc/IV** – _not_ resectable (definitive chemo-XRT)
- **Non–small cell** CA chemotherapy (stage II or higher) – carboplatin, Taxol
- **Small cell lung** CA chemotherapy – cisplatin, etoposide
- Lung CA overall 5-year survival rate 10% (30% with resection for cure)
- **Postop follow-up** (after resection for cure) – H and P plus chest CT every 6 month for 2 years, then annually thereafter

- **Pancoast tumor** – tumor invades apex of chest wall and patients have **Horner's syndrome** (invasion of sympathetic chain → ptosis, miosis, anhidrosis) or **ulnar nerve** symptoms
- **Superior vena cava** (SVC) **syndrome** – severe venous swelling of head, neck, and upper extremities; can also get laryngeal/tracheobronchial compression
  - Most commonly due to lung CA (MC small cell) invading SVC; 2nd – lymphoma
  - Nonmalignant causes – indwelling devices (pacemaker lead, HD catheter), sarcoid, substernal thyroid, fibrosing mediastinitis
  - Can be associated with **Horner's syndrome**
  - Dx: chest CT (venous phase contrast best)
  - If due to lung CA, the tumor is unresectable since it invades the mediastinum.
  - Initial Tx: Elevate head of bed, diuretics, hydrocortisone.
  - Tx: **emergent XRT** if severe and due to malignancy; endovascular stent if that fails
    - If <u>not</u> due to malignancy – endovascular stent (open bypass if that fails)
- **Mesothelioma**
  - Most malignant lung tumor
  - Aggressive local invasion, nodal invasion, and distant metastases common at the time of diagnosis
  - Asbestos exposure
- **Asbestos exposure** increases lung CA risk 90×.
- **Metastases to the lung** – if isolated and <u>not</u> associated with any other systemic disease, may be resected for colon, renal cell CA, sarcoma, melanoma, ovarian, and endometrial CA

CARCINOIDS

- **Neuroendocrine** tumor, usually central
  - 5% have metastases at time of diagnosis; 50% have symptoms (cough, hemoptysis).
- **Typical** carcinoid – 90% 5-year survival
- **Atypical** carcinoid – 60% 5-year survival
- Tx: resection; treat like cancer; outcome closely linked to histology
- Recurrence increased with positive nodes or tumors > 3 cm.

BRONCHIAL ADENOMAS

- Upper airway usual
- MC – **carcinoid** (90%)
- Others – **mucoepidermoid adenoma, mucous gland adenoma,** and **adenoid cystic adenoma** → *all are **malignant** tumors*
- **Mucoepidermoid adenoma** and **mucous gland adenoma**
  - Slow growth, <u>no</u> metastases
  - Tx: resection (1-cm margin)
- **Adenoid cystic adenoma**
  - From submucosal glands; spreads along **perineural lymphatics**, well beyond endoluminal component; *very XRT sensitive*
  - Slow growing; can get 10-year survival with incomplete resection
  - Tx: resection; if unresectable, XRT can provide good palliation

HAMARTOMAS

- Most common **benign** adult lung tumor
- Composed of fat, cartilage, and connective tissue
- Have **calcifications** and can appear as a **popcorn lesion** on chest CT
- Diagnosis can be made with CT.
- **Do not require resection**
- Repeat chest CT in 6 months to confirm diagnosis.

MEDIASTINAL TUMORS IN ADULTS

- Most are asymptomatic; can present with chest pain, cough, dyspnea
- MCC of mediastinal adenopathy – **lymphoma**
- **Neurogenic tumors** – most common mediastinal tumor in adults and children, usually in posterior mediastinum
- 50% of symptomatic mediastinal masses are malignant.
- 90% of asymptomatic mediastinal masses are benign.
- **Location** (adult)
  - **Anterior** (thymus) – most common site for mediastinal tumor; **T's** →
    - Thymoma (#1 anterior mediastinal mass in adults)
    - Thyroid CA and goiters
    - T-cell lymphoma
    - Teratoma (and other germ cell tumors)
    - Parathyroid adenomas
  - **Middle** (heart, trachea, ascending aorta)
    - Bronchiogenic cysts
    - Pericardial cysts
    - Enteric cysts
    - Lymphoma
  - **Posterior** (esophagus, descending aorta)
    - Enteric cysts
    - Neurogenic tumors
    - Lymphoma
- **Thymoma**
  - All thymomas require resection.
  - Thymus too big or associated with refractory myasthenia gravis → resection
  - 50% of thymomas are **malignant**.
  - 50% of patients with thymomas have **symptoms**.
  - 50% of patients with thymomas have **myasthenia gravis**.
  - 10% of patients with myasthenia gravis have thymomas.
  - *Are rare in children*
- **Myasthenia gravis** – fatigue, weakness, diplopia, ptosis (ocular symptoms most common)
  - Antibodies to acetylcholine receptors
  - Tx: anticholinesterase inhibitors (neostigmine); steroids, plasmapheresis
  - 80% get improvement with thymectomy, including patients who do not have thymomas.
- **Germ cell tumors**
  - If open biopsy is required, perform **anterior thoracotomy** (parasternal mediastinotomy [Chamberlain procedure]).
  - Mediastinoscopy will <u>not</u> reach these lesions if they are in the anterior or posterior mediastinum.
  - Need to check testicles in males and pelvic U/S in females to look for **primary tumor**
  - **Teratoma** – most common germ cell tumor in mediastinum
    - Can be benign or malignant
    - Tx: resection; possible chemotherapy
  - **Seminoma** – most common <u>malignant</u> germ cell tumor in mediastinum
    - 10% are beta-HCG positive; should <u>not</u> have AFP (alpha-fetoprotein)
    - Tx: **XRT** (*extremely sensitive*); chemotherapy reserved only for metastases or bulky nodal disease; surgery for residual disease after that
  - **Non-seminoma** – 90% have elevated beta-HCG and AFP
    - Tx: **chemo** (**cisplatin**, **bleomycin**, **etoposide**); surgery for residual disease

- **Cysts**
  - **Bronchiogenic** – usually posterior to carina. Tx: **resection**
  - **Pericardial** – usually at right costophrenic angle. Tx: **can leave alone** (benign)
- **Neurogenic tumors** – have pain, neurologic deficit. Tx: resection
  - 10% have intra-spinal involvement that requires simultaneous spinal surgery.
  - **Neurolemmoma** (schwannoma) – most common
  - **Paraganglioma** – can produce **catecholamines**, associated with von Recklinghausen's disease
  - Can also get **neuroblastomas** and **neurofibromas**

TRACHEA

- MC benign tumors: adults – **papilloma**; children – **hemangioma**
- MC malignant – **squamous cell carcinoma** (adults), **carcinoid** (children)
- Most common late complication after tracheal surgery – granulation tissue formation
- Most common early complication after tracheal surgery – laryngeal edema
  - Tx: reintubation, racemic epinephrine, steroids
- **Post-intubation stenosis** – at stoma site with tracheostomy, at cuff site with ET tube
  - Serial dilatation, bronchoscopic resection, or laser ablation if minor
  - Tracheal resection with end-to-end anastomosis if severe or if it keeps recurring
- **Tracheo-innominate artery fistula** – occurs after **tracheostomy**, can have rapid exsanguination
  - **Small amount** of bleeding (sentinel bleed) – Dx: bronchoscopy to look for fistula
  - **Large amount** of bleeding – Tx: place finger in tracheostomy hole and hold pressure against back of sternum → **median sternotomy** with **ligation and resection of innominate artery** (no graft, just ligate); close hole in trachea primarily; strap muscle between ligated artery and trachea
  - This complication is avoided by keeping tracheostomy between the 2nd and 3rd tracheal rings.
- **Tracheo-esophageal fistula**
  - Usually occurs with prolonged intubation
  - Place large-volume cuff endotracheal tube below fistula.
  - May need decompressing gastrostomy
  - Attempt repair after the patient is weaned from ventilator.
  - Tx: tracheal resection, reanastomosis, close hole in esophagus, sternohyoid flap between esophagus and trachea

LUNG ABSCESS

- Necrotic area; most commonly associated with aspiration
- Most commonly in the **superior segment of RLL**
- MC organism – *staph aureus*
- Tx: *antibiotics alone* (95% successful); CT-guided drainage if that fails
  - Surgery if above fails or cannot rule out cancer (> 6 cm, failure to resolve after 6 weeks)
- Chest CT can help differentiate empyema from lung abscess.

EMPYEMA

- Usually secondary to **pneumonia** and **subsequent parapneumonic effusion** (staph, strep)
- Can also be due to esophageal, pulmonary, or mediastinal surgery
- Symptoms: pleuritic chest pain, fever, cough, SOB

- Pleural fluid often has WBCs > 500 cells/cc, bacteria, and a positive Gram stain.
- **Exudative phase** (1st week) – Tx: chest tube, antibiotics
- **Fibro-proliferative phase** (2nd week) – Tx: chest tube, antibiotics; possible VATS (video-assisted thoracoscopic surgery) deloculation if lung doesn't re-expand
- **Organized phase** (3rd–4th week) – Tx: likely need **decortication**; fibrous peel occurs around lung (lung trapping)
  - Some are using **intra-pleural tPA** (tissue plasminogen activator) to try and dissolve the peel.
  - May need **Eloesser flap** (open thoracic window – direct opening to external environment) in frail/elderly

CHYLOTHORAX

- Milky white fluid; has ↑ lymphocytes and TAGs (> 110 mL/μL); Sudan red stains fat.
- **Fluid is resistant to infection.**
- 50% secondary to trauma or iatrogenic injury (symptoms start after oral intake)
- 50% secondary to tumor (**lymphoma** most common, due to tumor burden in the lymphatics)
- Injury **above T5–6** results in **left**-sided chylothorax.
- Injury **below T5–6** results in **right**-sided chylothorax.
- Tx: 2–3 weeks of conservative therapy (chest tube, octreotide, low-fat diet or TPN without lipids [or use medium chain fatty acids, _not_ long chain])
  - If above fails and chylothorax secondary to **trauma** or **iatrogenic injury**, need **ligation of thoracic duct** on **right side** low in mediastinum (80% successful).
  - For **malignant causes**, need **talc pleurodesis** and possible **chemo and/or XRT** (less successful than above).

MASSIVE HEMOPTYSIS

- **> 600 cc/24 h**; bleeding usually from high-pressure **bronchial arteries**
- Most commonly secondary to **infection**, death is due to asphyxiation.
- Tx: place bleeding side down; mainstem intubation to side opposite of bleeding to prevent drowning in blood; rigid bronchoscopy to identify site and possibly control bleeding; may need lobectomy or pneumonectomy to control; bronchial artery embolization if not suitable for surgery

SPONTANEOUS PNEUMOTHORAX

- Tall, healthy, thin, young males; more common on the **right**; RF – **smoking**
- Chest pain, dyspnea, tachycardia
- Primary pneumothorax – <u>no</u> preexisting disease
- Secondary pneumothorax – preexisting disease (eg COPD [MC], asthma, infection)
- Recurrence risk after 1st pneumothorax is 20%, after 2nd pneumothorax is 60%, after 3rd pneumothorax is 80%.
- Results from rupture of a bleb usually in the apex of the upper lobe of the lung
- For clinically stable PTX that is < 10% (< 3 cm) – can observe with serial CXRs
- Tx: **chest tube**
- Surgery for: recurrence, persistent air leak > 5 days, non-reexpansion (despite 2 chest tubes), high-risk profession (airline pilot, diver, mountain climber), patients who live in remote areas, tension PTX, hemothorax, bilateral PTX, previous pneumonectomy, large bleb on CT scan
- Surgery – VATS **apical blebectomy** and **mechanical pleurodesis** (use Bovie scratch pad)
  - If blebs <u>not</u> found in OR – proceed with apical wedge resection of upper lobe
  - Pleurodesis causes inflammatory reaction between pulmonary and parietal pleura getting them to stick/scar together.

OTHER CONDITIONS

- **Pleural effusion CXR** – lose costophrenic angle first; then starts to layer when > 300 cc
  - Appears homogenous on CT scan
- **Malignant pericardial effusion:** MCC – **lung CA**; Tx: **pericardial window**
- **Malignant pleural effusion:** MCC – **lung CA**; Tx: **drainage** and **talc pleurodesis**
- **Tension pneumothorax** – most likely to cause arrest after <u>blunt</u> trauma; impaired venous return
- **Catamenial pneumothorax** – occurs in temporal relation to menstruation
  - Caused by **endometrial implants** in the visceral lung pleura
- **Residual hemothorax despite 2 good chest tubes** → OR for thoracoscopic drainage
- **Clotted hemothorax** – surgical drainage if > 25% of lung, air–fluid levels, or signs of infection (fever, ↑ WBCs); surgery in 1st week to avoid peel; risk of empyema if not removed
- **Broncholiths** – usually secondary to infection
- **Mediastinitis** – usually occurs after cardiac surgery
- **Whiteout on chest x-ray**
  - Midline shift toward whiteout – most likely collapse → need bronchoscopy to remove plug
  - No shift – CT scan to figure it out
  - Midline shift away from whiteout – most likely effusion → place chest tube
- **Bronchiectasis** – acquired from infection, tumor, **cystic fibrosis**
  - Diffuse nature prevents surgery in most patients.
- **Tuberculosis** – lung apices; get calcifications, **caseating granulomas**
  - Ghon complex → parenchymal lesion + enlarged hilar nodes
  - Tx: INH, rifampin, pyrazinamide
- **Sarcoidosis** – has **non-caseating granulomas**

Evaluation of Pleural Fluid

Test	Transudate	Exudate	Empyema
WBC	< 1,000	> 1,000	> 1,000 > 50,000 most specific
pH	7.45–7.55	≤ 7.45	< 7.30
Pleural fluid protein to serum ratio	< 0.5	> 0.5	> 0.5
Pleural fluid LDH to serum ratio	< 0.6	> 0.6	> 0.6

- **Recurrent pleural effusions** can be treated with mechanical pleurodesis.
  - Talc pleurodesis for malignant pleural effusions
- **Airway fires** – usually associated with the laser
  - Tx: stop gas flow, remove ET tube, reintubate for 24 hours; bronchoscopy
- **AVMs** – connections between the pulmonary arteries and pulmonary veins; usually in **lower lobes**; can occur with Osler–Weber–Rendu disease
  - Symptoms: hemoptysis, SOB, neurologic events
  - Tx: **embolization**
- **Chest wall tumors**
  - **Benign** – **osteochondroma** most common
  - **Malignant** – **chondrosarcoma** most common

CONGENITAL HEART DISEASE

- **R → L shunts** cause **cyanosis**.
  - Children squat to *increase* SVR and *decrease* R → L shunts.
  - **Cyanosis** – can lead to polycythemia, strokes, brain abscess, endocarditis
  - **Eisenmenger's syndrome**: shift from **L → R shunt** to **R → L shunt**
    - Sign of increasing pulmonary vascular resistance (PVR) and **pulmonary HTN**; this condition is generally <u>irreversible.</u>
- **L → R shunts** cause **CHF** – manifests as failure to thrive, ↑ HR, tachypnea, hepatomegaly, pulmonary edema; CHF in **children** – *hepatomegaly* 1st sign
- **L → R shunts** (CHF) – VSD, ASD, PDA
- **R → L shunts** (cyanosis) – tetralogy of Fallot
- **Ductus arteriosus** – connection between descending aorta and left pulmonary artery (PA); blood shunted away from lungs in utero
- **Ductus venosum** – connection between portal vein and IVC; blood shunted away from liver in utero
- **Foramen ovale** – shunts blood away from lungs
- **Fetal circulation to placenta** – 2 umbilical arteries
- **Fetal circulation from placenta** – 1 umbilical vein

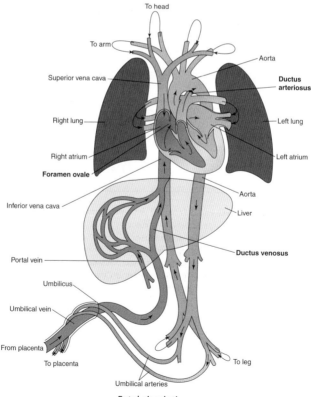

Fetal circulation.

- **Ventricular septal defect** (VSD)
  - **Most common congenital heart defect**
  - **L → R shunt**
  - **80% close spontaneously** (usually by age 6 months).
  - Large VSDs – usually cause symptoms after 4-6 weeks of life, as PVR ↓ and shunt ↑
  - Can get **CHF** (tachypnea, tachycardia) and **failure to thrive**
  - Medical Tx: diuretics and digoxin
  - <u>Usual timing of repair:</u>
    - **Large** VSDs (shunt > 2.5) – **1 year** of age
    - **Medium** VSDs (shunt 2-2.5) – **5 years** of age
    - *Failure to thrive* – *most common reason for earlier repair*
- **Atrial septal defect** (ASD)
  - **L → R shunt**
  - **Ostium secundum** – most common (80%); centrally located
  - **Ostium primum** (or atrioventricular canal defects or endocardial cushion defects); can have mitral valve and tricuspid valve problems; frequent in **Down's syndrome**
  - Usually symptomatic when **shunt > 2** → CHF (SOB, recurrent respiratory infections)
  - Can get **paradoxical emboli** in adulthood
  - Medical Tx: diuretics and digoxin
  - <u>Usual timing of repair</u> – **1–2 years** of age (age 3-6 months with canal defects)
- **Tetralogy of Fallot** (4 parts)
  - VSD, pulmonic stenosis, overriding aorta, right ventricular (RV) hypertrophy
  - **R → L shunt**; child is small for age; clubbing; spells of cyanosis relieved by squatting
  - **Most common congenital heart defect that results in cyanosis**
  - Have decreased pulmonary perfusion
  - Medical Tx: **β-blocker**
  - <u>Usual timing of repair</u> – 3-6 months of age
  - Repair: RV outflow tract obstruction (RVOT) removal, RVOT enlargement, and VSD repair

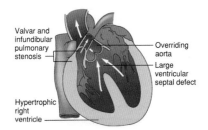

The four anatomic features of the tetralogy of Fallot. The primary morphologic abnormality, anterior and superior displacement of the infundibular septum, results in a malalignment ventricular septal defect, overriding of the aortic valve, and obstruction of the right ventricular outflow. Right ventricular hypertrophy is a secondary occurrence.

- **Patent ductus arteriosus** (PDA)
  - **L → R shunt**; bounding peripheral pulses, widened pulse pressure; machinelike murmur
  - **Indomethacin** – causes the PDA to close; rarely successful beyond neonatal period
  - Requires surgical ligation through left thoracotomy if it persists
- **Aortic coarctation**
  - Generally young patients with HTN in arms and low blood pressure in lower extremities
  - CXR – rib scalloping (erosion of large intercostal vessels into ribs)
  - Dx: CT angiogram
  - Tx: surgical resection

- **Vascular ring**
  - Difficulty swallowing, episodes of respiratory distress (stridor, crowing respirations), neck hyperextension
  - Trachea and esophagus are encircled by 2 aortic arches.
  - Dx: barium swallow, bronchoscopy
  - Tx: surgery to divide the smaller of the 2 aortic arches

ADULT CARDIAC DISEASE

- **Coronary artery disease**
  - Most common cause of death in the United States
  - Risk factors – smoking, HTN, male gender, family history, hyperlipidemia, diabetes
  - Medical Tx: nitrates, smoking cessation, weight loss, statin drugs, ASA
  - Left main coronary artery branches into left anterior descending (LAD) and circumflex (Cx) arteries.
  - Most atherosclerotic lesions are **proximal**.
  - **Complications of myocardial infarction**:
    - **VSR** (ventricular septal rupture) – hypotension, pansystolic murmur, usually occurs **3–7 days** after MI; have a **step-up in oxygen content** between right atrium and pulmonary artery secondary to L → R shunt; Dx: **echo**; Tx: IABP to temporize, **patch over septum**
    - **Papillary muscle rupture** – get severe mitral regurgitation with hypotension and pulmonary edema; usually occurs **3–7 days** after MI; Dx: **echo**; Tx: IABP to temporize, **replace valve**
  - **Drug-eluting stent** – restenosis in 20% at 1 year
  - **Saphenous vein graft** – 80% 5-year patency
  - **Internal mammary artery** – off subclavian artery
    - **Best conduit for CABG** (> 95% 20-year patency when placed to **LAD**)
    - Collateralizes with **superior epigastric artery**
  - **CABG procedure**
    - **Potassium** and **cold solution cardioplegia** – causes arrest of the heart in diastole; keeps the heart protected and still while grafts are placed
  - **Best indications for CABG** (> 70% stenosis significant for most areas except left main disease)
    - Left main disease (> 50% stenosis considered significant)
    - 3-vessel disease (LAD, Cx, and right coronary artery)
    - 2-vessel disease involving the LAD
    - Lesions not amenable to stenting
  - **High mortality risk factors**: *preop cardiogenic shock* (#1 risk factor), emergency operations, age, low EF

VALVE DISEASE

- **Bioprosthetic tissue valves** (do not require anticoagulation)
  - For patients who want pregnancy, have contraindication to anticoagulation, are older (> 65) and unlikely to require another valve in their lifetime, or have frequent falls
  - Tissue valves **last 10–15 years** – not as durable as mechanical valves
  - Because of rapid calcification in children and young patients, use of tissue valves is contraindicated in those populations.
- **Aortic stenosis** (AS) – most from degenerative calcification; most common valve lesion
  - **Cardinal symptoms**:
    - **Dyspnea** on exertion – mean survival 5 years
    - **Angina** – mean survival 4 years
    - **Syncope** (*worst of the cardinal symptoms*) – mean survival 3 years
  - Indications for operation – when **symptomatic** (usually have a peak gradient > 50 mm Hg and a valve area < 1.0 cm2)

- **Mitral regurgitation** (MR) – commonly caused by leaflet prolapse
  - Dyspnea, fatigue, pulmonary edema; can develop atrial fibrillation
  - Left ventricle becomes dilated.
  - **Ventricular function** – key index of disease progression in patients with MR
  - **Atrial fibrillation** is common; in end-stage disease, **pulmonary congestion** occurs.
  - Indications for operation – when **symptomatic** or if **severe mitral regurgitation**
- **Mitral stenosis** – rare now; most from rheumatic fever
  - **Pulmonary edema** and **dyspnea**; can get atrial fibrillation and hemoptysis as it progresses
  - Indications for operation – when **symptomatic** (usually have valve area $< 1 \text{ cm}^2$)
  - **Balloon commissurotomy** to open valve often used as 1st procedure (not as invasive)
  - **Constrictive pericarditis**
    - Dyspnea on exertion, hepatomegaly, ascites
    - Inflammation of the pericardium causes constriction of the heart.
    - Square root sign on right heart catheterization (equalization of right atrial, right ventricular diastolic, pulmonary artery diastolic, wedge, and left ventricular diastolic pressures)
    - Tx: pericardiectomy

ENDOCARDITIS

- Fever, chills, sweats
- **Aortic valve** – most common site of prosthetic valve infections
- **Mitral valve** – most common site of native valve infections
- *Staphylococcus aureus* responsible for 50% of cases
- Most commonly left sided except in **drug abusers** (*Staph aureus also* most common organism for drug abusers)
- Medical therapy first – successful in 75%; sterilizes valve in 50%
- Indications for surgery – **failure of antimicrobial therapy, severe valve failure, perivalvular abscesses, pericarditis**

OTHER CARDIAC CONDITIONS

- **Most common tumors of heart**
  - Most common benign tumor – **myxoma**; 75% in LA
  - Most common malignant tumor – **angiosarcoma**
  - Most common metastatic tumor to the heart – **lung CA**
- Coming off cardiopulmonary bypass and aortic root vent blood is dark and aortic perfusion cannula blood is red.
  - Tx: **Ventilate the lungs.**
- Coronary veins have the **lowest oxygen tension** of any tissue in the body due to high oxygen extraction by myocardium.
- **Mediastinal bleeding** – > 500 cc for 1st hour or > 250 cc/h for 4 hours → need to re-explore after cardiac procedure
- **Risk factors for mediastinitis** – obesity, use of bilateral internal mammary arteries, diabetes
  - Tx: sternal debridement, drain mediastinitis; eventually need pectoralis flaps; can also use omentum
- **Post-pericardiotomy syndrome** – pericardial friction rub, fever, chest pain, SOB
  - EKG – diffuse ST-segment elevation in multiple leads
  - Tx: **NSAIDs, steroids**

INTRODUCTION

- **Most common congenital hypercoagulable disorder** – resistance to activated protein C (Leiden factor)
- **Most common acquired hypercoagulable disorder** – smoking

ATHEROSCLEROSIS STAGES

- **1st – foam cells** → macrophages that have absorbed fat and lipids in the vessel wall
- **2nd – smooth muscle cell proliferation** → caused by growth factors released from macrophages; results in wall injury
- **3rd – intimal disruption** (from smooth muscle cell proliferation) → leads to exposure of collagen in vessel wall and eventual **thrombus formation** → fibrous plaques then form in these areas with underlying atheromas
- Risk factors: smoking, HTN, hypercholesterolemia, DM, hereditary factors

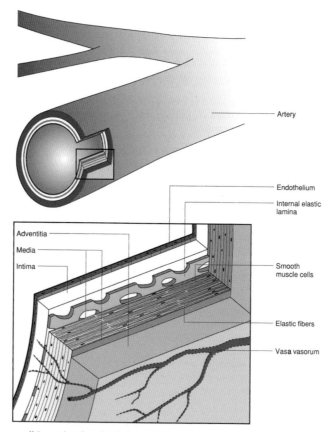

The artery wall is made of multiple layers (intima, media, and adventitia) that vary in composition depending on the artery.

CEREBROVASCULAR DISEASE

- Stroke 5th most common cause of death in the United States
- **HTN** – most important risk factor for stroke and cerebrovascular disease
- Carotid sheath contains carotid artery, internal jugular vein, and vagus nerve.
- Carotids supply 85% of blood flow to brain.
  - **Carotid bifurcation** – most common site of stenosis
- Normal internal carotid artery (ICA) has **continuous forward flow** (biphasic signal, fast antegrade, then slower diastolic antegrade signal).
  - 1st branch of internal carotid artery – **ophthalmic artery**
- Normal external carotid artery (ECA) has **triphasic flow** (antegrade, retrograde, then antegrade again).
  - 1st branch of external carotid artery – **superior thyroid artery**
- Communication between the ICA and ECA occurs through the **ophthalmic artery** (off ICA) and **internal maxillary artery** (off ECA).
- **Middle cerebral artery** – most commonly diseased intracranial artery
- **Cerebral ischemic events** (eg stroke, TIA) – most commonly from **arterial embolization** from the ICA (not thrombosis)
  - Can also occur from a **low-flow state** through a severely stenotic lesion
  - **Heart** is the 2nd most common source of cerebral emboli.
- **Anterior cerebral artery events** – mental status changes, release, slowing
- **Middle cerebral artery events** – contralateral motor and speech (if dominant side); contralateral facial droop
- **Posterior cerebral artery events** – vertigo, tinnitus, drop attacks, incoordination
- **Amaurosis fugax** – occlusion of the ophthalmic branch of the ICA (visual changes → shade coming down over eyes); visual changes are transient.
  - See **Hollenhorst plaques** on ophthalmologic exam.
- **Carotid traumatic injury with major fixed deficit**
  - If occluded, do not repair → can exacerbate injury with bleeding
  - If not occluded – repair with carotid stent or open procedure
- **Carotid endarterectomy** (CEA)
  - **Repair indications**: symptomatic > 50% stenosis, asymptomatic > 70% stenosis
    - Symptomatic < 50% Tx: Plavix, ASA, statin, optimize meds (not CEA)
    - Asymptomatic 50%–70% Tx: Plavix, ASA, statin, optimize meds
  - **Emergent CEA** may be of benefit with fluctuating neurologic symptoms or crescendo/evolving/increasing TIAs.
  - Timing of operation after **stroke**:
    - **Small** non-hemorrhagic stroke – 2 weeks
    - **Large** non-hemorrhagic stroke – 3 weeks
    - **Hemorrhagic stroke** – 6–8 weeks
  - Repair the **tightest side first** if the patient has bilateral stenosis.
  - Repair the **dominant side first** if the patient has equally tight carotid stenosis bilaterally.
  - Removing the **intima and part of the media** with CEA
  - Most important technical concern – getting a **good distal end point**
  - Use a **shunt** if the **back pressure is < 50 mm Hg** or if the **contralateral side is tight or occluded**.
  - **Occluded ICA** – do not repair (no benefit); **heparin** or Plavix to prevent clot propagation if acute
  - **Facial vein** – branch off internal jugular vein; overlies carotid bifurcation; can routinely divide safely
  - **Complications from repair**
    - **Vagus nerve injury** – *most common cranial nerve injury with CEA* → secondary to **vascular clamping** during endarterectomy; patients get *hoarseness* (recurrent laryngeal nerve comes off vagus)
    - **Hypoglossal nerve injury** – tongue deviates to the side of injury → *speech and mastication difficulty* (nerve is cephalad to carotid bifurcation)

- **Glossopharyngeal nerve injury** – rare; occurs with really high carotid dissection → causes *difficulty swallowing* (*dysphagia*; nerve is deep to posterior belly of digastric muscle)
- **Ansa cervicalis** – innervation to strap muscles; no serious deficits
- **Marginal mandibular branch of facial nerve** – affects corner of mouth (smile); from the retractor at the angle of the jaw
- **Acute event immediately after CEA** → back to OR to check for flap or thrombosis (use intraop U/S)
- **Pseudoaneurysm** – pulsatile, bleeding mass after CEA; Tx: drape and prep before intubation, intubate, then repair
- **20% have hypertension following CEA** – caused by injury to carotid body; Tx: **Nipride** to avoid bleeding
- **Myocardial infarction** – most common cause of non-stroke morbidity and mortality following CEA
- **15% restenosis** rate after CEA
- **Carotid stenting** – for high-risk patients (eg patients with previous CEA, multiple medical comorbidities [eg severe cardiac disease], previous neck XRT, previous neck dissection)
- **TCAR** (transcarotid artery revascularization) – carotid stenting procedure that has a lower stroke rate by using a distal carotid to femoral artery shunt that redirects blood flow (and debris) away from the head and into the femoral artery

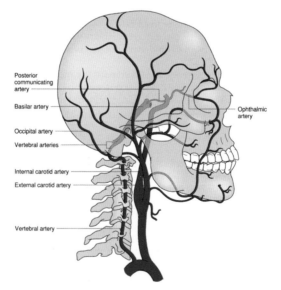

Posterior communicating artery

Basilar artery

Occipital artery

Vertebral arteries

Internal carotid artery

External carotid artery

Vertebral artery

Ophthalmic artery

The paired carotid and vertebral arteries supply blood to the brain. Extensive extracranial collaterals between the external carotid and vertebral systems allow for antegrade perfusion when a proximal occlusion develops in either vessel. Likewise, periorbital collaterals allow for retrograde flow through the ophthalmic artery to the internal carotid artery in the presence of a cervical internal carotid artery occlusion. Extensive side-to-side collaterals are found between the right and left external carotid arteries and right and left vertebral arteries.

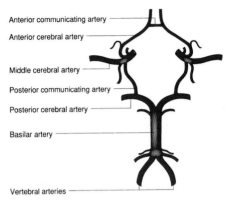

Anterior communicating artery

Anterior cerebral artery

Middle cerebral artery

Posterior communicating artery

Posterior cerebral artery

Basilar artery

Vertebral arteries

The circle of Willis is a highly efficient intracranial collateral network; however, multiple important variations occur, and an incomplete circle producing an isolated hemisphere is not uncommon.

- **Vertebrobasilar artery disease**
  - Anatomy: The two **vertebral arteries** arise from the **subclavian arteries** and combine to form a single **basilar artery**; the basilar then splits into two **posterior cerebral arteries**.
  - Usually need basilar artery or bilateral vertebral artery disease to have symptoms
  - Caused by atherosclerosis, spurs, bands; get vertebrobasilar insufficiency
  - Symptoms: diplopia, vertigo, tinnitus, drop attacks, incoordination
  - Tx: PTA with stent
- **Carotid body tumors** – present as a painless neck mass, usually near bifurcation, neural crest cells; are *extremely vascular* (consider preop embolization); can secrete **catecholamines**; Tx: all need resection

THORACIC AORTIC DISEASE

- Anatomy – aortic arch vessels include the **innominate artery** (which branches into the right subclavian and right common carotid arteries), the **left common carotid artery**, and the **left subclavian artery**
- **Ascending aortic aneurysms**
  - Often asymptomatic and picked up on routine CXR
  - Can get compression of vertebra (back pain), RLN (voice changes), bronchi (dyspnea or PNA), or esophagus (dysphagia)
  - Indications for repair: **acutely symptomatic**, $\geq$ **5.5 cm** (with Marfan's > 5.0 cm), or **rapid ↑ in size** (> 0.5 cm/yr)
- **Descending aortic aneurysms** (also thoracoabdominal aneurysms)
  - Indications for repair
    - If **endovascular** repair possible: > 5.5 cm
    - If **open** repair needed: > 6.5 cm
  - Risk of **paraplegia** is a major concern with repair.
    - Less with **endovascular repair** (< 5%) compared to open repair (20%)
    - **Prevention** – place **lumbar drain** to remove CSF fluid and **reduce spinal pressure**; **increase systemic BP** with Neo-Synephrine to **increase spinal perfusion**
    - **Spinal perfusion pressure** = MAP – spinal pressure (similar to ICP)
  - Reimplant **intercostal arteries below T8** to help prevent paraplegia with open repair.

- **Aortic dissections**
  - **Stanford classification** – based on presence or absence of involvement of ascending aorta
    - **Class A** – any ascending aortic involvement
    - **Class B** – descending aortic involvement only
  - **DeBakey classification** – based on the site of tear and extent of dissection
    - **Type I** – ascending and descending
    - **Type II** – ascending only
    - **Type III** – descending only
  - Most dissections start in the **ascending aorta.**
  - Can mimic myocardial infarction
  - Symptoms: tearing-like chest pain; can have unequal pulses (or BP) in upper extremities
  - 95% of patients have **severe HTN** at presentation.
  - Other risk factors: Marfan's syndrome, previous aneurysm, atherosclerosis
  - CXR – usually normal; may have wide mediastinum
  - Dx: chest CT with contrast
  - Dissection occurs in **medial layer** of blood vessel wall.
  - **Aortic insufficiency** occurs in 70%, caused by annular dilatation or when aortic valve cusp is sheared off.

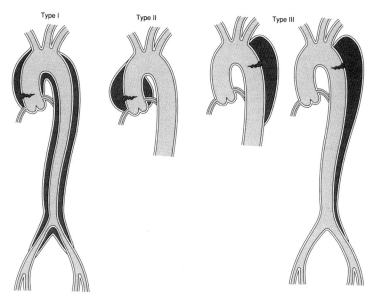

DeBakey classification of aortic dissection.

- Can also have occlusion of the coronary arteries and major aortic branches
- Death with ascending aortic dissections usually secondary to **cardiac failure** from aortic insufficiency, **cardiac tamponade**, or **rupture**
- Medical Tx initially → **control BP** with IV **beta-blockers** (eg esmolol) and **Nipride**
- Tx:
  - Operate on *all ascending* aortic dissections – Tx: need **open repair**; graft is placed to eliminate flow to the false lumen (median sternotomy).
  - Only operate on **descending** aortic dissections with **visceral** or **extremity ischemia** or if **contained rupture** – Tx: **endograft** or **open repair** (left thoracotomy); can

also just place **fenestrations** in the dissection flap to restore blood flow to viscera or extremity if ischemia is the problem
- Follow these patients with lifetime serial scans (MRI to decrease radiation exposure); 30% eventually get aneurysm formation requiring surgery.
- Postop complications for thoracic aortic surgery – **MI**, **renal failure**, **paraplegia** (descending thoracic aortic surgery)
- **Paraplegia** caused by spinal cord ischemia due to occlusion of intercostal arteries and artery of Adamkiewicz that occurs with descending thoracic aortic surgery

ABDOMINAL AORTIC DISEASE

- **Abdominal aortic aneurysms** (AAAs)
  - Normal aorta 2-3 cm
  - MCC – **atherosclerosis** (results in degeneration of the **medial layer**)
  - Risk factors: males, age, smoking, family history
  - Usually found incidentally
  - Can present with rupture, distal embolization, or compression of adjacent organs
  - **Rupture**
    - Leading cause of death without an operation
    - **50% mortality with rupture** if patient reaches hospital alive
    - Symptoms: back or abdominal pain; can have profound hypotension

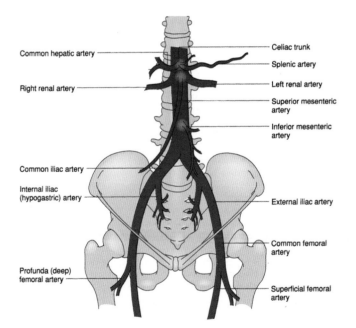

Common hepatic artery

Right renal artery

Common iliac artery

Internal iliac (hypogastric) artery

Profunda (deep) femoral artery

Celiac trunk

Splenic artery

Left renal artery

Superior mesenteric artery

Inferior mesenteric artery

External iliac artery

Common femoral artery

Superficial femoral artery

Anatomy of the abdominal aorta and iliac arteries.

- Dx: **CT angio**
- CT shows **fluid** in retroperitoneal space and **extraluminal contrast** with rupture.
- Most likely to rupture on **left posterolateral wall**, **2-4 cm below renals**
- More likely to rupture in presence of diastolic **HTN** or **COPD** (predictors of expansion)
- Allow **permissive hypotension** (SBP 80-100) until you get proximal control.

- **Emergency proximal control** – compress aorta against spine through **gastrohepatic ligament** (supraceliac aorta; underneath crus of diaphragm)
  - Divide gastrohepatic ligament (enters lesser sac) to place cross-clamp.
  - Can divide posterior crus of diaphragm if necessary to place clamp
- **Surveillance intervals** (duplex U/S):
  - 3.0–3.9 cm   **every 3 years**
  - 4.0–4.9 cm   **yearly**
  - > 5.0 cm   **every 6 months**
- **Repair** indications:
  - **≥ 5.5 cm** for average male patient
  - **≥ 5.0 cm** for **women** or those with **high rupture risk** (eg severe COPD, numerous relatives with rupture, poorly controlled HTN, eccentric shape)
  - **Growth > 1.0 cm/yr**
  - **Symptomatic**
  - **Infected** (mycotic)
  - **EVAR** *better* than open surgery for the **elderly**, for **high-risk** patients (ie multiple comorbidities), or those with **"hostile" abdomens**
  - For **high-risk patients**, delay in repair until **5.5 cm** is warranted (non-symptomatic patients), especially if EVAR is not an option.
- **Technical aspects:**
  - **Reimplant inferior mesenteric artery** (IMA) if: backpressure < 40 mm Hg (ie poor back-bleeding), previous colonic surgery (disrupts collaterals [eg Arc of Riolan, Marginal Artery of Drummond]), patient has SMA stenosis, or flow to left colon appears inadequate (colon looks dusky).
  - **Ligate bleeding lumbar arteries.**
  - Usually use a straight tube Dacron graft for repair of AAAs
  - If performing an aorto-bifemoral repair instead of a straight tube graft, you should ensure flow to at least **one internal iliac artery** (hypogastric; should see back-bleeding) to avoid **vasculogenic impotence** and **buttock claudication**.
    - Can **reimplant internal iliac artery** into distal limb of graft
  - **EVAR** – has less peri-op mortality, ICU stay, and hospital stay; requires more reviews and late interventions; no change in late survival
- **Complications**
  - **Major vein injury with proximal cross-clamp** – retro-aortic left renal vein
  - **Impotence** in ⅓ secondary to disruption of autonomic nerves and blood flow to the pelvis
  - 5% mortality with elective repair
  - **#1 cause of <u>acute</u> death after surgery** – MI
  - **#1 cause of <u>late</u> death after surgery** – renal failure
  - RFs for **mortality** - **creatinine > 1.8** (#1), CHF, EKG ischemia, pulmonary dysfunction, older age, females
  - **Graft infection rate** – 1% (*staph epidermidis* #1; *staph aureus, E. coli*)
  - **Pseudoaneurysm** after graft placement – 1%
  - **Atherosclerotic occlusion** – most common late complication after aortic graft placement
  - **Diarrhea** (especially **bloody**) after AAA repair worrisome for **ischemic colitis**:
    - **Inferior mesenteric artery** (IMA) often sacrificed with AAA repair and can cause ischemia (most commonly the **left colon**)
    - Other RF for ischemic colitis – preop or intraop **hypotension**
    - Dx: **lower endoscopy** (*best test*) or abdominal CT; middle and distal rectum are spared from ischemia (middle and inferior rectal arteries are branches off internal iliac artery)
    - Initial Tx: **fluid resuscitation** and **antibiotics**
    - If diffuse peritonitis, sepsis, mucosa is black on endoscopy, or part of the colon looks necrotic on CT scan → take to OR for **colectomy** and colostomy placement

- **Chylous ascites** – due to lymphatic disruption; resumption of oral intake leads to **abdominal distension** and **milky white fluid** on paracentesis
  - Tx: **low-fat**, **high-protein diet** (use short or medium chain fatty acids); can also keep patient **NPO** and use **TPN** _without_ lipids (or _avoid_ lipids with long chain fatty acids)

Ideal Criteria for Abdominal Aortic Aneurysm (AAA) Endovascular Repair

AAA Morphology	Criteria
Neck length	> 10 mm
Neck diameter	< 32 mm
Neck angulation	< 60 degrees
Common iliac artery length	> 10 mm
Common iliac artery diameter	7–18 mm
Other	Non-tortuous, noncalcified iliac arteries
	Lack of neck thrombus/calcification

Endoleak Type	Failure Site	Tx
Type I	Proximal or distal graft **attachment sites**	**Extension cuffs**
Type II	**Collaterals** (eg patent lumbar, IMA, intercostals, accessory renal)	**Observe** most; percutaneous coil embolization if pressurizing aneurysm
Type III	**Overlap sites** when using multiple grafts or fabric tear	**Secondary endograft** to cover overlap site or tear
Type IV	**Graft wall porosity** or suture holes	**Observe**; can place nonporous stent if that fails
Type V (endotension)	**Expansion of aneurysm without evidence of leak**	**Repeat EVAR** or **open repair**

- **Inflammatory aneurysms**
  - Occurs in 10% of patients with AAA; males
  - <u>Not</u> secondary to infection – just an inflammatory process
  - Can get adhesions to the 3rd and 4th portions of the **duodenum**
  - **Ureteral entrapment** in 25%
  - Weight loss, ↑ ESR, thickened rim above calcifications on CT scan
  - May need to place preoperative **ureteral stents** to help avoid injury
  - Inflammatory process resolves after aortic graft placement.
- **Mycotic aneurysms**
  - *Staphylococcus* #1, *Salmonella* #2
  - Bacteria infect atherosclerotic plaque, cause aneurysm.
  - Pain, fevers, positive blood cultures in 50%
  - Periaortic fluid, gas, retroperitoneal soft tissue edema, lymphadenopathy
  - Usually need extra-anatomic bypass (axillary-femoral with femoral-to-femoral crossover) and resection of infrarenal abdominal aorta to clear infection
- **Aortic graft infections**
  - *Staphylococcus #1* (staph epidermidis #1), *E. coli* #2
  - See fluid, gas, thickening around graft.
  - Blood cultures negative in many patients
  - Tx: Bypass through non-contaminated field (eg axillary to bifemoral bypass) and then resect the infected graft.
  - More common with grafts going to the **groin** (eg aorto-bifemoral grafts)
- **Aortoenteric fistula**
  - Usually occurs > 6 months after abdominal aortic surgery
  - **Herald bleed with hematemesis**, then blood per rectum, then exsanguination

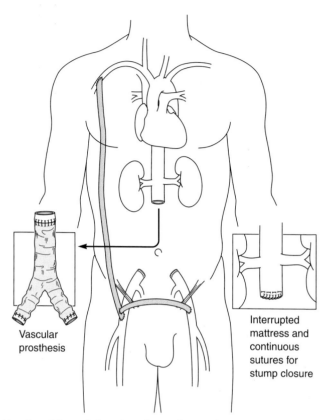

Vascular
prosthesis

Interrupted
mattress and
continuous
sutures for
stump closure

Standard treatment for an infected aortic vascular prosthesis. An axillobifemoral bypass is performed first. This is followed a few days later by removal of the infected aortic prosthesis and careful oversewing of the aortic stump as illustrated.

- Graft erodes into 3rd or 4th portion of **duodenum** near proximal suture line.
- Tx: Bypass through non-contaminated field (eg axillary-femoral bypass with femoral-to-femoral crossover), resect graft, and then close hole in the duodenum.

PERIPHERAL ARTERIAL DISEASE (PAD)

- **Leg compartments**
  - **Anterior** – deep peroneal nerve (dorsiflexion, sensation between 1st and 2nd toes), anterior tibial artery
  - **Lateral** – superficial peroneal nerve (eversion, lateral foot sensation)
  - **Deep posterior** – tibial nerve (plantar flexion), posterior tibial artery, peroneal artery
  - **Superficial posterior** – sural nerve
- **Signs/symptoms of PAD** – extremity pain, pallor with dependent rubor, hair loss, shiny atrophic skin, slow capillary refill, ulcers (usually start in toe tips)
  - Most commonly due to **atherosclerosis**
- **Statin drugs** (lovastatin) – #1 preventive agent for atherosclerosis
- **Homocystinuria** can ↑ risk of atherosclerosis; Tx: **folate** and B_{12}

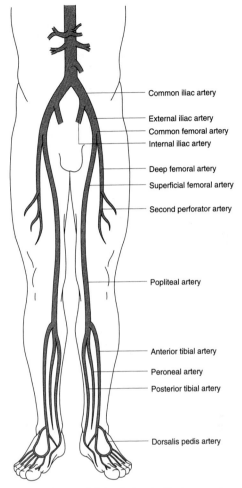

Anatomy of the arterial circulation to the lower extremity.

- **Claudication** (pain): medical therapy first → smoking cessation (#1), ASA, statin, exercise until pain occurs to improve collaterals
- **Symptoms** occur at **one level below** occlusion:
  - **Buttock** claudication – aortoiliac disease
  - **Mid-thigh** claudication – external iliac
  - **Calf** claudication – superficial femoral artery
  - **Foot** claudication – popliteal artery
- **Lumbar stenosis** can mimic claudication.
- **Diabetic neuropathy** can mimic rest pain.
- **Leriche syndrome**
  - No femoral pulses
  - Buttock or thigh claudication
  - Impotence (from ↓ flow in the internal iliacs)

- Lesion at aortic bifurcation or above
- Tx: aorto-bifemoral bypass graft
- **Most common atherosclerotic occlusion in lower extremities** – Hunter's canal (**distal superficial femoral artery** exits here); the **sartorius muscle** covers Hunter's canal
- **Collateral circulation** – forms from abnormal pressure gradients
  - Circumflex iliacs to subcostals
  - Circumflex femoral arteries to gluteal arteries
  - Geniculate arteries around the knee
- **Postnatal angiogenesis** – budding from preexisting vessels; angiogenin involved
- **Ankle–brachial index** (ABI)
  - Highest pedal pressure (DP or PT) divided by highest brachial pressure (left or right)
  - **< 0.9** – start to get **claudication** (typically occurs at same distance each time)
  - **< 0.5** – start to get **rest pain** (usually calf and foot)
  - **< 0.4** – **ulcers** (usually starts in toes)
  - **< 0.3** – **tissue loss** (gangrene)
  - **Noncompressible vessels** (due to **calcification**; often in diabetics) – can give **falsely elevated** ABIs; need to use **toe pressures** (less likely to be calcified) or go off **Doppler waveforms** in these patients
  - In patients with claudication, the ABI in the extremity drops with walking (ie resting ABI may be 0.9 but can drop to < 0.6 with exercise, resulting in pain).
  - Diabetics tend to have disease of **trifurcation vessels** and feet **microvasculature** (often *not* able to intervene with stent/bypass as there are no distal targets).
- **Pulse volume recordings** (PVRs; noninvasive flow study) – used to find significant occlusion and at what level
- **Arteriogram** is indicated if PVRs suggest significant disease – can also at times treat the patient with percutaneous intervention; gold standard for vascular imaging
  - Can use CO_2 **angiogram** if poor renal function
- **Surgical indications for PAD** – rest pain, ulceration or gangrene, severe lifestyle limitation despite medical therapy, atheromatous embolization
  - **PTFE** (Gore-Tex) – *only* for bypasses **above the knee** (have reduced patency below knee); need to use **saphenous vein** for below the knee bypasses
  - **Dacron** – good for aorta and large vessels
  - Best predictor of long-term patency – **vein quality**
  - **ASA** after lower extremity bypass is the best treatment for **patency** and **reducing cardiovascular events**.
  - **Duplex U/S** – best technique for graft surveillance
  - **Aortoiliac occlusive disease** – most get aorto-bifemoral repair
    - Need to ensure flow to at least **1 internal iliac artery** (hypogastric artery; want to see **good back-bleeding** from at least 1 of the arteries, otherwise need a bypass to an internal iliac artery) when performing aorto-bifemoral repair to prevent **vasculogenic impotence** and **pelvic ischemia**
  - **Isolated iliac lesions** – PTA with stent 1st choice; if that fails, consider femoral-to-femoral crossover
  - **Femoropopliteal grafts**
    - 75% 5-year patency
    - Improved patency rate with surgery for claudication as opposed to limb salvage
    - Popliteal artery exposure below knee – posterior muscle is **gastrocnemius** and anterior muscle is **popliteus**
  - **Femoral-distal grafts** (peroneal, anterior tibial, or posterior tibial artery)
    - 50% 5-year patency; patency not influenced by level of distal anastomosis
    - Distal lesions more limb threatening because of lack of collaterals
    - Bypasses to **distal vessels** are usually used only for **limb or tissue salvage** (eg nonhealing ulcer).
    - Bypassed vessel needs to have **run-off below the ankle** for this to be successful.

- Synthetic grafts have **decreased patency below the knee** → need to use saphenous vein
- **Extra-anatomic grafts** can be used to avoid hostile conditions in the abdomen (multiple previous operations in a frail patient).
- **Femoral-to-femoral crossover graft** – doubles blood flow to donor artery; can get vascular steal in donor leg
- Swelling following lower extremity bypass:
  - **Early** – **reperfusion injury** and **compartment syndrome** (Tx: fasciotomies)
  - **Late** – DVT (Dx: **U/S**, Tx: **heparin, Coumadin**)
- Complications of reperfusion of ischemic tissue – **compartment syndrome, lactic acidosis, hyperkalemia, myoglobinuria**
- **Technical problem** – #1 cause of early failure of reversed saphenous vein grafts
- **Vein atherosclerosis** – #1 cause of late failure of reversed saphenous vein grafts
- **Patients with heel ulceration to bone** → Tx: amputation
- **Dry gangrene** – noninfectious; can allow to autoamputate if small or just toes
  - Large lesions should be amputated.
  - See if patient has correctable vascular lesion.
- **Wet gangrene** – infectious; remove infected necrotic material; keep moist; non-weight bearing; antibiotics
  - Can be a surgical emergency if **extensive infection** (eg swollen red toe with pus coming out and red streaks up leg) or **systemic complications** occur (eg septic) – *may need **emergency amputation***
- **Diabetic foot ulcer**
  - Usually at the **metatarsal heads** (2nd MTP joint most common) or **heel**
  - Arises due to **neuropathy**; fails to heal due to diabetic **microvascular disease**
  - Can have **osteomyelitis**
  - Dx: **MRI** of foot
  - Tx: non-weight bearing, bone debridement if osteomyelitis (usually metatarsal head; also need to remove cartilage), antibiotics (6 weeks); assess need for revascularization (start with ABIs and PVRs).
- **Endovascular therapy** (generally a covered stent used)
  - Excellent for common iliac artery stenosis
  - Best for short stenoses that are not heavily calcified
  - *Not* used at **joint sites** (eg common femoral artery, popliteal artery) as they are prone to **kinking**
  - Intima usually ruptured and media stretched, pushes the plaque out
  - Requires passage of wire first
- **Compartment syndrome**
  - Is caused by **reperfusion injury** to the extremity (mediated by **PMNs**; occurs with cessation of blood flow to extremity and reperfusion > 4–6 hours later)
  - Consider **prophylactic fasciotomy** for ischemia > 4–6 hours to avoid.
  - Reperfusion injury leads to **swelling of the muscle compartments** → raising compartment pressures, which can lead to **ischemia** and **rhabdomyolysis**
  - Symptoms: **pain with passive motion**; extremity feels tight and swollen.
  - Most likely to occur in the **anterior compartment** of leg (get foot drop)
  - Dx: often based on clinical suspicion; compartment pressure > 20–30 mm Hg abnormal
  - Tx: **fasciotomies** (get all 4 compartments if in lower leg) → leave open 5–10 days
  - Risk of **superficial peroneal nerve** injury with **lateral incision** (affects foot eversion)
  - Untreated compartment syndrome can lead to rhabdomyolysis.
- **Rhabdomyolysis** (muscle necrosis)
  - Can lead to hyperkalemia, myoglobinemia, myoglobinuria, and renal failure
  - Tx: aggressive IVFs and alkalinization of urine; treatment of hyperkalemia

- **Lower extremity fasciotomy**
  - Medial incision: 2 cm posterior to the tibia; open **superficial posterior space** and then **soleus muscle** incised to enter the **deep posterior space**
  - Lateral incision: 2 cm anterior to the fibula opens **anterior/lateral compartments** (open both sides of the **intramuscular septum**)
- **Popliteal entrapment syndrome**
  - Most present with mild **intermittent claudication**; can be **bilateral**.
  - Men; *loss of pulses with plantar flexion*
  - Have medial deviation of artery around medial head of **gastrocnemius muscle**
  - Tx: **resection of medial head of gastrocnemius muscle**; may need arterial reconstruction
- **Adventitial cystic disease**
  - Men; **popliteal fossa** most common area
  - Ganglia originate from adjacent joint capsule or tendon sheath.
  - Symptoms: intermittent claudication; changes in symptoms with **knee flexion/extension**
  - Dx: angiogram
  - Tx: **resection of cyst**; vein graft if the vessel is occluded
- **Arterial autografts** – radial artery grafts for CABG, IMA for CABG

AMPUTATIONS

- For gangrene, large nonhealing ulcers, or unrelenting rest pain not amenable to surgery
- 50% mortality within 3 years for leg amputation
- **BKA** – 80% heal, 70% walk again, 5% mortality
- **AKA** – 90% heal, 30% walk again, 10% mortality
- Emergency amputation for **systemic complications** or **extensive infection**

ACUTE ARTERIAL EMBOLI

Clinical Distinctions Between Acute Arterial Embolism and Acute Arterial Thrombosis	
Embolism	**Thrombosis**
Arrhythmia	No arrhythmia
No prior claudication or rest pain	History of claudication or rest pain
Normal contralateral pulses	Contralateral pulses absent
No physical findings of chronic limb ischemia	Physical findings of chronic limb ischemia

- Usually do <u>not</u> have collaterals, signs of chronic limb ischemia, or history of claudication with emboli
- Contralateral leg usually has no chronic signs of ischemia and pulses are usually normal.
- Symptoms: sudden onset of pain, paresthesia, poikilothermia, paralysis
- Extremity ischemia evolution: pallor (white) → cyanosis (blue) → marbling
- **Most common cause** – *atrial fibrillation*, recent MI with left ventricular thrombus, myxoma, aortoiliac disease
- *Common femoral artery* at **bifurcation** of SFA and profunda is the most common site of peripheral obstruction from emboli.
- Tx: *embolectomy usual*; need to get pulses back; postop angiogram
  - Consider prophylactic fasciotomy if ischemia > 4–6 hours.
  - Aortoiliac emboli (loss of both femoral pulses) can be treated with bilateral femoral artery cutdowns and retrograde bilateral transfemoral embolectomies.

- **Atheroma embolism** – cholesterol clefts that can lodge in small arteries
  - **Renals** most common site of atheroma embolization
  - **Blue toe syndrome** – flaking atherosclerotic emboli off abdominal aorta or branches
    - Patients typically have good distal pulses.
    - **Aortoiliac disease** most common source
  - Dx: **chest/abdomen/pelvis CT scan** (look for aneurysmal source) and **ECHO** (clot or myxoma in heart)
  - Tx: may need aneurysm repair or arterial exclusion with bypass

ACUTE ARTERIAL THROMBOSIS

- These patients usually do <u>not</u> have arrhythmias.
- Do have a history of claudication and have signs of chronic limb ischemia and poor pulses in the contralateral leg
- Tx: **threatened limb** (loss of sensation or motor function) → give heparin and go to OR for ***thrombectomy***; if **limb is not threatened** → angiography for ***thrombolytics***
- **Thrombosis of PTFE graft** → thrombolytics and anticoagulation; if limb threatened → OR for thrombectomy

RENAL VASCULAR DISEASE

- Right renal artery runs posterior to IVC.
- Accessory renal arteries in 25%
- **Renovascular HTN** (renal artery stenosis) – bruits, diastolic blood pressure > 115, HTN, in children or premenopausal women, HTN resistant to drug therapy
  - **Renal atherosclerosis** – left side, proximal ⅓, men
  - **Fibromuscular dysplasia** – right side, distal ⅓, women
  - Dx: CT angiogram
  - Tx: **PTA** <u>without</u> stent if due to FMD (percutaneous transluminal angioplasty); place **stent** if due to atherosclerotic disease.
- **Indications for nephrectomy with renal HTN** → atrophic kidney < 6 cm with persistently high renin levels

UPPER EXTREMITY

- **Upper extremity embolic disease** – most likely to occur in **brachial artery** at **bifurcation** of radial and ulnar arteries
- **Occlusive disease** – proximal lesions usually asymptomatic secondary to ↑ collaterals
  - **Subclavian artery** most common site of upper extremity stenosis
  - Tx: **covered stent**; common carotid to subclavian artery bypass if that fails
- **Subclavian steal syndrome** – proximal subclavian artery stenosis resulting in reversal of flow through ipsilateral vertebral artery into the subclavian artery
  - Dx – duplex U/S shows reversal of flow in the vertebral artery
  - Operate for limb (claudication) or neurologic symptoms (usually vertebrobasilar – visual or equilibrium problems); symptoms can worsen with exertion.
  - Tx: **covered stent** to **subclavian artery**; common carotid to subclavian artery bypass if that fails
- **Thoracic outlet syndrome** (TOS)
  - **Normal anatomy**
    - **Subclavian vein** – passes over the 1st rib <u>anterior</u> to the anterior scalene muscle, then behind clavicle
    - **Brachial plexus** and **subclavian artery** – pass over the 1st rib <u>posterior</u> to the anterior scalene muscle and anterior to the middle scalene muscle
      - Brachial plexus is <u>posterior</u> to the subclavian artery.
    - **Phrenic nerve** – runs on top of **anterior scalene muscle**

- General symptoms: back, neck, arm, and/or hand pain/weakness/tingling/numbness (often worse with palpation/manipulation)
- Dx: cervical spine and chest MRI (check for cervical ribs)
- **Neurologic involvement** – much more common than vascular
- **#1 anatomic abnormality** – cervical rib
- **#1 cause of pain** – brachial plexus irritation (90%)
- **Brachial plexus irritation**
  - Usually have normal neurologic exam; tapping can reproduce symptoms (Tinsel's test).
  - **Ulnar nerve** distribution (C8–T1) most common (inferior portion of brachial plexus) → weakness of intrinsic muscles of hand, weak wrist flexion
  - Medical Tx first line – **physical therapy**
  - If physical therapy fails – get **nerve conduction study** or perform **anterior scalene muscle block** (symptoms should improve) to confirm diagnosis
  - Surgical Tx: cervical rib and 1st rib resection, divide anterior scalene muscle, neurolysis (free up brachial plexus)
- **Subclavian vein**
  - Usually presents as **effort-induced thrombosis** of subclavian vein (Paget–von Schrötter disease; baseball pitchers) – **acutely painful**, **swollen**, **blue limb**
  - Venous thrombosis – much more common than arterial
  - Dx: **Venography** is the gold standard for diagnosis, but **duplex U/S** makes the diagnosis and is quicker to get.
  - 80% have associated thoracic outlet problem.
  - Tx: **catheter directed thrombolytics** initially; **repair at that admission** (cervical rib and 1st rib resection, divide anterior scalene muscle).

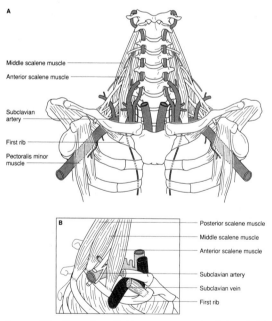

The normal anatomy of the thoracic outlet in anteroposterior **(A)** and oblique **(B)** views. The brachial plexus and subclavian artery traverse the narrow triangle formed by the anterior and middle scalene muscles and the first rib. The subclavian vein lies anteriorly.

- **Subclavian artery**
  - Compression usually secondary to **anterior scalene hypertrophy** (weight lifters); least common cause of TOS; can cause an **aneurysm** with **embolic risk**
  - Symptoms – hand pain from ischemia; **thrombosis** – cold, white hand
  - Absent radial pulse with head turned to ipsilateral side (Adson's test)
  - Dx: duplex U/S or angiogram (gold standard)
  - Tx: **surgery** → cervical rib and 1st rib resection, divide anterior scalene muscle; interposition bypass graft usual (artery usually aneurysmal or too damaged for primary repair)
- **Motor function can remain in digits** after prolonged **hand ischemia** because motor groups are in the proximal forearm.

MESENTERIC ISCHEMIA

- Overall mortality 60%; usually involves the **superior mesenteric artery** (SMA)
- Findings on **abdominal CTA** (*best test*) that suggest intestinal ischemia – vascular occlusion, bowel wall thickening, intramural gas, portal venous gas
- Most common causes of visceral ischemia:
  - **Embolic occlusion** – 50% (most common type; most commonly from heart)
  - **Thrombotic occlusion** – 25% (MC from atherosclerotic disease)
  - **Nonocclusive mesenteric ischemia (NOMI)** – 15% (MC from low cardiac output state)
  - **Venous thrombosis** – 5% (MC from hypercoagulable state)
- **SMA embolism**
  - Most commonly occurs **2–10 cm distal** to origin of SMA – <u>heart</u> #1 source (atrial fibrillation)
  - Pain out of proportion to exam; pain usually of sudden onset; hematochezia and peritoneal signs are late findings (followed by sepsis and acidosis).
  - May have a history of atrial fibrillation, endocarditis, recent MI, recent angiography
  - **Heparin** given initially to prevent **clot propagation**
  - Embolus is often distal to the **first jejunal branch** – can get **proximal jejunal sparing** (unlike SMA thrombosis which usually occurs at SMA origin)
  - Tx: OR for **open embolectomy**, resect infarcted bowel if present
  - **SMA exposure** – divide ligament of Treitz, SMA is to the right of this near the base of the transverse colon mesentery
  - **Planned 2nd look laparotomy** – best to <u>*not*</u> resect questionable (marginally perfused) bowel, leave abdomen open, and reexplore in 24 hours to reinspect and decide on resection
- **SMA thrombosis**
  - Often history of chronic problems (abdominal pain, food fear, and weight loss over months to years)
  - Symptoms: similar to embolism; may have developed **collaterals**
  - Usually occurs at **SMA ostium** (flush with SMA take-off from aorta)
  - **Heparin** given initially to prevent **clot propagation**
  - Tx: **thrombectomy** (open thrombectomy or catheter directed thrombolytics); may need **covered stent** or **open bypass** after the vessel is opened for any residual stenosis; resection of infarcted bowel
- **Mesenteric vein thrombosis**
  - Usually short segments of intestine involved
  - Usually **subacute** – multiple days of bloody diarrhea and crampy abdominal pain
  - May have a history of vasculitis, hypercoagulable state, or portal HTN
  - Dx: abdominal CTA with venous phase – small bowel wall thickening, mesenteric edema, clot in SMV
  - Tx: **heparin only** usual; *rarely* need resection of infarcted bowel

- **Nonocclusive mesenteric ischemia (NOMI)**
  - Patients are usually in a **critically ill state** (eg multiple inotropes/pressors, CHF, sepsis).
  - Spasm, low-flow states, hypovolemia, hemoconcentration, pressors → final common pathway is **low cardiac output** to visceral vessels
  - Risk factors: prolonged shock, CHF, prolonged cardiopulmonary bypass
  - Symptoms: bloody diarrhea, pain
  - **Watershed areas** (Griffith's – splenic flexure and Sudeck's – upper rectum) most vulnerable
  - Tx: **volume** resuscitation and **improve cardiac output**; resection of infarcted bowel if present
- **Median arcuate ligament syndrome**
  - Causes **celiac artery** compression
  - **Bruit near epigastrium**, chronic pain, weight loss, diarrhea
  - Tx: transect **median arcuate ligament**; may need arterial reconstruction
- **Chronic mesenteric angina**
  - Weight loss secondary to **food fear** (visceral angina 30 minutes after meals)
  - Dx: **CTA** to see origins of **celiac** and **SMA** (can also use mesenteric duplex)
  - Tx: **PTA and stent**; bypass if that fails
- **Arc of Riolan** is an important collateral between the SMA and IMA.

VISCERAL AND PERIPHERAL ANEURYSMS

- **Rupture** – most common complication of aneurysms above inguinal ligament (external iliac and above)
- **Emboli** (MC) and **thrombosis** – most common complications of aneurysms below inguinal ligament (common femoral artery and below)
- **Visceral artery aneurysms**
  - Risk factors: medial fibrodysplasia, portal HTN, arterial disruption secondary to inflammatory disease (eg pancreatitis)
  - **Repair all splanchnic artery aneurysms** (> 2 cm) when diagnosed (50% risk for rupture) *except* **splenic** (see indications below)
    - **Splenic artery aneurysm** – most common visceral aneurysm (more common in women; 2% risk of rupture)
      - Repair splenic artery aneurysms if **symptomatic**, if patient is **pregnant**, if occurs in **women of childbearing age**, or is > **3 cm**.
      - High rate of pregnancy-related rupture – usually in **3rd trimester** (up to 70%)
  - Tx: **covered stent** (*best*) and/or **coil embolization**
  - Splenic artery aneurysms can just be **ligated** if open procedure is required (spleen has good collaterals); if near hilum (very distal) may require splenectomy if coil embolization fails
  - Surgery for **rupture** (patient unstable) – **splenectomy** (ligate splenic artery proximal to aneurysm)
- **Renal** (> 1.5 cm) artery aneurysm – Tx: **covered stent**
- **Iliac** (> 3.5 cm) artery aneurysms – Tx: **covered stent**
  - Often associated with **abdominal aortic aneurysms**
- **Femoral** (> 3.5 cm) artery aneurysms – Tx: **resection with interposition bypass graft** (*avoid* using covered stents across joint lines – tendency to kink off)
- **Popliteal artery aneurysm**
  - Most common peripheral aneurysm
  - MCC – atherosclerosis
  - Rarely rupture
  - Leg exam reveals prominent popliteal pulses.
  - ½ are **bilateral**.
  - ½ have **another aneurysm elsewhere** (AAA, femoral, etc – get abdominal/pelvic CT scan).

- Most likely to get **emboli (MC)** or **thrombosis** with **limb ischemia**
- Can also get leg pain from compression of adjacent structures
- Dx: ultrasound
- Surgical indications: **symptomatic, > 2 cm,** or **mycotic**
- Tx: **exclusion** and **vein bypass graft** (*avoid* PTFE below knee) of all popliteal aneurysms; 25% have complication that requires amputation if not treated; *covered stent not recommended for these unless not a candidate for open surgery*
- **Pseudoaneurysm**
  - Collection of blood in continuity with the arterial system but <u>not</u> enclosed by all 3 layers of the arterial wall; most common location is the **femoral artery.**
  - Can result from percutaneous interventions or from disruption of a suture line between graft and artery
  - If it occurs after **percutaneous intervention** → Tx: ultrasound-guided **compression with thrombin injection** (surgical repair if flow remains in the pseudoaneurysm after thrombin injection)
  - If it occurs at a **suture line** early after surgery → ***need surgical repair***
  - Pseudoaneurysms that occur at suture lines late after surgery (months to years) → ***suggests graft infection***

OTHER VASCULAR DISEASES

- **Fibromuscular dysplasia**
  - Young women; **HTN** if renals involved, **headaches** or **stroke** if carotids involved
  - **Renal artery** (renal artery stenosis) most commonly involved vessel, followed by carotid and iliac
  - String of beads appearance (stenotic regions followed by dilated areas)
  - **Medial fibrodysplasia** most common variant (85%)
  - Tx: **balloon angioplasty** (*best*); bypass if that fails.
- **Buerger's disease**
  - Young men, smokers
  - Severe rest pain with bilateral ulceration; gangrene of digits, especially fingers
  - **Corkscrew collaterals** on angiogram and severe distal disease; normal arterial tree proximal to popliteal and brachial vessels (is a <u>small vessel</u> disease)
  - Tx: **Stop smoking** or will require continued amputations.
- **Marfan's disease**
  - **Fibrillin defect** (connective tissue elastic fibers) causes cystic medial necrosis.
  - Marfanoid habitus, retinal detachment, aortic root dilatation, mitral valve prolapse
- **Temporal arteritis** (large artery immune arteritis)
  - Women, age > 55, headache, fever, blurred vision (risk of **blindness**), fatigue
  - Temporal artery biopsy → **giant cell** arteritis, **granulomas**
  - Inflammation of large vessels (aorta and branches)
  - Long segments of **smooth stenosis** alternating with segments of larger diameter
  - Tx: **steroids,** bypass of large vessels if needed; <u>no</u> endarterectomy
- **Radiation arteritis**
  - **Early** – sloughing and thrombosis (obliterative endarteritis)
  - **Late** (1–10 years) – fibrosis, scar, stenosis
  - **Late late** (3–30 years) – advanced atherosclerosis
- **Raynaud's disease** – young women; ***pallor* → *cyanosis* → *rubor***
  - Tx: **calcium channel blockers,** warmth

DIALYSIS ACCESS

- **Temporary dialysis catheters** (eg Quinton, Vascath)
  - Nontunneled, noncuffed, temporary central line used for dialysis or infusion
  - **IJ** and **subclavian** sites – can remain for **3 weeks** (infection risk)
  - **Femoral** site – can remain for **5 days**

- **Permanent dialysis catheters** (eg permacath)
  - Tunneled, cuffed central line; can stay in for **1 year**; **lower infection rate** compared to temporary catheters although not as good as fistula or graft
  - **Right IJ** site usually best – less dialysis flow issues; more direct access to right atrium
  - *Avoid* using side with preexisting or expected A-V fistula/graft (can cause central venous stenosis and fistula/graft failure).
- **Dialysis fistulas/grafts**
  - Try to always start with **a nondominant arm distal fistula** (eg Cimino) for dialysis access (try and conserve sites; go more proximal or in legs only when you have to).
    - Increases life expectancy; decreases need for central line access
    - Some patients with **limited life-expectancy** may be better off with **permacath**.
  - **Cimino fistula** – radial artery to cephalic vein
    - Wait 6 weeks to use → allows vein to mature
    - Rule of "6's" – at **6 weeks** need fistula of **6 mm diameter**, **6 cm length** (to allow 2 needle access), **depth < 6 mm**, and flow rate **> 600 cc/min**
  - **Interposition graft** (eg brachiocephalic loop graft) – wait 6 weeks to allow fibrous scar to form
  - Most common failure of A-V fistula/grafts for dialysis – **venous obstruction** secondary to *intimal hyperplasia*
  - **Failure of fistula to form** – can be arterial inflow or venous outflow problem
    - Dx: **angiogram with shunt run-off** (*best*) although usually start with **U/S** to look for inflow/outflow/anastomosis problems
    - May need better **arterial inflow** (subclavian stenosis usual problem – place covered stent) or better **venous outflow** (venous hyperplasia usual problem – see below)
    - Can have **anastomotic issues** that may need revision/angioplasty
    - Competing **venous side branches** can be a problem (Tx: ligate or coil).
  - **Venous obstruction** – can present with high venous return pressures, increased recirculation, or bleeding problems after dialysis
    - Dx: **fistulogram with shunt run-off** (best); U/S may show obstruction/poor flow.
    - Tx: **balloon angioplasty** of stenotic site
  - **Bleeding** from graft/fistula (hold pressure first)
    - **Pinpoint bleeding** from **needle access site** can be controlled with a stitch; U/S and fistulogram within next 24 hours
    - Bleeding at a **graft ulcer** site suggests **erosion into graft** – is a surgical emergency usually requiring **graft excision** (partial graft excision with jump-graft placement may be an option)
    - Bleeding at a **fistula ulcer** site suggests **vein damage** – is a surgical emergency usually requiring **vein repair**

VENOUS DISEASE

- **Greater saphenous vein** – joins femoral vein near groin; runs medially
- <u>No</u> clamps on IVC → will tear
- **Left renal vein** can be ligated near the IVC in emergencies because of collaterals (left gonadal vein, left adrenal vein); right renal vein does <u>not</u> have these collaterals.
- **Acquired A-V fistula** – usually secondary to trauma; can get peripheral arterial insufficiency, CHF, aneurysm, limb-length discrepancy
  - Dx: **U/S**
  - Most need repair → **lateral venous suture**; arterial side may need patch or bypass graft; try to place interposing tissue so it does not recur
- **Varicose veins**
  - Smoking, obesity, low activity
  - Tx: **sclerotherapy**

- **Venous ulcers**
  - Secondary to venous valve incompetence (90%)
  - Ulceration occurs above and posterior to medial malleoli.
  - Ulcers < 3 cm often heal without surgery.
  - **Brawny edema** – hemosiderin deposition
  - Tx: **Unna boot** (zinc oxide and calamine) compression wraps cure 90%.
  - May need to ligate perforators or have vein stripping of greater saphenous vein (see below)
  - DVT is a contraindication to vein stripping.
- **Venous insufficiency**
  - Aching, swelling, night cramps, brawny edema, venous ulcers
  - **Edema** – secondary to incompetent perforators and/or valves
  - Elevation brings relief.
  - Dx: **U/S**
  - Tx: leg wraps, ambulation with avoidance of long standing, D/C smoking, weight loss
    - Greater saphenous **vein stripping** (for saphenofemoral valve incompetence) or **removal of perforators** (if just perforator valves are incompetent; stab avulsion technique) for severe symptoms or recurrent ulceration despite medical Tx
- **Superficial thrombophlebitis** – nonbacterial inflammation
  - Tx: NSAIDs, warm packs, ambulation, arm elevation, +/− antibiotics
- **Suppurative thrombophlebitis** – pus fills vein; fever, ↑ WBCs, erythema, fluctuance; usually associated with infection following a peripheral IV; *staph aureus* most common
  - Tx: Resect entire vein for continued purulence or sepsis despite antibiotics.
- **Migrating thrombophlebitis** – pancreatic CA
- **Normal venous Doppler ultrasound** – augmentation of flow with distal compression or release of proximal compression
- **Sequential compression devices** (SCDs) – help prevent blood clots by ↓ venous stasis and ↑ tPA release
- **Deep venous thrombosis** (DVT)
  - Most common in **calf** (some say ilio-femoral although combining sites)
  - Pain, tenderness, calf swelling
  - **Left leg 2×** more involved than right (longer left iliac vein compressed by right iliac artery)
  - Risk factors: **Virchow's triad** → venous stasis, hypercoagulability, venous wall injury
  - **Calf** DVT – minimal swelling
  - **Femoral** DVT – ankle and calf swelling
  - **Iliofemoral** DVT – leg swelling
  - DVT Tx: **heparin, Coumadin**
  - **Phlegmasia alba dolens** (painful, swollen **white** leg) – less severe than below
  - **Phlegmasia cerulea dolens** (painful, swollen **blue** leg extending up to buttocks) – more severe; can lead to **gangrene**; usually occurs with acute **iliofemoral** DVT
    - Tx: **catheter-directed thrombolytics**
    - Emergent **thrombectomy** if extremity **threatened** (ie loss of sensation or motor function)
    - 50% of these patients have a **malignancy** somewhere.
- **Venous thrombosis with central line** – pull out central line if not needed, then heparin; can try to treat with systemic heparin or TPA down line if the access site is important
- **Contraindications to vein stripping** – DVT, venous outflow obstruction, pregnancy

LYMPHATICS

- Do **not** contain a basement membrane
- **Not** found in bone, muscle, tendon, cartilage, brain, or cornea
- Deep lymphatics have valves.
- **Lymphedema**
  - Occurs when lymphatics are obstructed, too few in number, or nonfunctional
  - Is usually **secondary lymphedema** (MCC – previous ALND for breast CA)
  - Leads to woody edema secondary to fibrosis in subcutaneous tissue – toes, feet, ankle, leg
  - **Cellulitis** and **lymphangitis** secondary to minor trauma are big problems.
  - **Strep** most common infection
  - Congenital lymphedema L > R
  - Tx: leg elevation, compression, antibiotics for infection
- **Lymphangiosarcoma**
  - Raised blue/red coloring; early metastases to lung
  - **Stewart–Treves syndrome** – lymphangiosarcoma associated with breast axillary dissection and chronic lymphedema
- **Lymphocele** following surgery
  - Usually after dissection in the groin (eg after femoral to popliteal bypass)
  - Leakage of **clear fluid**
  - Tx: percutaneous drainage (can try a couple of times); resection if that fails
  - Can inject **isosulfan blue dye** into foot to identify the lymphatic channels supplying the lymphocele if having trouble locating

28 Gastrointestinal Hormones

- **Gastrin** – produced by G cells in stomach **antrum**
  - Secretion stimulated by amino acids, vagal input (acetylcholine), calcium, ETOH, antral distention, pH > 3.0
  - Secretion inhibited by pH < 3.0, somatostatin, secretin, CCK
  - Target cells – **parietal cells** and **chief cells**
  - Response – ↑ HCl, intrinsic factor, and pepsinogen secretion (gastrin is the strongest stimulator for all)
  - **Omeprazole** blocks H/K ATPase of parietal cell (**final pathway for H^+ release**).
- **Somatostatin** – mainly produced by D (somatostatin) cells in stomach **antrum**
  - Secretion stimulated by acid in duodenum
  - Target cells – many; is the great inhibitor
  - Response – inhibits gastrin and HCl release (primary role); inhibits release of insulin, glucagon, secretin, CCK, and motilin; ↓ pancreatic and biliary output; slows gastric emptying
  - **Octreotide** (somatostatin analogue) – can be used to ↓ pancreatic fistula output
- **CCK** – produced by I cells of **duodenum**
  - Secretion stimulated by amino acids and fatty acid chains
  - Response – gallbladder contraction, relaxation of sphincter of Oddi, ↑ **pancreatic enzyme secretion** (acinar cells)
- **Secretin** – produced by S cells of **duodenum**
  - Secretion stimulated by fat, bile, pH < 4.0
  - Secretion inhibited by pH > 4.0, gastrin
  - Response – ↑ **pancreatic HCO_3^- release** (ductal cells), inhibits gastrin release (this is reversed in patients with gastrinoma), and inhibits HCl release
    - High pancreatic duct output – ↑ HCO_3^-, ↓ Cl^-
    - Slow pancreatic duct output – ↑ Cl^-, ↓ HCO_3^- (carbonic anhydrase in duct exchanges HCO_3^- for Cl^-)
- **Vasoactive intestinal peptide** – produced by cells in **pancreas and gut**
  - Secretion stimulated by fat, acetylcholine
  - Response – ↑ **intestinal secretion** (water and electrolytes) and **motility**
- **Glucagon** – mainly released by alpha cells of **pancreas** (starvation state)
  - Secretion stimulated by ↓ glucose, ↑ amino acids, acetylcholine
  - Secretion inhibited by ↑ glucose, ↑ insulin, somatostatin
  - Response – glycogenolysis, gluconeogenesis, ↓ gastric acid secretion, ↓ gastrointestinal motility, relaxes sphincter of Oddi, ↓ pancreatic secretion
- **Insulin** – released by beta cells of the **pancreas** (fed state)
  - Secretion stimulated by glucose, glucagons, CCK
  - Secretion inhibited by somatostatin
  - Response – cellular glucose uptake; promotes protein synthesis
- **Pancreatic polypeptide** – secreted by islet cells in **pancreas**
  - Secretion stimulated by food, vagal stimulation, other GI hormones
  - Response – ↓ **pancreatic** and **gallbladder secretion**
- Motilin – released by intestinal cells of gut
  - Primarily released from the **duodenum**
  - Primary target is the **stomach antrum**.
  - Secretion stimulated by duodenal acid, food, vagus input
  - Secretion inhibited by gastrointestinal motility, relaxes sphincter of Oddi somatostatin, secretin, pancreatic polypeptide, duodenal fat
  - Response – ↑ **intestinal motility** (small bowel; phase III peristalsis) → **erythromycin** acts on this receptor

- **Bombesin** (gastrin-releasing peptide) – ↑ intestinal motor activity, ↑ pancreatic enzyme secretion, ↑ gastric acid secretion
- **Peptide YY** – released from terminal ileum following a fatty meal → inhibits acid secretion and stomach contraction; inhibits gallbladder contraction and pancreatic secretion
- **Anorexia** – mediated by hypothalamus
- **Causes of B_{12} deficiency** – **gastric bypass** (needs acidic environment to bind intrinsic factor), **terminal ileum resection** (is absorbed there)
- **Bowel recovery**
  - Small bowel 24 hours
  - Stomach 48 hours
  - Large bowel 3–5 days
- **Peristalsis phases**
  - I – resting
  - II – accelerating
  - III – peristalsis
  - IV – decelerating

29 Esophagus

ANATOMY AND PHYSIOLOGY

- Mucosa (squamous epithelium), submucosa, and muscularis propria (longitudinal muscle layer); **_no serosa_**
- Upper ⅓ esophagus – **striated muscle**
- Middle ⅓ and lower ⅓ esophagus – **smooth muscle**
- **Thoracic esophagus** – vessels directly off the **aorta** are the major blood supply

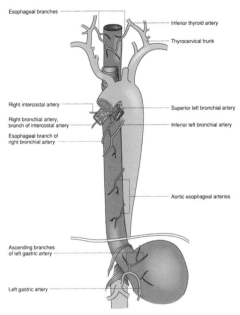

Arterial blood supply of the esophagus.

- **Cervical esophagus** – supplied by **inferior thyroid artery**
- **Abdominal esophagus** – supplied by **left gastric** and inferior phrenic arteries
- **Venous drainage** – hemi-azygous and azygous veins in chest
- **Lymphatics** – upper ⅔ drains cephalad, lower ⅓ caudad
- **Right vagus nerve** – travels on posterior portion of stomach as it exits chest; becomes **celiac plexus**; also has the criminal nerve of Grassi → can cause persistently high acid levels postoperatively if left undivided after vagotomy
- **Left vagus nerve** – travels on anterior portion of stomach; goes to **liver** and **biliary tree**
- **Thoracic duct** – travels from right to left at **T4–5** as it ascends mediastinum; inserts into left subclavian vein
- **Upper esophageal sphincter** (UES; 15 cm from incisors) – is the **cricopharyngeus muscle** (circular muscle, prevents air swallowing); recurrent laryngeal nerve innervation
  - Normal UES pressure at rest: 60 mm Hg
  - Normal UES pressure with food bolus: 15 mm Hg

- **Cricopharyngeus muscle** – most common site of esophageal perforation (usually occurs with EGD); also most common site for esophageal foreign body
- **Aspiration with brainstem stroke** – failure of cricopharyngeus to relax
- **Lower esophageal sphincter** (<u>40</u> cm from incisors) – relaxation mediated by inhibitory neurons; normally contracted at resting state (prevents reflux); is an anatomic zone of high pressure, <u>not</u> an anatomic sphincter (not visible on EGD)
  - Normal LES pressure at rest: 15 mm Hg
  - Normal LES pressure with food bolus: 0 mm Hg
- **Anatomic areas of esophageal narrowing** (prone to iatrogenic injury)
  - Cricopharyngeus muscle
  - Compression by the left mainstem bronchus and aortic arch
  - Diaphragm (near lower esophageal sphincter)
- **Swallowing stages** – CNS initiates swallow
  - **Primary peristalsis** – occurs with food bolus and swallow initiation
  - **Secondary peristalsis** – occurs with incomplete emptying and esophageal distention; propagating waves
  - **Tertiary peristalsis** – non-propagating, non-peristalsing (dysfunctional)
  - UES and LES are normally contracted between meals.
- Swallowing mechanism – soft palate occludes nasopharynx, larynx rises and airway opening is blocked by epiglottis, cricopharyngeus relaxes, pharyngeal contraction moves food into esophagus; **LES relaxes** soon after initiation of swallow (**vagus** mediated)

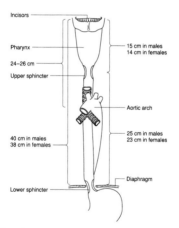

Important clinical endoscopic measurements of the esophagus in adults.

- **Surgical approach**
  - Cervical esophagus – **left** neck incision
  - Upper ⅔ thoracic – **right** thoracotomy (avoids the aorta)
  - Lower ⅓ thoracic – **left** thoracotomy (left-sided course in this region)
- **Hiccoughs**
  - Causes – gastric distention, temperature changes, ETOH, tobacco
  - Reflex arc – vagus, phrenic, sympathetic chain T6–12
- **Esophageal dysfunction**
  - **Primary** – achalasia, diffuse esophageal spasm, nutcracker esophagus
  - **Secondary** – GERD (most common), scleroderma
- **Endoscopy** – best initial test for **heartburn** (can visualize esophagitis)
- **Barium swallow** – best initial test for **dysphagia** or **odynophagia** (better at picking up masses)

- **Meat impaction** – Dx and Tx: endoscopy
- **Foreign body** – Dx and Tx: endoscopy
- **Perforation** – Dx: Gastrografin swallow

PHARYNGOESOPHAGEAL DISORDERS

- Trouble in transferring food from mouth to esophagus
- Most commonly neuromuscular disease – myasthenia gravis, muscular dystrophy, stroke
- **Liquids** worse than solids.
- **Plummer–Vinson syndrome** – can have upper esophageal web; Fe-deficient anemia. Tx: **dilation**, Fe; need to screen for **oral CA**

DIVERTICULA

- **Zenker's diverticulum** – caused by increased pressure during swallowing
  - Is a **false diverticulum** (cervical pulsion diverticulum) located **posteriorly**
  - Occurs between superior **pharyngeal constrictors** and inferior **cricopharyngeus** (Killian's triangle)
- Caused by **failure of the cricopharyngeus to relax**
- Symptoms: upper esophageal dysphagia, choking, halitosis; regurgitation of non-digested food
- Dx: **barium swallow studies**, manometry; risk for perforation with EGD and Zenker's
- Tx: *cricopharyngeal myotomy* (key point); Zenker's itself can either be resected or suspended (removal of diverticula is *not* necessary); left cervical incision; leave drains in; esophagogram POD #1
- **Endoscopic division of cricopharyngeus muscle** also an option for diverticulum **> 3 cm** (creates common channel between esophagus and diverticulum; diverticulum needs to be 3 cm to fit stapler)

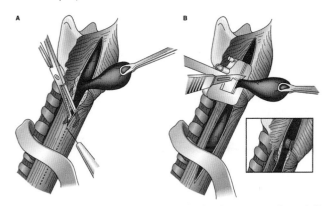

Cricopharyngomyotomy and concomitant resection of a pharyngoesophageal diverticulum. **(A)** A cricopharyngomyotomy is performed. **(B)** After completion of the cricopharyngomyotomy, the base of the pouch is crossed with a TA-30 stapler and amputated.

- **Traction diverticulum**
  - Is a **true diverticulum** (involves all 3 esophageal layers)
  - Due to inflammation, granulomatous disease, tumor
  - Usually found in the **lateral mid-esophagus**
  - Symptoms: regurgitation of undigested food, dysphagia
  - If asymptomatic, leave alone.
  - Tx: VATS excision and primary closure (with contralateral myotomy) if symptomatic; may need palliative therapy (ie XRT) if due to invasive CA

- **Epiphrenic diverticulum**
  - Rare pulsion diverticulum (false diverticulum)
  - Associated with **esophageal motility disorders** (eg <u>achalasia</u>)
  - Most common in the **distal 10 cm** of the esophagus
  - Most are asymptomatic; can have dysphagia and regurgitation
  - Dx: esophagogram and esophageal manometry
  - Tx if symptomatic: **diverticulectomy**, **Heller myotomy** (on the side opposite the diverticulectomy), and **partial Nissen**

ACHALASIA

- **Dysphagia** (worse for liquids), **regurgitation**, **weight loss**, respiratory symptoms
- Caused by **lack of peristalsis** and **failure of LES to relax** after food bolus
- Secondary to destruction of **inhibitory neuronal ganglion cells** in muscle wall (autoimmune [#1], infectious, genetic)
- Manometry – high/normal basal LES pressure, **incomplete LES relaxation**, and **_poor_ or _no_ peristalsis**
- Can get tortuous dilated esophagus and epiphrenic diverticula; bird's beak appearance
- Need EGD to rule out esophageal CA (**pseudoachalasia**)
- Tx: **laparoscopic Heller myotomy** for good surgical candidates (considered definitive therapy with better long-term results compared to balloon dilatation)
  - **Myotomy** of <u>lower</u> esophagus only (6 cm up esophagus, 2 cm onto stomach)
  - Also need **partial Nissen** fundoplication
- **Balloon dilatation of LES** → effective in 80% <u>however</u> high incidence of repeat procedures and complications
- Can get **esophageal CA** late (squamous cell most common)
- *Trypanosoma cruzi* can produce similar symptoms (Chagas' disease).

ISOLATED HYPERTENSIVE LES

- Have **high basal LES pressure**, normal LES relaxation, and normal peristalsis
- Often have associated **GERD**
- Tx: calcium channel blocker, nitrates; heterogenous group (some may benefit from Heller)

DIFFUSE ESOPHAGEAL SPASM

- **Dysphagia**; may have psychiatric history
- Manometry – frequent **high amplitude, non-peristaltic, unorganized contractions**, normal basal LES pressure, normal LES relaxation
- **> 20%** of wet swallows with simultaneous contractions **> 30 mm Hg**
- Tx: calcium channel blocker, nitrates, trazodone; **Heller myotomy** if those fail (myotomy of <u>upper</u> and <u>lower</u> esophagus; right thoracotomy)
- Surgery usually less effective for diffuse esophageal spasm than for achalasia

NUTCRACKER ESOPHAGUS

- **Chest pain** (can be severe) +/− dysphagia
- Manometry – **high-amplitude peristaltic contractions** (**> 180 mm Hg**); normal basal LES pressure, normal LES relaxation
- Tx: calcium channel blocker, nitrates, trazodone; **Heller myotomy** if those fail (myotomy of <u>upper</u> and <u>lower</u> esophagus; right thoracotomy)
- Surgery usually less effective for nutcracker than for achalasia

SCLERODERMA

- Heartburn, massive reflux, dysphagia
- Esophagus is the most common organ involved in scleroderma.
- **Fibrous replacement** of esophageal **smooth muscle**

- Causes **dysphagia** and loss of LES tone with **massive reflux** and **strictures**
- Manometry – low LES pressure and aperistalsis
- Tx: **PPI** and **Reglan**; esophagectomy usual if severe

GASTROESOPHAGEAL REFLUX DISEASE (GERD)

- **Normal anatomic protection from GERD** – need LES competence (most common defect in GERD), normal esophageal body, normal gastric reservoir
- GERD caused by ↑ acid exposure to esophagus from loss of gastroesophageal barrier
- Sx: **heartburn** (burning retrosternal chest pain) 30–60 minutes after meals; worse lying down, with tight clothing, or bending over
- Can also have asthma symptoms (cough), choking, aspiration
- Make sure patient does not have another cause for pain (check for unusual symptoms):
  - **Dysphagia/odynophagia/weight loss/anemia** – need to worry about esophageal tumors (Dx: upper endoscopy)
  - **Bloating** – suggests aerophagia and delayed gastric emptying (Dx: gastric emptying study)
  - **Epigastric pain** – suggests peptic ulcer, gastric tumor (Dx: upper endoscopy)
- Most treated empirically with **PPI** (omeprazole, 99% effective)
  - Weight loss, avoid instigating foods, elevate head of bed
- If **long-standing**, consider upper endoscopy to check for **Barrett's esophagus**.
- Failure of PPI despite escalating doses (give it 3–4 weeks) → need diagnostic studies (usually start with EGD)
- Dx: 24-hour **pH probe** (*best test*), **endoscopy**, **histology**, **manometry** (need to rule out motility disorder; resting LES < 6 mm Hg suggests GERD)
  - pH probe most sensitive indicator (impedance probe): > **4.5%** of total time with **pH < 4**
- **Surgical indications**: failure of medical Tx, avoidance of lifetime meds, young patients, refractory complications (eg bleeding, esophagitis, stricture, ulcer), respiratory symptoms (eg cough, asthma, aspiration, hoarseness, congestion)
- Tx: **Nissen fundoplication** → divide **short gastrics**, mobilize and pull **esophagus** into abdomen (restores normal GE junction; need ≥ **2 cm** of esophagus in abdomen), **approximate crura** (permanent suture), 270- (partial) or 360-degree **gastric fundus** wrap (creates antireflux valve; completely mobilize fundus, **2 cm** floppy wrap over large bougie)
  - Phrenoesophageal membrane is an extension of the **transversalis fascia**.
  - Key maneuver for **dissection** is finding the **right crura**.
  - Key maneuver for **wrap** is identification of the **left crura**.
  - Complications – injury to spleen, diaphragm, esophagus, or capnothorax (CO_2 PTX)
  - **Belsey** – approach is through the chest
  - **Collis gastroplasty** – when not enough esophagus exists to pull down into abdomen, can staple along stomach cardia and create a "new" esophagus (neo-esophagus)
  - Most common cause of dysphagia following Nissen – *wrap is too tight* (generally resolves on its own; give clears for 1st week; can dilate after 1 week)
- Postop Tx:
  - Scheduled **antiemetics** (eg Zofran; avoid postop retching/vomiting)
  - **Liquids** first day or 2, then **Nissen soft diet** for 4–6 weeks (eat 6 small meals/day)
  - *Avoid* (4–6 weeks) – bread, raw fruits/vegetables, meat, carbonated beverages, spicy foods
  - **Preferred diet** – pureed foods, soups
- **Dysphagia**
  - Common after Nissen
  - Stay with **clears** until edema improves and wrap loosens up (give it 1 week)
  - If not able to **handle saliva** (patient keeps spitting) – back to OR to **loosen wrap**
  - **Persistent or late dysphagia** – get **esophagogram** to look for slipped Nissen or recurrent hiatal hernia; if no mechanical problem can bougie dilate (wait 1 week after surgery)

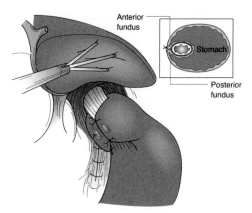

Fixation of the fundoplication. The fundoplication is sutured in place with a single U-stitch of 2-0 Prolene pledgeted on the outside. A 60-French mercury-weighted bougie is passed through the gastroesophageal junction prior to fixation of the wrap to assure a floppy fundoplication. Inset illustrates the proper orientation of the fundic wrap.

HIATAL HERNIA

- **Type I** – **sliding hernia** from dilation of hiatus (most common type); often associated with GERD; GE junction rises above the diaphragm
- **Type II** – **paraesophageal**; hole in the diaphragm alongside the esophagus; normal GE junction
- **Type III** – **combined** sliding and paraesophageal
- **Type IV** – **sliding** with entire stomach in the chest plus **another organ** (ie colon, spleen)
- *For type I* – repair is not indicated unless the patient has GERD
- *For type II* – still need **Nissen** as diaphragm repair can affect LES; also helps anchor stomach
- *For types II–IV* – all need repair; mobilize and **excise hernia sac** to help prevent recurrence (+/− mesh to repair diaphragm if large hernia)

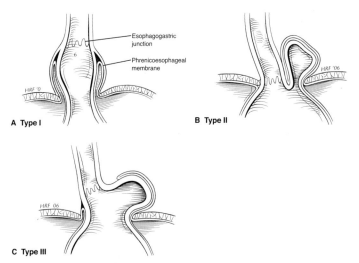

Classification of hiatal hernia. **(A)** Type I, sliding. **(B)** Type II, pure paraesophageal. **(C)** Type III, mixed hernia.

PARAESOPHAGEAL HERNIA (TYPES II AND III)

- Chest pain, retching without vomiting, can't pass NG tube, dysphagia, early satiety
- All usually need repair even if asymptomatic → at risk for gastric **incarceration**
- **Type IV** hiatal hernias are also at risk for organ incarceration and need repair.
- May want to avoid repair in the elderly and frail if minimal symptoms

SCHATZKI'S RING

- Almost all patients have an associated **sliding hiatal hernia** (ring caused by **GERD**).
- Symptoms: **dysphagia**
- Narrowed ring of **mucosa/submucosa** found at **squamocolumnar junction** (just <u>above</u> EGJ)
- Dx: barium esophagogram (*best*)
- Tx: **dilatation of the ring** and **PPI** usually sufficient; *do <u>not</u> resect.*

BARRETT'S ESOPHAGUS

- **Squamous** changes to **columnar** epithelium (**metaplasia**; raised, pink lesion)
- Occurs with long-standing exposure to **gastric reflux** (is acquired)
- **Intestinal type** columnar metaplasia is the only type predisposed to esophageal CA.
  - Pathology shows **goblet cells**.
  - CA risk is increased 50 times compared to general population (adenocarcinoma; relative risk [RR] 50)
- **Barrett's** surveillance:
  - EGD **annually** for **2 years** (4 quadrant Bx's at 1-cm intervals for entire length of involved segment and Bx of any suspicious areas)
  - If EGD **negative** for dysplasia for **2 years**, get EGD with biopsies **every 3 years**.
- **Low-grade dysplasia** (LGD)
  - Needs to be confirmed by **2 experienced pathologists**
  - **Repeat EGD** with Bx's in 3–6 months.
  - If repeat biopsy again shows **LGD** – Tx: **endoscopic resection** <u>or</u> **continued annual surveillance**
- **High-grade dysplasia** (HGD) – considered carcinoma in situ
  - Needs to be confirmed by **2 experienced pathologists**
  - Tx: **endoscopic mucosal resection** (need mucosa and submucosa)
  - Cell types other than Barrett's (eg squamous cell carcinoma in situ) – follow above as well
- **Uncomplicated Barrett's** (ie no dysplasia) can be treated like GERD (ie PPI or Nissen) – Tx will decrease esophagitis and further metaplasia
  - Need EGD surveillance for lifetime, even after Nissen
  - *Barrett's CA risk is <u>not</u> reversed with PPI or fundoplication.*

ESOPHAGEAL CANCER

- Esophageal tumors are almost always **malignant**; early invasion of nodes
- Spreads quickly along **submucosal lymphatic channels** (often advanced at Dx)
- Symptoms: **dysphagia** (especially solids), **weight loss**
- Risk factors **squamous cell CA: ETOH, tobacco**, achalasia, caustic injury, nitrosamine, men
- Risk factors **adenocarcinoma: GERD, obesity**, Barrett's, men
- Workup (staging):
  - **EGD** with biopsy, **CT chest/abdomen** (*best single test for resectability*), **bronchoscopy** if above carina to look for airway invasion; **PET-CT**
  - **Suspicious nodes** – EUS with FNA
- **Unresectability** – hoarseness (RLN invasion), Horner's syndrome (brachial plexus invasion), phrenic nerve invasion, malignant pleural effusion, malignant fistula, invasion of another structure (T4b; eg airway, vertebra, lung, aorta)

- Invasion of **pleura, pericardium,** or **diaphragm** (T4a) – still **resectable**
- **Adenocarcinoma** is the #1 esophageal cancer – not squamous
  - **Adenocarcinoma** – usually in **lower** ⅓ of esophagus; **liver** metastases most common
  - **Squamous cell carcinoma** – usually in **upper** ⅔ of esophagus; **lung** metastases MC
- **Cervical esophageal CA** (for tumors up to **5 cm** below cricopharyngeus muscle) – all get definitive chemo-XRT (_not surgery_); consider surgery only for non-complete responders
- **Esophagogastric junction (EGJ) CA** – treated like thoracic **esophageal CA** (for tumors up to **5 cm** below EGJ)
- Most important prognostic factor in patient devoid of systemic metastases – **nodal spread**
- **Thoracic esophageal CA**
  - **Nodal disease outside area of resection** (ie supraclavicular or celiac nodes – considered M1 disease) – contraindication to esophagectomy
  - **High-grade dysplasia, carcinoma in situ,** and select **T1a tumors** (invades lamina propria or muscularis <u>mucosa</u> only, < 2 cm, well moderately differentiated, and no nodal metastases). Tx: **endoscopic resection**
  - **T1b** (invades submucosa) or greater – **esophagectomy** if resectable
  - **Neoadjuvant chemo-XRT** (**cisplatin** and **5FU** _or_ **carboplatin** and **Taxol**)
    - **Improves survival** for resectable tumors
    - Can **downstage tumors** and make them **resectable**
    - Indicated for ≥ **T2** (invades muscularis <u>propria</u> or more) or **positive periesophageal nodes**
    - **Adjuvant chemo** also **improves survival.**
  - **Esophagectomy** – 5% mortality from surgery; curative in 20%
    - No difference in long-term survival between approaches
    - Need **6–8 cm margins**
    - **Right gastroepiploic artery** – primary blood supply to stomach after replacing esophagus (have to divide left gastric and short gastrics)
    - **Transhiatal approach** – abdominal and neck incisions; bluntly dissect intrathoracic esophagus
      - May have **lower morbidity** from esophageal leaks with cervical anastomosis
      - May miss some lymph nodes; may be difficult for large tumors
    - **Ivor Lewis** – abdominal incision and right thoracotomy → exposes all of the intrathoracic esophagus; intrathoracic anastomosis
    - **3-Hole esophagectomy** – abdominal, thoracic, and cervical incisions
    - Need **pyloromyotomy** with these procedures
    - **Colonic interposition** – may be choice in young patients when you want to preserve gastric function; 3 anastomoses required; blood supply depends on colon marginal vessels; also good if patient had previous gastric resection
    - After esophagectomy → need contrast study on postop day 7 to rule out leak
    - **Postoperative strictures** – most can be dilated
    - Need for **preop enteral nutrition** (eg severe dysphagia or malnutrition and undergoing neoadjuvant Tx) – place **laparoscopic J tube** (_avoid_ PEG tube in stomach conduit)
    - **Chylothorax** – white to clear fluid; high in **lymphocytes** and **TAGs**
      - Tx: drainage, NPO, TPN, short- or medium-chain fatty acids (_avoid_ long-chain); conservative Tx for 1–3 weeks
      - **Thoracic duct ligation** (right side, low in the mediastinum) if drainage is > **2 L/day** or is **refractory to medical Tx**
- **Adjuvant chemo-XRT** – indicated for ≥ **T2** or **positive nodes**
- **Unresectable tumors** – get definitive chemo-XRT
- **Malignant fistulas** – most die within 3 months due to aspiration; Tx – esophageal stent for palliation

FANCONI ANEMIA

- Mutation in FA genes (**DNA repair genes**)
- Pancytopenia, fatigue
- At risk for **leukemia**, **aplastic anemia** and **squamous cell CA** of oral cavity and esophagus

TYLOSIS

- Mutation in RHBDF2 suppressor gene (autosomal dominant)
- **Hyperkeratosis** of the palms and soles of feet
- 70% lifetime risk of **squamous cell esophageal CA**
- **Upper endoscopy screening** starting at **age 20**

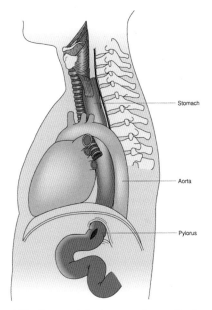

Final position of the mobilized stomach in the posterior mediastinum after transhiatal esophagectomy and cervical esophagogastric anastomosis. The gastric fundus has been suspended from the cervical prevertebral fascia, and an end-to-side cervical esophago-gastrostomy has been performed. The pylorus is now located several centimeters below the level of the diaphragmatic hiatus.

LEIOMYOMA

- Most common benign esophageal tumor; located in **muscularis propria**
- Symptoms: **dysphagia**; usually in **lower ⅔** of esophagus (<u>smooth muscle cells</u>)
- Dx: **esophagogram** (tumor has smooth contour, is well circumscribed), EUS, CT scan (need to rule out CA)
- **Do _not_ biopsy** → can form **mucosal scar** and make subsequent **enucleation** difficult
- Tx: **> 5 cm** or **symptomatic** → excision (extra-mucosal enucleation; leave mucosa intact) via thoracotomy/VATS
- **Leiomyosarcoma Tx**: esophagectomy

ESOPHAGEAL POLYPS

- Symptoms: dysphagia, hematemesis
- 2nd most common benign tumor of the esophagus; usually in the cervical esophagus
- Small lesions can be resected with endoscopy; larger lesions require cervical incision.

CAUSTIC ESOPHAGEAL INJURY

- **No NG tube. Do not induce vomiting. Nothing to drink**
- **Alkali** – causes deep liquefaction necrosis, especially liquid (eg Drano)
  - Worse injury than acid; also more likely to cause cancer
- **Acid** – causes coagulation necrosis; mostly causes gastric injury
- **Chest** and **abdominal CT scan** to look for free air and signs of perforation
- **Endoscopy** to assess lesion (best test)
  - Do not use with suspected perforation and do not go past a site of severe injury.
- Serial exams and plain films required
- **Degree of injury**:
  - **Primary burn** – hyperemia
    - Tx: observation and conservative therapy
    - **Conservative Tx**: IVFs, spitting, antibiotics, oral intake after 3–4 days; may need future serial dilation for strictures (usually cervical)
    - Can also get shortening of esophagus with GERD (Tx: PPI)
  - **Secondary burn** – ulcerations, exudates, and sloughing
    - Tx: prolonged observation and conservative therapy as above; TPN
    - **Indications for esophagectomy** – sepsis, peritonitis, mediastinitis, free air, mediastinal or stomach wall air, crepitance, contrast extravasation, pneumothorax, large effusion
  - **Tertiary burn** – deep ulcers, charring, and lumen narrowing
    - Tx: as above; **esophagectomy** usually necessary
    - Alimentary tract not restored until after patient recovers from the caustic injury
- **Caustic esophageal perforations** require esophagectomy (are not repaired due to extensive damage).

PERFORATIONS

- Usually **iatrogenic** (caused by **EGD** procedures)
- Most common site – left posterior lateral **intrathoracic esophagus** 2–4 cm above **EGJ**
- Most common iatrogenic site – **cervical esophagus** near **cricopharyngeus muscle**
- Symptoms: pain, dysphagia, tachycardia, subcutaneous air in lower neck
- Dx: CXR initially (look for extraluminal air, pleural effusion)
  - **Gastrografin swallow** (*best test*) followed by barium swallow; *no EGD*
  - *Avoid* Gastrografin if patient is **aspiration risk** and use dilute barium.
- **Initial Tx**: IVFs, NPO, broad-spectrum antibiotics (including yeast)
- **Criteria for nonsurgical management** – contained perforation by contrast, self-draining, no systemic effects
- **Noncontained perforations**:
  - If quick to diagnose it (< **24 hours**) and area has **minimal contamination** → **primary repair** with drains
    - Need **longitudinal myotomy** to see the full extent of injury
    - Repair in **2 layers** (**mucosa/submucosa** – absorbable suture; **muscularis propria** – permanent suture)
    - Buttress repair with **intercostal muscle flaps**
    - Place drains.

- If late to diagnose it (**> 48 hours**) or area has **extensive contamination** →
  - **Neck** – just place **drains** (_no esophagectomy_) → will eventually heal
  - **Chest** – need 1) **resection** (esophagectomy, cervical esophagostomy) _or_
    2) **exclusion and diversion** (cervical esophagostomy, staple across distal
    esophagus, washout mediastinum, place chest tubes – late esophagectomy at
    time of gastric replacement)
  - Gastric replacement of esophagus late when patient fully recovers
- **Perforation after dilatation for achalasia** – need **contralateral myotomy** if
  undergoing primary repair
- **Esophagectomy** – may be needed for any perforation (contained or noncontained)
  in patients with **severe intrinsic disease** (eg burned out esophagus from achalasia,
  esophageal CA)
- **Boerhaave's syndrome**
  - **Forceful vomiting** followed by **chest pain**; often history of **ETOH**
  - Perforation most likely at left lateral wall of esophagus, 2–4 cm above GE junction
  - **Hartmann's sign** – mediastinal crunching on auscultation
  - Fever, leukocytosis, and sepsis occur as **mediastinitis** develops.
  - *Highest mortality of all perforations* – early diagnosis and treatment improve survival
  - Dx: Gastrografin swallow (*best test*)
  - Tx: fluid resuscitation, surgery as above for esophageal perforations

30 Stomach

ANATOMY AND PHYSIOLOGY

- Stomach transit time 3–4 hours
- **Peristalsis** – occurs only in distal stomach (**antrum**)
- Gastroduodenal pain sensed through afferent sympathetic fibers T5–10
- **Blood supply**
  - **Celiac trunk** – left gastric, common hepatic artery, splenic artery
    - Left gastroepiploic and short gastric are branches of splenic artery.
  - **Greater curvature** – right and left gastroepiploics, short gastrics
    - Right gastroepiploic is a branch of gastroduodenal artery.
  - **Lesser curvature** – right and left gastrics
    - **Right gastric** is a branch off the proper hepatic artery *after* the GDA takeoff.
  - **Pylorus** – gastroduodenal artery
- Mucosa – lined with **simple columnar** epithelium

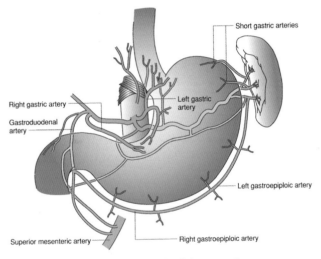

Arterial blood supply of the stomach.

- **Cardia glands** – mucus secreting
- **Fundus and body glands**
  - **Chief cells** – pepsinogen (1st enzyme in proteolysis)
  - **Parietal cells** – release H^+ and **intrinsic factor**
  - **Acetylcholine** (vagus nerve), **gastrin** (from G cells in antrum), and **histamine** (from mast cells) cause H^+ release.
  - **Acetylcholine** and **gastrin** activate *phospholipase* ($PIP \rightarrow DAG + IP_3$ to $\uparrow Ca$); Ca-calmodulin activates **phosphorylase kinase** $\rightarrow \uparrow H^+$ release
  - **Histamine** activates *adenylate cyclase* $\rightarrow cAMP \rightarrow$ activates **protein kinase A** $\rightarrow \uparrow$ H^+ release
  - **Phosphorylase kinase** and **protein kinase A** phosphorylate H^+/K^+ **ATPase** to $\uparrow H^+$ secretion and K^+ absorption

- **Omeprazole** blocks H^+/K^+ ATPase in parietal cell membrane (**final pathway for H^+ release**).
- **Inhibitors of parietal cells** – somatostatin, prostaglandins (PGE_1), secretin, CCK
- **Intrinsic factor** – binds B_{12} and the complex is reabsorbed in the terminal ileum
- **Antrum and pylorus glands**
  - **Mucus** and **HCO_3^-** secreting glands – protect stomach
  - **G cells** release **gastrin** – reason why antrectomy is helpful for ulcer disease
    - *Inhibited* by **H^+ in duodenum**
    - *Stimulated* by **amino acids, acetylcholine**
  - **D cells** – secrete **somatostatin**; inhibit gastrin and acid release
- **Brunner's glands** – in <u>duodenum</u>; secrete **alkaline mucus**
- **Somatostatin, CCK,** and **secretin** – released with antral and duodenal acidification
- **Rapid gastric emptying** – previous surgery (#1), ulcers
- **Delayed gastric emptying** – diabetes, opiates, anticholinergics, hypothyroidism
- **Trichobezoars** (hair) – hard to pull out
  - Tx: EGD generally inadequate; likely need gastrostomy and removal
- **Phytobezoars** (fiber) – often in diabetics with poor gastric emptying
  - Tx: enzymes, EGD, diet changes
- **Dieulafoy's ulcer** – vascular malformation; can bleed
- **Ménétrier's disease** – mucous cell hyperplasia, ↑ rugal folds

GASTRIC VOLVULUS

- Associated with types II–IV hiatal hernias; high morbidity/mortality
- Nausea without vomiting; severe pain
- Usually **organoaxial volvulus** (along axis between EGJ and pylorus)
- Tx: emergent reduction, repair hernia, Nissen (helps anchor stomach) may need partial gastrectomy if devitalized

MALLORY–WEISS TEAR

- Secondary to forceful vomiting
- Presents as hematemesis following severe retching
- Bleeding often stops spontaneously.
- Dx/Tx: **EGD** with **hemoclips**; tear is usually on lesser curvature (near GE junction).
- If continued bleeding, may need gastrostomy and oversewing of the vessel

VAGOTOMIES

- **Vagotomy** – both truncal and proximal forms ↓ **liquid emptying** → **vagally mediated receptive relaxation is removed** (results in ↑ gastric pressure that accelerates liquid emptying)
- **Truncal vagotomy** – divides vagal trunks at level of esophagus; ↑ **emptying of solids**
- **Proximal vagotomy** (highly selective) – divides individual fibers, preserves "crow's foot"; **normal emptying of solids**
- Addition of **pyloroplasty** to truncal vagotomy results in ↑ **solid emptying**.
- Other alterations caused by **truncal vagotomy**:
  - **Gastric effects** – ↓ acid output by 90%, ↑ gastrin, gastrin cell hyperplasia
  - **Nongastric effects** – ↓ exocrine pancreas function, ↓ postprandial bile flow, ↑ gallbladder volumes, ↓ release of vagally mediated hormones
  - **Diarrhea** (40%) – most common problem following vagotomy
    - Caused by **sustained MMCs** (migrating motor complex) forcing bile acids into the colon
    - Tx: **cholestyramine** and **loperamide**

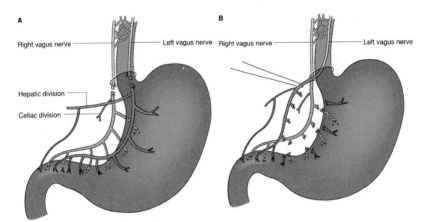

Truncal vagotomy and proximal gastric vagotomy. **(A)** With truncal vagotomy, both nerve trunks are divided at the level of the diaphragmatic hiatus. **(B)** Proximal gastric vagotomy involves division of the vagal fibers that supply the gastric fundus. Branches to the antropyloric region of the stomach are not transected, and the hepatic and celiac divisions of the vagus nerves remain intact.

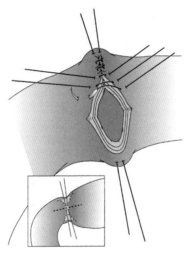

Pyloroplasty formation. A Heineke–Mikulicz pyloroplasty involves a longitudinal incision of the pyloric sphincter followed by a transverse closure.

UPPER GASTROINTESTINAL BLEEDING (UGI BLEEDING)

- Symptoms – hematemesis; can also present with anemia, melena, or red blood per rectum
- Bleeding can be anywhere from the nose to the ligament of Treitz.
- More common than lower GI bleeding
- **Risk factors**: previous UGI bleed, peptic ulcer disease, NSAID use, smoking, liver disease, esophageal varices, splenic vein thrombosis, sepsis, burn injuries, trauma, severe vomiting
- Initial Tx: 2 large-bore IVs T and C for 6 pRBCs (transfuse as necessary), ICU care

- Dx/Tx: **EGD** (confirm bleeding is from ulcer); can potentially treat with hemoclips, Epi injection, cautery
  - EGD 90% effective in controlling initial bleed
  - Biggest risk factor for **rebleeding** at the time of initial EGD – #1 ***spurting blood vessel*** (60% chance of rebleed), #2 visible blood vessel (40% chance), #3 diffuse oozing (30% chance), #4 adherent clot (20% chance), #5 clean base (< 5%)
  - **Rebleed Tx**: need **repeat EGD** (*usually best option*)
    - If ulcer, **angioembolization** an option if EGD fails again and patient is stable
  - **Surgical indications** (non-variceal bleeding) – **failed repeat** EGD, **unstable** patient after 1st EGD, or **rebleed** with **ulcer > 2 cm** after 1st EGD
  - **Highest risk factor for mortality** with non-variceal UGI bleed – ***continued or rebleeding***
  - Place **NG tube** after procedure to monitor **bleeding**.
  - Slow bleeding and having trouble localizing source → **tagged RBC scan**
  - Patient with **liver failure** is likely bleeding from **esophageal varices**, <u>not</u> an ulcer → Tx: EGD with **variceal bands** or **sclerotherapy**; **TIPS** if that fails

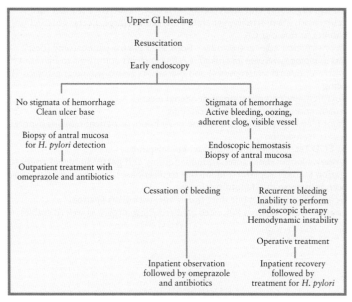

Treatment of bleeding ulceration.

DUODENAL ULCERS

- From ↑ **acid production** and ↓ **defense**: **H. pylori** present in **95%** (#1 risk factor)
- **Most common peptic ulcer**; more common in men
- Usually in 1st part of the duodenum; **usually anterior**
  - **Anterior** ulcers <u>perforate</u>.
  - **Posterior** ulcers <u>bleed</u> from <u>gastroduodenal artery</u>.
- Symptoms: epigastric pain radiating to the back; abates with eating but recurs 30 minutes after
- Dx: **endoscopy**
- Dx of *H. pylori* – **histologic exam of antral biopsies**
- Tx: **proton pump inhibitor** (PPI; omeprazole) and Tx of ***Helicobacter pylori*** – **amoxicillin**, and **metronidazole** or **tetracycline** (vast majority heal)
- Surgery for ulcers rarely indicated since **PPIs**

- Need to rule out **gastrinoma** in patients with complicated ulcer disease (Zollinger–Ellison syndrome – **gastric acid hypersecretion**, **peptic ulcers**, and **gastrinoma**)
- **Surgical indications**:
  - **Perforation**
  - **Protracted bleeding** despite EGD therapy
  - **Obstruction**
  - **Intractability** despite medical therapy
  - **Inability to rule out cancer** (ulcer remains despite treatment) → requires resection of ulcer
  - *If patient has been on a PPI, an acid-reducing surgical procedure is required in addition to above.*
- **Surgical options** (acid-reducing surgery)
  - **Highly selective vagotomy** – lowest rate of complications, preserves motor to pylorus (no need for antral or pylorus procedure); 10%–15% ulcer recurrence; 0.1% mortality
  - **Truncal vagotomy** and **pyloroplasty** – 5% ulcer recurrence, 1% mortality
  - **Truncal vagotomy** and **antrectomy** – 1% ulcer recurrence (lowest rate of recurrence), 2% mortality; generally reserved for large ulcers, obstruction, or inability to rule out CA
  - Reconstruction after antrectomy – **Roux-en-Y gastro-jejunostomy** (best)
  - *Less dumping syndrome and alkaline reflux gastritis* compared to Billroth I (gastro-duodenal anastomosis) and Billroth II (gastro-jejunal anastomosis)
- **Bleeding**
  - Most frequent complication of duodenal ulcers
  - Usually minor but can be life threatening
  - Major bleeding – > 6 units of blood in 24 hours or patient remains hypotensive despite transfusion
  - Tx: **EGD 1st** – hemoclips, cauterize, Epi injection
  - **Surgery** – longitudinal anterior duodenotomy and **gastroduodenal artery** (GDA) **ligation** (sutures superior and inferior to ulcer base); approximate tissue over ulcer, transverse duodenotomy closure
  - Avoid hitting common bile duct (posterior) with GDA ligation.
  - If patient has been on a PPI, need acid-reducing surgery as well (if stable)

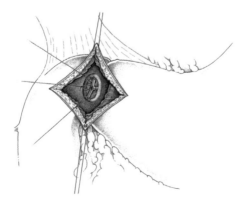

Proper suture ligation of a bleeding ulcer arising from the gastroduodenal artery requires a 3-suture ligation. The proximal and distal branches of the gastroduodenal artery are transfixed. A third suture, U type in configuration, is necessary to transfix the transverse pancreatic branch of the artery.

- **Obstruction**
  - **PPI** and **serial dilation** initial treatment of choice (NG tube, IVF resuscitation, and TPN up to 1 week; majority open up with conservative Tx)
  - Get **metabolic alkalosis** (hypochloremic, hypokalemic).
  - Surgical options – **antrectomy** and **truncal vagotomy** (best); include ulcer in resection if it's located proximal to ampulla of Vater
  - Need to Bx area of resection to rule out CA
- **Perforation**
  - 80% will have free air.
  - Patients usually have sudden sharp epigastric pain; can have generalized peritonitis
  - Pain can radiate to the pericolic gutters with dependent drainage of gastric content.
  - Initial Tx: fluid resuscitation, PPI, broad spectrum antibiotics (including yeast), NG tube
  - Tx: **Graham patch** (place **omentum** over the perforation)
    - Also need acid-reducing surgery if the patient has been on a PPI

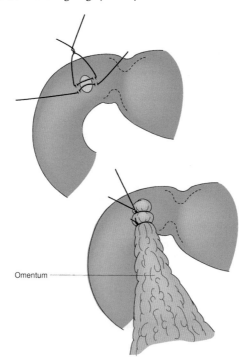

Omental patching of perforated duodenal ulcer.

- **Intractability**
  - > 3 months without relief while on escalating doses of PPI
  - Based in EGD **mucosal findings**, not symptoms
  - Tx: acid-reducing surgery

GASTRIC ULCERS

- Older men; slow healing; **H. pylori** present in **75%** (#1 risk factor)
- Other risk factors: **NSAIDs** (#2), male, tobacco, ETOH, uremia, stress (burns, sepsis, trauma), steroids, chemotherapy

- 80% on **lesser curvature** of the stomach
- **Hemorrhage** is associated with **higher mortality** than duodenal ulcers.
- Need to get **biopsy** to rule out CA – 5% of gastric ulcers are **gastric CA**
- Symptoms: epigastric pain radiating to the back; relieved with eating but recurs 30 minutes later; melena or guaiac-positive stools
- *Best test for H. pylori* – **histologic examination of biopsies from antrum**
- CLO test (rapid urease test) – test for *H. pylori*, detects urease released from *H. pylori*
- **Types**:
  - **Type I** – **lesser curve low along body of stomach**; due to ↓ mucosal protection
  - **Type II** – **2 ulcers** (lesser curve and duodenal); similar to duodenal ulcer with high acid secretion
  - **Type III** – **pre-pyloric ulcer**; similar to duodenal ulcer with high acid secretion
  - **Type IV** – **lesser curve high along cardia** of stomach; ↓ mucosal protection
  - **Type V** – **diffuse ulcers** associated with **NSAIDs**
- Tx: **proton pump inhibitor** (PPI; omeprazole) and Tx of ***Helicobacter pylori*** – **amoxicillin**, and **metronidazole** or **tetracycline** (vast majority heal)
- *Best test for H. pylori **eradication*** – urea breath test
- **Surgical indications** (initial Tx of these the same as duodenum) – perforation, bleeding not controlled with EGD, refractory obstruction, cannot exclude malignancy, intractability (> 3 months without relief – based on mucosal findings)
- Surgery: **truncal vagotomy** and **antrectomy** (*best*; pylorus removed with antrectomy); try to **include the ulcer** with resection (extended antrectomy) – need **separate ulcer excision** if that is not possible (Gastric ulcers are resected at time of surgery due to high risk of **gastric CA**.)
  - Omental patch and ligation of bleeding vessels are poor options for gastric ulcers due to **high recurrence of bleeding** and **risk of gastric CA** in the ulcer.
  - If **damage control** – anterior gastrotomy and over-sew ulcer (biopsy); definitive surgery when stabilized
- **Cushing's ulcer** – head trauma and gastric ulcer
- **Curling's ulcer** – burn patients and duodenal ulcer

STRESS GASTRITIS

- Occurs 3–10 days after event (eg multiple trauma, burns, complicated postop)
- Lesions appear in **fundus** first; can progress to **ulcers**
- Tx: **PPI**
- EGD with cautery of specific bleeding point may be effective.

CHRONIC GASTRITIS

- Type A (fundus) – associated with pernicious anemia, autoimmune disease
- Type B (antral) – associated with ***H. pylori***
- Tx: **PPI**

GASTRIC ADENOCARCINOMA

- Symptoms: **pain** unrelieved by eating and **weight loss**
- **Antrum** – 40% of gastric cancers (most common area)
- **Japan** – accounts for 50% of cancer-related deaths
- 85% sporadic
- **Risk factors** – significant ETOH, tobacco, *H. pylori*, adenomatous polyps, previous gastric operations, intestinal metaplasia, atrophic gastritis, pernicious anemia, type A blood, nitrosamines
  - **Adenomatous polyps** – 15% risk of cancer. Tx: endoscopic resection
- **Krukenberg tumor** – metastases to ovaries
- **Virchow's nodes** – metastases to supraclavicular node

- Tumors crossing within **5 cm of EGJ** are treated as **esophageal CA.**
- Workup (staging) – **EGD** with **biopsy,** CT chest/abdomen/pelvis, PET-CT
  - **Suspicious nodes** – EUS with FNA
- Unresectable disease – peritoneal or distant metastases, SMA or celiac encasement, positive para-aortic lymph nodes (EUS-FNA), root of mesentery involvement
  - **Spleen** or **splenic vessel** involvement still resectable (*resect spleen en bloc*)
- **Diagnostic laparoscopy** (staging) with peritoneal washings indicated *before* **resection** or **neoadjuvant chemo-XRT** for ≥ **T2** (invades muscularis propria or greater)
- **Neoadjuvant chemo-XRT** – indicated for ≥ **T2** or **positive peri-gastric nodes**
- **Surgery** – need **5 cm margins**
  - *No* need for prophylactic splenectomy
  - **T4 tumors** require en bloc resection of involved structures (eg liver resection en bloc).
  - Want **R0 tumor resection** (negative microscopic margins) along with **D1 nodal resection en bloc** (peri-gastric nodes along the lesser/greater curves)
- **Intestinal-type gastric CA** – found in high-risk factor populations, older men; Japan; rare in United States; histology shows **glands**
  - **Proximal tumor** – **total gastrectomy** with esophago-jejunal anastomosis (need **5-cm margins**)
  - **Distal tumor** – **sub-total gastrectomy**
  - Overall 5-YS – 35%
- **Diffuse gastric cancer** (linitis plastica) – found in low-risk factor populations, women; most common type in the United States; often associated with genetic abnormalities
  - Diffuse lymphatic invasion; *no* glands
  - **Less favorable prognosis** than intestinal-type gastric CA (overall 5-YS – 25%)
  - Surgical Tx: **total gastrectomy** usual because of diffuse nature of linitis plastica
- **Chemotherapy:** **5FU** based; leucovorin, cisplatin
  - **Adjuvant chemo** indicated for ≥ **T3** (invades sub-serosa or greater) or **positive nodes**
- **Palliation of gastric CA**
  - **Obstruction** – proximal lesions can be **stented**; distal lesions can be bypassed with **gastrojejunostomy**
  - Low to moderate **bleeding** or **pain** – Tx: XRT; possible angioembolization for bleeding
  - If these fail, consider palliative gastrectomy for obstruction or bleeding.
- **Hereditary diffuse gastric cancer**
  - **CDH1** mutation (autosomal dominant)
  - **70%** lifetime risk of **gastric CA**
  - **40%** lifetime risk of **breast CA in women**
  - **Prophylactic gastrectomy** recommended between **ages 20 and 40**
- Other syndromes at risk for Gastric CA – FAP, Lynch, Peutz–Jeghers, juvenile polyposis, Li–Fraumeni

GASTROINTESTINAL STROMAL TUMORS (GISTS)

- Most common benign gastric neoplasm, although can be malignant
- Symptoms: usually asymptomatic, but obstruction and bleeding can occur
- Hypoechoic on ultrasound; smooth edges
- Dx: biopsy – are **C-KIT–positive**
- Considered malignant if > **5 cm** or > **5 mitoses/50 HPF** (high-powered field)
- Tx: **resection** with 1-cm margins; *no nodal dissection*
- *Chemotherapy with **imatinib*** (Gleevec; tyrosine kinase inhibitor) if malignant

MUCOSA-ASSOCIATED LYMPHOID TISSUE LYMPHOMA (MALT LYMPHOMA)

- Related to ***H. pylori*** infection
- Usually regresses after treatment for *H. pylori*
- Stomach most common location

- Marginal zone B cell lymphoma (biopsy shows many small lymphoid cells)
- Tx: *triple-therapy antibiotics for H. pylori* and surveillance; if MALT does not regress, need XRT

GASTRIC LYMPHOMAS

- Have ulcer symptoms; stomach is the most common location for **extra-nodal lymphoma**.
- Usually **non-Hodgkin's lymphoma** (B cell)
- Dx: EGD with biopsy
- Chemotherapy and XRT are primary treatment modalities; surgery for complications
- Surgery possibly indicated only for stage I disease (tumor confined to stomach mucosa) and then only partial resection is indicated
- Overall 5-year survival rate > 50%

MORBID OBESITY

> ### Criteria for Patient Selection for Bariatric Surgery (Need All 4)
>
> - Body mass index > 40 kg/m² or body mass index > 35 kg/m² with coexisting comorbidities
> - Failure of nonsurgical methods of weight reduction
> - Psychological stability
> - Absence of drug and alcohol abuse

- Central obesity – worse prognosis in general population
- Operative mortality is approximately 1%.
- **Gets better after surgery** – diabetes, cholesterol, sleep apnea, HTN, urinary incontinence, GERD, venous stasis ulcers, pseudotumor cerebri (intracranial hypertension), joint pain, migraines, depression, polycystic ovarian syndrome, nonalcoholic fatty liver disease
- Does <u>not</u> get better – peripheral arterial disease
- **Roux-en-Y gastric bypass**
  - Better weight loss than just banding
  - **Hiatal hernia** discovered at time of gastric weight loss surgery – **repair**
  - Risk of marginal ulcers, leak, necrosis, B_{12} deficiency (intrinsic factor needs acidic environment to bind B_{12}), iron-deficiency anemia (bypasses duodenum where Fe absorbed), gallstones (from rapid weight loss)
  - **10% failure rate** due to high-carbohydrate snacking
  - **Leak**
    - **Ischemia** – most common cause of leak
    - **Signs of leak** – ↑ RR, ↑ HR, fever, elevated WBCs; often do <u>not</u> have abdominal pain
    - Tx: **early leak** (not contained) → emergent re-op; **late leak** (weeks out from surgery, likely contained) → percutaneous drain, antibiotics
  - **Marginal ulcers** (on the jejunum) – develop in 10%. Tx: PPI
    - **Marginal ulcer perforation Tx**: Place Graham patch.
  - **Stenosis** – usually responds to serial dilation
  - **Dilation of excluded stomach postop** – hiccoughs, large stomach bubble
    - Dx: **AXR**; Tx: **G-tube** (gastrostomy tube)
  - **Small bowel obstruction** – nausea and vomiting, intermittent abdominal pain; AXR shows dilated small bowel; this is a *surgical emergency* in patients with gastric bypass due to the high risk of **small bowel herniation**, **strangulation**, **infarction**, and subsequent **necrosis**; Tx: emergent surgical exploration

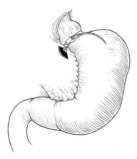

Laparoscopic adjustable gastric band.

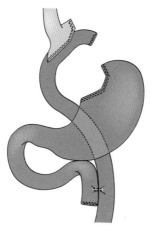

Laparoscopic proximal Roux-en-Y gastric bypass (retrocolic, retrogastric).

- **Jejunoileal bypass**
  - These operations are no longer done.
  - Associated with **liver cirrhosis**, **kidney stones**, and **osteoporosis** ($\downarrow$ Ca)
  - Need to correct these patients and perform Roux-en-Y gastric bypass if ileojejunal bypasses are encountered

POSTGASTRECTOMY COMPLICATIONS

- **Dumping syndrome**
  - Can occur after gastrectomy or after vagotomy and pyloroplasty
  - Occurs from rapid entering of **carbohydrates** into small bowel
  - 90% of cases resolve with medical therapy.
  - 2 **phases** (**early** and **late**)
    - Hyperosmotic load causes **fluid shift** into small bowel (**20 minutes** after meal).
      - Diarrhea, dizziness, diaphoresis, bloating, flushing
    - **Hypoglycemia** from rapid carbohydrate load and reactive $\uparrow$ **insulin** (**2 hours** after meal)
      - Tachycardia, weakness (*2nd phase rarely occurs*)
  - Can almost always be treated medically (*avoid* sugary drinks)
  - Dx: gastric emptying study

- Tx: small, low-fat, low-carbohydrate, **high-protein meals**; no liquids with meals, no lying down after meals; **octreotide**
- **Surgical options** (rarely needed)
  - Conversion of Billroth I or Billroth II to Roux-en-Y gastrojejunostomy
  - Operations to ↑ gastric reservoir (jejunal pouch) or ↑ emptying time (reversed jejunal loop)
- **Alkaline reflux gastritis** (bile reflux gastritis)
  - Occurs with Billroth I or Billroth II
  - Postprandial epigastric pain associated with N/V; pain not relieved with vomiting
  - Dx: **pH probe** (impedance probe; *best test*); EGD – shows evidence of **bile reflux** into stomach, histologic evidence of **gastritis**
  - Tx: PPI, cholestyramine, metoclopramide
  - Surgical option: conversion of Billroth I or Billroth II to Roux-en-Y gastrojejunostomy with afferent limb 60 cm distal to gastrojejunostomy
- **Chronic gastric atony**
  - Delayed gastric emptying (gastroparesis)
  - Symptoms: nausea, vomiting, pain, early satiety
  - Dx: gastric emptying study
  - Tx: metoclopramide, prokinetics
  - Surgical options: near-total gastrectomy with Roux-en-Y; pyloroplasty if not already done; **gastric electric stimulator**
- **Small gastric remnant** (early satiety)
  - Actually want this for gastric bypass patients
  - Dx: UGI
  - Tx: small meals
  - Surgical option: jejunal pouch construction
- **Blind-loop syndrome**
  - With Billroth II or Roux-en-Y; caused by **poor motility**
  - Symptoms: **pain, steatorrhea** (bacterial deconjugation of bile), **B$_{12}$ deficiency** (megaloblastic anemia; bacteria use it up), malabsorption, malnutrition
  - Caused by **bacterial overgrowth** (**E. coli**, GNRs) from stasis in afferent limb
  - Dx: **EGD of afferent limb** with **aspirate and culture** for organisms
  - Tx: tetracycline and Flagyl, metoclopramide to improve motility
  - Surgical option: reanastomosis with shorter (40-cm) afferent limb
- **Afferent-loop obstruction**
  - With Billroth II or Roux-en-Y; caused by **mechanical obstruction** of afferent limb
  - Symptoms: RUQ pain; nonbilious vomiting, pain relieved with bilious emesis
    - Can also cause obstructive jaundice, cholangitis, and pancreatitis from back pressure into biliary system
  - Risk factors – long afferent limb with Billroth II or Roux-en-Y
  - Dx: **CT scan** – shows dilated afferent limb
  - Tx: Balloon dilation may be possible.
  - Surgical option: reanastomosis with shorter (40-cm) afferent limb to relieve obstruction
- **Efferent-loop obstruction**
  - With Billroth II or Roux-en-Y
  - Symptoms of obstruction – nausea, vomiting, abdominal pain
  - Dx: CT scan
  - Tx: **emergency surgery** (same as gastric bypass with internal hernia)
- **Post-vagotomy diarrhea**
  - Secondary to nonconjugated **bile salts** in the colon (osmotic diarrhea)
  - Caused by **sustained postprandial organized MMCs**
  - Tx: cholestyramine, loperamide
  - Surgical option: reversed interposition jejunal graft

- **Retained antrum**
  - With Billroth II or Roux-en-Y; retained antrum located in **duodenal stump**
  - Causes **stomach ulcers** after gastric resection
  - Antral **G cells** secrete gastrin due to **alkaline environment**; acid is persistently released from proximal stomach.
  - Rule out a gastrinoma.
  - Tx: retained antrum resection and vagotomy (if not already performed)
- **Duodenal stump blow-out** (after gastrectomy) – Dx: CT scan; Tx: place lateral duodenostomy tube and drains; these patients can be really sick.
- **PEG complications** – insertion into the liver or colon

31 Liver

ANATOMY AND PHYSIOLOGY

- **Hepatic artery variants**
  - **Right hepatic artery** off **superior mesenteric artery** (#1 hepatic artery variant; 20%) courses behind pancreas, posterolateral to the common bile duct.
  - **Left hepatic artery** off **left gastric artery** (about 20%) – found in gastrohepatic ligament medially
- **Falciform ligament** – separates medial and lateral segments of the left lobe; attaches liver to anterior abdominal wall; extends to umbilicus and carries remnant of the umbilical vein
- **Ligamentum teres** – carries the obliterated umbilical vein to the undersurface of the liver; extends from the falciform ligament
- Line drawn from the middle of the **gallbladder fossa** to **IVC** (portal fissure or Cantlie's line) separates the right and left liver lobes.

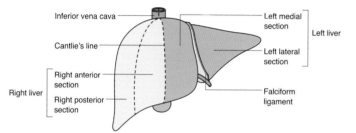

Anatomic division of the liver into right and left halves by a line extending from the gallbladder fossa posteriorly to the inferior vena cava.

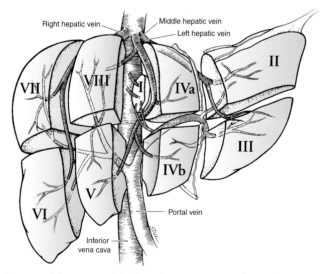

Couinaud's segmental anatomy of the liver. Segments II, III, and IV make up the left lobe and segments V, VI, VII, and VIII constitute the right lobe. Segment I is the caudate lobe.

- **Segments**
  - I – caudate
  - II – superior left lateral segment
  - III – inferior left lateral segment
  - IV – left medial segment (quadrate lobe)
  - V – inferior right anteromedial segment
  - VI – inferior right posterolateral segment
  - VII – superior right posterolateral segment
  - VIII – superior right anteromedial segment
- Glisson's capsule – peritoneum that covers the liver
- Bare area – area on the posterior-superior surface of liver not covered by Glisson's capsule
- Triangular ligaments – lateral and medial extensions of the coronary ligament on the posterior surface of the liver; made up of peritoneum
- **Portal triad** enters **segments IV** and **V**.
- **Gallbladder** lies under **segments IV** and **V**.

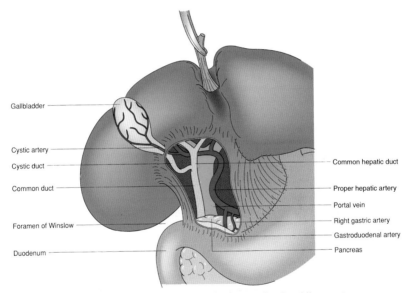

Relationship of structures within the hepatoduodenal ligament.

- **Kupffer cells** – **liver macrophages**
- **Portal triad** – **common bile duct** (lateral), **portal vein** (posterior), and **proper hepatic artery** (medial); come together in the **hepatoduodenal ligament** (porta hepatis)
- **Pringle maneuver** – porta hepatis clamping; will not stop hepatic vein bleeding
- **Foramen of Winslow** (entrance to lesser sac)
  - Anterior – portal triad
  - Posterior – IVC
  - Inferior – duodenum
  - Superior – liver (caudate lobe)
- **Portal vein**
  - Forms from **superior mesenteric vein** joining **splenic vein** (no valves)
  - **Inferior mesenteric vein** – enters splenic vein

- **Portal veins** – 2 in liver; ⅔ of hepatic blood flow
  - <u>Left</u> – goes to segments II, III, and IV
  - <u>Right</u> – goes to segments V, VI, VII, and VIII
- **Arterial blood supply**
  - Right, left, and middle hepatic arteries (follows hepatic vein system below)
  - Middle hepatic artery MC a branch off the left hepatic artery
  - Most primary and secondary **liver tumors** are supplied by the <u>hepatic artery.</u>
- **Hepatic veins** – 3 hepatic veins; drain into IVC
  - <u>Left</u> – II, III, and superior IV
  - <u>Middle</u> – V and inferior IV
  - <u>Right</u> – VI, VII, and VIII
  - **Middle hepatic vein** merges with left hepatic vein in 80% before going into IVC; other 20% goes directly into IVC.
  - **Accessory right hepatic veins** – drain medial aspect of right lobe directly to IVC
  - **Inferior phrenic veins** – also drain directly into the IVC
- **Caudate lobe** – receives separate right and left portal and arterial blood flow; drains directly into IVC via separate hepatic veins
- **Extended right hepatectomy** – take **5–8 + 4**
- **Extended left hepatectomy** – take **2–4** (+/− caudate lobe) + **5 and 8**
- **Alkaline phosphatase** – normally located in <u>canalicular</u> membrane
- **Nutrient uptake** – occurs in <u>sinusoidal</u> membrane
- **Ketones** – usual energy source for liver; glucose is converted to glycogen and stored
  - Excess glucose converted to fat
- **Urea** – synthesized in the liver
- <u>Not</u> **made in the liver** – von Willebrand factor and factor VIII (endothelium)
- Liver stores large amount of **fat-soluble vitamins**.
- **B$_{12}$** – the only water-soluble vitamin stored in the liver
- **Bleeding** and **bile leak** – most common problems with hepatic resection
- **Hepatocytes most sensitive to ischemia** – central lobular (acinar zone III)
- 75% of normal liver can be safely resected.

BILIRUBIN

- A breakdown product of **hemoglobin** (Hgb → heme → biliverdin → bilirubin)
- Conjugated to **glucuronic acid** (glucuronyl transferase) in the liver → improves water solubility
- Conjugated bilirubin is actively secreted into bile.
- **Urobilinogen**
  - Breakdown of conjugated bilirubin by bacteria in the terminal ileum occurs.
  - **Free bilirubin** is reabsorbed, converted to **urobilinogen**, and eventually released in the urine as **urobilin** (yellow color).
  - Excess urobilinogen turns urine dark like cola.

BILE

- Contains **bile salts** (85%), proteins, phospholipids (lecithin), cholesterol, and bilirubin
- Final bile composition determined by passive (Na/K ATPase) reabsorption of water in gallbladder
- **Cholesterol** – used to make bile salts/acids
- **Bile salts** are conjugated to **taurine** or **glycine** (improves water solubility).
  - <u>Primary bile acids</u> (salts) – **cholic** and **chenodeoxycholic**
  - <u>Secondary bile acids</u> (salts) – **deoxycholic** and **lithocholic** (dehydroxylated primary bile acids by bacteria in gut)

- **Lecithin** – main biliary phospholipid (emulsifies fat, solubilizes cholesterol)
- **Bile** solubilizes cholesterol and emulsifies fats in the intestine, forming **micelles**, which enter enterocytes by fusing with membrane.

JAUNDICE

- Occurs when total bilirubin > 2.5; 1st evident under the tongue
- Maximum bilirubin is 30 unless patient had underlying renal disease, hemolysis, or bile duct–hepatic vein fistula.
- Elevated **unconjugated bilirubin** (indirect; usually with **normal** or mildly elevated conjugated bilirubin) – prehepatic causes (hemolysis); hepatic deficiencies of uptake or conjugation
- Elevated **conjugated bilirubin** (direct; accompanied by **elevated** unconjugated bilirubin) – secretion defects into bile ducts (eg hepatitis); excretion defects into GI tract (obstructive jaundice; eg gallstones, cancer, benign stricture)
  - **Hepatitis** – very high transaminases, modest alkaline phosphatase
  - **Obstructive jaundice** – modest transaminases, very high alkaline phosphatase
- Syndromes
  - **Gilbert's disease** – abnormal conjugation; mild defect in **glucuronyl transferase**
  - **Crigler–Najjar disease** – inability to conjugate; severe deficiency of **glucuronyl transferase**; high unconjugated bilirubin → life-threatening disease
  - **Physiologic jaundice of newborn** – immature glucuronyl transferase; high unconjugated bilirubin
  - **Rotor's syndrome** – deficiency in storage ability; high conjugated bilirubin
  - **Dubin–Johnson syndrome** – deficiency in secretion ability; high conjugated bilirubin

VIRAL HEPATITIS

- All hepatitis viral agents can cause **acute hepatitis** (no surgery in setting of acute hepatitis).
- **Fulminant hepatic failure** can occur with hepatitis B, D, and E (very rare with A and C).
- Hepatitis B, C, and D can cause **chronic hepatitis** and **hepatoma**.
- **Hepatitis A** (RNA) – serious consequences uncommon
- **Hepatitis B** (DNA) – MC hepatitis worldwide
  - Anti-HBc-IgM (c = core) is elevated in the first 6 months; IgG then takes over.
  - Vaccination – have ↑ anti-HBs (s = surface) antibodies only
  - ↑ anti-HBc and ↑ anti-HBs antibodies and no HBs antigens (HBsAg) → patient had infection with recovery and subsequent immunity
- **Hepatitis C** (RNA) – can have long incubation period; currently most common viral hepatitis leading to liver TXP; Tx: **Sovaldi** (95% cure rate)
- **Hepatitis D** (RNA) – cofactor for hepatitis B (worsens prognosis)
- **Hepatitis E** (RNA) – fulminant hepatic failure in pregnancy, most often in 3rd trimester
- **Hepatitis B + D** has the **highest overall mortality**.

LIVER FAILURE

- **Most common cause of liver failure** – cirrhosis (palpable liver, jaundice, ascites)
- Best indicator of synthetic function in patient with cirrhosis – **prothrombin time** (PT)
- **Acute liver failure** (fulminant hepatic failure) – 80% mortality
- Outcome determined by the course of **encephalopathy**
- Consider **urgent liver TXP listing** if King's College criteria are met.

King's College Criteria of Poor Prognostic Indicators		
Acetaminophen-Induced ALF		

Arterial pH < 7.3 irrespective of coma grade
OR all of the following:
INR > 6.5, creatinine > 3.4 mg/dL (300 μmol/L), grade III/IV encephalopathy

Non–Acetaminophen-Induced ALF

INR > 6.5
OR any three of the following:
Age < 10 or > 40, drug toxicity or undetermined etiology, jaundice > 7 days before
    encephalopathy, INR > 3.5, bilirubin > 17 mg/dL (300 μmol/L)

ALF, acute liver failure; INR, international normalized ratio.

- **Hepatic encephalopathy**
  - Liver failure leads to inability to metabolize → get buildup of ammonia, mercantanes, and false neurotransmitters
  - Causes other than liver failure for encephalopathy – GI bleeding, infection (spontaneous bacterial peritonitis [SBP]), electrolyte imbalances, drugs
  - May need to embolize previous therapeutic shunts or other major collaterals
  - Tx: **lactulose** – **cathartic** that gets rid of bacteria in the gut and acidifies colon (preventing NH_3 uptake by converting it to ammonium), titrate to 2–3 stools/day
    - **Limit protein intake** (< 70 g/day)
    - **Branched-chain amino acids** – metabolized by skeletal muscle, may be of some value
    - <u>No</u> antibiotics unless for a specific infection
    - **Neomycin** (gets rid of ammonia-producing bacteria from gut)
- **Cirrhosis mechanism** – hepatocyte destruction → fibrosis and scarring of liver → ↑ hepatic pressure → portal venous congestion → lymphatic overload → leakage of splanchnic and hepatic lymph into peritoneum → ascites
- **Paracentesis for ascites** – replace with albumin (1 g for every 100 cc removed)
  - Albumin increases **oncotic pressure** and draws fluid **intravascular.**
- **Ascites** – from **hepatic/splanchnic** lymph
  - Tx: water restriction (1–1.5 L/d), ↓ NaCl (1–2 g/d), diuretics (spironolactone counteracts hyperaldosteronism seen with liver failure), paracentesis, TIPS if refractory, prophylactic antibiotics to prevent SBP (**norfloxacin**; used if previous SBP or current UGI bleed)
- **Aldosterone is elevated with liver failure** – secondary to impaired hepatic metabolism
- **Hepatorenal syndrome** – progressive renal failure; same lab findings as prerenal azotemia; usually a sign of **end-stage liver disease**; kidneys are normal but not perfused well.
  - Volume challenge does <u>not</u> work (unlike prerenal azotemia).
  - Tx: stop diuretics, give **albumin**, start **vasopressin**; no good therapy other than liver TXP
- **Neurological changes** – <u>asterixis</u>; sign that liver failure is progressing
- **Postpartum liver failure with ascites** – hepatic vein thrombosis (from ovarian vein source); has an infectious component (pelvic thrombophlebitis)
  - Dx: SMA arteriogram with venous phase contrast
  - Tx: **heparin** and **antibiotics**

SPONTANEOUS BACTERIAL PERITONITIS (PRIMARY BACTERIAL PERITONITIS)

- Patient with **ascites**
- Fever, abdominal pain, PMNs > 250 in fluid, positive cultures
- ***E. coli*** (#1), pneumococci, streptococci

- Most commonly mono-organism; if not, need to worry about bowel perforation
- Risk factors – prior SBP, UGI bleed (variceal hemorrhage), low-protein ascites, childhood nephrotic syndrome
- Tx: 3rd-generation cephalosporins; patients usually respond within 48 hours.

ESOPHAGEAL VARICES

- **Bleed** by rupture
- **Initial management** – T and C for 6 pRBCs (transfuse as necessary), intubate for airway protections, antibiotics
- Tx: **banding** and **sclerotherapy** (95% effective)
  - **Vasopressin** (splanchnic artery constriction) and **octreotide** (↓ portal pressure by ↓ blood flow) can be used to temporize.
  - Patients with history of CAD should receive NTG while on vasopressin.
  - Sengstaken–Blakemore esophageal tube – has a balloon used to control variceal bleeding; risk of rupture of the esophagus (hardly used anymore)
- **Propranolol** – good for patients with asymptomatic varices or with previous variceal bleed to help prevent rebleeding; no good role acutely
- Can get later strictures from sclerotherapy; usually easily managed with dilatation
- **TIPS** is needed for refractory variceal bleeding (continued bleeding after 2nd endoscopy).

PORTAL HYPERTENSION

- **Pre-sinusoidal obstruction** – schistosomiasis, portal vein thrombosis (50% of portal hypertension cases in children)
- **Sinusoidal obstruction** – cirrhosis (eg ETOH, viral)
- **Post-sinusoidal obstruction** – Budd–Chiari syndrome (hepatic vein occlusive disease), constrictive pericarditis, CHF
- For measurement of **portal vein pressure** – get **hepatic venous wedge pressure**
- Portal vein pressure > **10 mm Hg** considered significant
- Collateral splanchnic to systemic venous drainage:
  - **Coronary vein** (left gastric vein) and **pyloric vein** (right gastric vein) act as collaterals between the **portal vein** and the lower **esophagus submucosal venous system** (*esophageal varices*; this system eventually dumps into the <u>azygous vein</u>).
  - **Umbilicus** – **para-umbilical** veins and vestigial **umbilical** vein (ligamentum teres) to **epigastric veins** (*caput medusae*)
  - Rectum (**IMV** to **internal iliac** and **pudendal veins**)
- Portal HTN leads to esophageal variceal hemorrhage, ascites, splenomegaly, and hepatic encephalopathy.
- Shunts can decompress portal system.
- **TIPS** – used for protracted bleeding, progression of coagulopathy, visceral hypoperfusion, or refractory ascites, refractory hydrothorax
  - Allows antegrade flow from portal vein to the IVC
  - Complication of TIPS – *development of encephalopathy*
- **Splenorenal shunt** (considered selective shunt) – low rate of encephalopathy; need to ligate left adrenal vein, left gonadal vein, inferior mesenteric vein, coronary vein, and pancreatic branches of splenic vein; *do not need splenectomy*
  - Used only for Child's A cirrhotics who present with just **bleeding**
  - Contraindicated in patients with refractory ascites, as splenorenal shunts can worsen ascites
- **Partial portosystemic shunt** (considered a selective shunt; calibration based on size of graft used) – uses interposition graft between portal vein and IVC
  - Used if TIPS is not available and **refractory ascites** is the problem
- **Nonselective shunts** – not used anymore due to high rate of **encephalopathy**

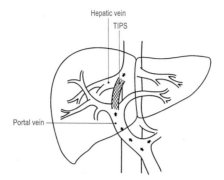

Transjugular intrahepatic portosystemic shunt (TIPS). A catheter is passed into the hepatic vein via the jugular vein. A needle, inserted through the catheter, is passed from the hepatic vein through the liver tissue into a major portal vein branch. The liver tract is dilated with an angioplasty balloon catheter, and the tract is kept open after deployment of an expandable metal stent.

- **Child's B or** C with indication for shunt → **TIPS**
- **Child's A** that just has **bleeding** as symptom → consider **splenorenal shunt** (more durable); otherwise TIPS
- **Child-Pugh Score** correlates with mortality after open shunt placement.

Child-Pugh Score	1 Point	2 Points	3 Points
Albumin	> 3.5	3–3.5	< 3.0
Bilirubin	< 2.5	2.5–4	> 4
Encephalopathy	None	Minimal	Severe
Ascites	None	Treatable with meds	Refractory
INR	< 1.7	1.7–2.3	> 2.3

- Child's A (5–6 pts)   2% mortality with shunt
- Child's B (7–9 pts)   10% mortality with shunt
- Child's C (10 pts or greater)   50% mortality with shunt

- **MELD score** (model for end-stage liver disease) – uses INR, creatinine, and total bilirubin to grade liver failure; often preferred compared to Child's
  - Need **MELD score ≥ 15** to get survival benefit from **liver TXP**
- Portal HTN in **children**
  - Usually from **extrahepatic portal vein thrombosis**
  - Most common cause of **massive hematemesis** in children

BUDD–CHIARI SYNDROME

- Occlusion of hepatic veins or IVC
- RUQ pain, hepatosplenomegaly, ascites, fulminant hepatic failure, variceal bleeding
- RF – **polycythemia vera**
- Dx: angiogram with venous phase, CT angiogram; liver biopsy shows sinusoidal dilatation, congestion, centrilobular congestion.
- Tx: **porta-caval shunt** (needs to connect to the IVC above the obstruction); can try catheter-directed tPA if acute

SPLENIC VEIN THROMBOSIS

- Can lead to **isolated gastric varices** without elevation of pressure in the rest of the portal system
- These gastric varices can **bleed.**
- **Splenic vein thrombosis** is most often caused by **pancreatitis.**
- Tx: **splenectomy** if symptomatic

PORTAL VEIN THROMBOSIS

- Usually **extrahepatic**
- RF – **hypercoagulable states**
- Get ascites _without_ liver failure
- Can get **esophageal varices** (MCC of massive hematemesis in children)
- Tx: **heparin** indicated if acute thrombosis (avoid if UGI bleeding present); may eventually need a shunt

LIVER ABSCESSES

- **Pyogenic abscess**
  - Most common type (account for 80% of all liver abscesses); can be multiple
  - Symptoms: fever, chills, weight loss, RUQ pain, ↑ LFTs, ↑ WBCs, sepsis
  - ↑ in right lobe; 15% mortality with sepsis
  - GNRs – #1 organism (**E. coli**)
  - Most commonly secondary to **contiguous infection** from **biliary tract** (eg cholangitis)
  - Can occur following **bacteremia** from other types of infections (eg diverticulitis, appendicitis)
  - Dx: aspiration
  - Tx: **CT-guided drainage** and **antibiotics**; surgical drainage for unstable condition and continued signs of sepsis
- **Amebic**
  - ↑ LFTs; ↑ in **right lobe** of liver, usually single
  - Primary infection occurs in the colon → **amebic colitis**
  - Risk factors – travel to Mexico, ETOH; fecal–oral transmission
  - Diagnosis – serology for _Entamoeba histolytica_ (90% have infection)
  - Symptoms: fever, chills, RUQ pain, ↑ WBCs, jaundice, hepatomegaly
  - Reaches liver via **portal vein**
  - Cultures of abscess often sterile → protozoa exist only in peripheral rim
  - Can usually diagnose based on CT characteristics
  - Tx: **Flagyl** (_rarely needs drainage_); aspiration _only_ if refractory (rare); surgery _only_ if free rupture (rare)
- _**Echinococcus**_
  - Forms cyst (hydatid cyst)
  - Positive **Casoni skin test**, positive **serology**
  - **Sheep** – carriers; **dogs** – human exposure; ↑ in **right lobe** of the liver
  - Do _not_ aspirate → can leak out and cause **anaphylactic shock**
  - Abdominal CT shows ectocyst (calcified) and endocyst (double-walled cyst).
  - Preop ERCP for _jaundice_, ↑ _LFTs_, or _cholangitis_ to check for communication with the biliary system
  - Tx: **preop albendazole** (2 weeks) and **surgical removal** (intraop can inject cyst with alcohol to kill organisms, then aspirate out); **need to get all of cyst wall**
  - Do not spill cyst contents – can cause anaphylactic shock
- **Schistosomiasis**
  - Maculopapular rash, ↑ eosinophils
  - Contact through the **skin**; acquired in **water**
  - Can cause variceal bleeding
  - Tx: **praziquantel** and control of variceal bleeding

BENIGN LIVER TUMORS

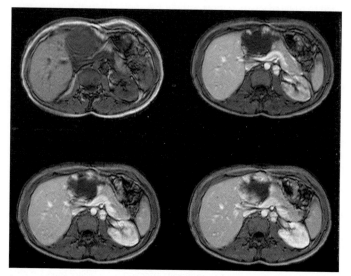

Magnetic resonance imaging of a hepatic hemangioma, demonstrating hypointensity on unenhanced images (*upper left*) and peripheral nodular enhancement with centripetal progression of enhancement on contrast-enhanced images (*upper right, lower left, lower right*).

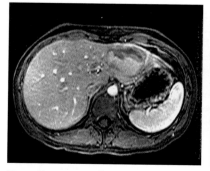

Magnetic resonance imaging of a hepatic adenoma consuming much of segments II and III, with intratumoral hemorrhage.

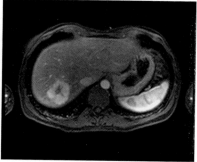

Gadolinium-enhanced magnetic resonance imaging of the liver, revealing a mass consistent with focal nodular hyperplasia.

- **Hepatic adenomas**
  - Women, steroid use, OCPs
  - 80% are symptomatic; 50% risk of significant bleeding (**Rupture risk** increases with **size**.)
  - Can become malignant (10%)
  - More common in **right lobe**
  - Symptoms: pain, ↑ LFTs, ↓ BP (from rupture), palpable mass
  - Dx: <u>no Kupffer cells</u> in adenomas, thus **no uptake on sulfur colloid scan** (cold)

- Tx:
  - <u>Asymptomatic</u> and < 4 cm – stop OCPs; if regression, no further therapy is needed; if no regression, patient needs resection of the tumor
  - <u>Symptomatic</u> or > 4 cm – tumor resection for bleeding and malignancy risk; embolization if multiple and unresectable
  - <u>Rupture</u> – emergent angioembolization, recovery, then resection
- **Focal nodular hyperplasia**
  - Has **central stellate scar** on imaging (diagnostic); more common in women
  - No malignancy risk; very unlikely to rupture; usually asymptomatic
  - Dx: abdominal CT; <u>has Kupffer cells</u>, so **will take up sulfur colloid on liver scan**
  - Tx: conservative therapy (*no resection*)
- **Hemangiomas**
  - Most common benign hepatic tumor
  - Rupture rare; most asymptomatic; more common in women
  - *Avoid* biopsy → risk of hemorrhage
  - Dx: MRI and CT scan show **peripheral to central enhancement**.
    - Appears as a *very **hypervascular** lesion on T2 MRI* (*very bright*)
    - Tagged RBC scan (*best test*)
  - Tx: conservative (regardless of size) unless symptomatic, then **resection ± preop embolization**; steroids (possible XRT) for unresectable disease
  - **Rare complications of hemangioma** – consumptive **coagulopathy** (Kasabach–Merritt syndrome) and **CHF**; these complications are usually seen in children
- **Simple cysts**
  - Congenital; women, right lobe more common; walls have a characteristic blue hue.
  - Complications from these cysts are rare; most can be left alone.
  - Will **always recur** if aspirated
  - **Laparoscopic fenestration** if **symptomatic** (send capsule to pathology to rule out CA)

MALIGNANT LIVER TUMORS

- **Metastases:primary ratio** is **20:1**.
- **Hepatocellular CA** (hepatoma)
  - **Most common cancer worldwide**
  - Symptoms – RUQ discomfort and weight loss; usually occurs in setting of **cirrhosis**
  - Risk factors – **HepB** (#1 cause worldwide), HepC, ETOH, hemochromatosis, alpha-1-antitrypsin deficiency, primary sclerosing cholangitis, aflatoxins, hepatic adenoma, steroids, inflammation, pesticides
  - **Fibrolamellar** type (adolescents and young adults; usually <u>not</u> in the setting of cirrhosis; neurotensin marker) – best prognosis
  - **Diffuse nodular** type – worst prognosis
  - **AFP level** correlates with tumor size.
  - Most common site of metastasis – **lung**
  - **CT scan** – shows **mosaic pattern** (non-homogenous necrotic areas mixed with hypervascular sections)
  - Characteristic **CT findings** and **elevated AFP** makes diagnosis (*no biopsy needed*).
  - Few hepatic tumors are resectable due to **cirrhosis** (Child's B/C), **portohepatic lymph node** involvement, **major vascular invasion**, or **metastases** (only 15% resectable).
  - **Early stage**, resectable liver CA and **Child's A** cirrhosis – proceed with **resection**
  - **Early stage** liver CA and **Child's B/C** cirrhosis – liver TXP evaluation
  - If tumor looks resectable, need to make sure to leave adequate liver behind to sustain life (**termed future liver remnant** [FLR])
    - **No cirrhosis** – FLR needs to be **25%** (of preop liver)
    - **Child's A** – FLR needs to be **40%** (of preop liver)
    - If **FLR does <u>not</u> look adequate** – consider preop **portal vein embolization** of tumor side lobe (contralateral lobe will hypertrophy) and reassess FLR

- Need **1-cm margin**
- 5-year survival rate with resection – 30%
- Tumor recurrence most likely to occur in the liver after resection
- **Palliation** based on **lesion size**:
  - **< 5 cm** – <u>ablation</u> (radiofrequency, microwave, or cryotherapy)
  - **> 5 cm** – <u>TACE</u> (transarterial chemoembolization)
  - Consider **radiation therapy** (XRT) if not amenable to above.
- **Hepatic sarcoma**
  - Risk factors – PVC, Thorotrast, arsenic → rapidly fatal
- **Isolated colon CA metastases to liver** – can resect if you leave enough liver for the patient to survive; 35% 5-year survival rate after resection for cure
- **Primary liver tumors** – generally hypervascular
- **Metastatic liver tumors** – generally hypovascular

UMBILICAL HERNIA REPAIR WITH ASCITES

- Should be repaired electively to avoid **rupture** and other complications
  1. Remove and control **preop ascites** (diuretics, paracentesis if necessary, consider TIPS if refractory).
  2. Correct **coagulopathy** (vitamin K if you have time; consider FFP [or PCC] and platelets).
  3. Repair hernia with **mesh** if **elective** (<u>*no*</u> drains; close peritoneum to avoid adhesions).
  4. Need **urgent** repair for **perforation**, **infection**, or **bowel incarceration** (<u>*without*</u> mesh if perforation, infection, or bowel resection)
  5. Control postop ascites (intermittent paracentesis if necessary).

32 Biliary System

ANATOMY AND PHYSIOLOGY

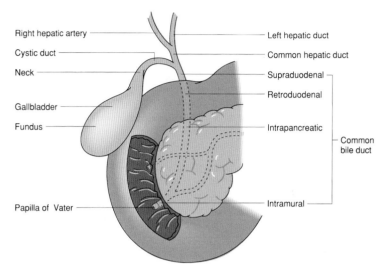

Right hepatic artery — — Left hepatic duct
Cystic duct — — Common hepatic duct
Neck — — Supraduodenal
— Retroduodenal
Gallbladder — — Intrapancreatic — Common bile duct
Fundus —
Papilla of Vater — — Intramural

Anatomic divisions of the common bile duct.

- Gallbladder lies beneath **segments IV** and **V**.
- **Cystic artery** branches off right hepatic artery.
  - Is found in the **triangle of Calot** (**cystic duct** [lateral], **common hepatic duct** [medial], **liver** [superior])
- **Right hepatic** (lateral) and retroduodenal branches of the **gastroduodenal artery** (medial) supply the hepatic and common bile duct (9- and 3-o'clock positions when performing endoscopic retrograde cholangiopancreatography [ERCP]); considered longitudinal blood supply
- **Cystic veins** drain into the **right branch of the portal vein**.
- **Lymphatics** are on the **right side** of the common bile duct.
- Parasympathetic fibers come from **left** (anterior) **trunk of the vagus**.
- Sympathetic fibers from T7-10 (**splanchnic and celiac ganglions**)
- Gallbladder has **no submucosa**; mucosa is **columnar** epithelium.
- Common bile duct and common hepatic duct **do not have peristalsis**.
- Gallbladder normally fills by **contraction of sphincter of Oddi** at the ampulla of Vater.
  - **Morphine** – contracts the sphincter of Oddi
  - **Glucagon** – relaxes the sphincter of Oddi
- **Normal sizes**: common bile duct (CBD) ≤ **6 mm** (≤ **10 mm** after cholecystectomy), gallbladder wall ≤ 4 mm, pancreatic duct ≤ 4 mm
- After cholecystectomy, total bile salt pools ↓.
- Highest concentration of **CCK** and **secretin cells** are in the **duodenum**.
- **Rokitansky–Aschoff sinuses** – epithelial invaginations in the gallbladder wall; formed from ↑ gallbladder pressure
- **Ducts of Luschka** – biliary ducts that can leak after a cholecystectomy; lie in the gallbladder fossa

- **Bile excretion regulation**
  - ↑ **bile excretion** – CCK, secretin, and vagal input
  - ↓ **bile excretion** – somatostatin, sympathetic stimulation
  - **Gallbladder contraction** – CCK causes constant, steady, tonic contraction
- **Essential functions of bile:**
  - Fat-soluble vitamin absorption
  - Essential fat absorption
  - Bilirubin and cholesterol excretion
- **Gallbladder** – forms concentrated bile by **active resorption of NaCl** (ATPase) and **passive resorption of water**
  - Active resorption of **conjugated bile salts** occurs in the **terminal ileum** (50%).
  - Passive resorption of **nonconjugated bile salts** can occur in the **small intestine** (45%) and **colon** (5%).
  - Postprandial gallbladder emptying is maximum at 2 hours (80%).
  - Bile secreted by **hepatocytes** (80%) and **bile canalicular cells** (20%)
  - Color of bile is mostly due to **conjugated bilirubin**.
  - **Stercobilin** – breakdown product of conjugated bilirubin in gut; gives stool brown color
  - **Urobilinogen** – conjugated bilirubin is broken down in the gut and reabsorbed; gets converted to urobilinogen and eventually urobilin, which is released in the urine (yellow color)

	Na (mEq/L)	Cl (mEq/L)	Bile Salts (mEq/dL)	Cholesterol (mEq/dL)
Hepatic bile	140–170	50–120	1–50	50–150
Gallbladder bile	225–350	1–10	250–350	300–700

CHOLESTEROL AND BILE ACID SYNTHESIS

- HMG CoA → (**HMG CoA reductase**) → cholesterol → (**7-alpha-hydroxylase**) → bile salts (acids)
- **HMG CoA reductase** – rate-limiting step in cholesterol synthesis

GALLSTONES

- Occur in 10% of the population; vast majority are **asymptomatic** (Tx: observation *only*).
- Only 10% of gallstones are radiopaque.
- **Nonpigmented stones**
  - **Cholesterol stones** – caused by **stasis, calcium nucleation,** and ↑ **water reabsorption** from gallbladder
  - Also caused by ↓ **lecithin** and **bile salts**
  - Found almost exclusively in the gallbladder
  - Most common type of stone found in the United States (75%)
- **Pigmented stones** – most common worldwide
  - **Calcium bilirubinate stones** – caused by solubilization of unconjugated bilirubin with precipitation
  - Dissolution agents (monooctanoin) do <u>not</u> work on pigmented stones.
  - **Black stones**
    - Can be caused by **hemolytic disorders, cirrhosis, chronic TPN**
    - Factors for development – ↑ bilirubin load, ↓ hepatic function, and bile stasis → get **calcium bilirubinate stones**
    - Almost always form in gallbladder
    - Tx: **cholecystectomy** if symptomatic

- **Brown stones** (primary CBD stones, formed in ducts, Asians)
  - **Infection** causing deconjugation of bilirubin
  - *E. coli* most common – produces **beta-glucuronidase**, which deconjugates bilirubin with formation of **calcium bilirubinate**
  - Need to check for ampullary stenosis, duodenal diverticula, abnormal sphincter of Oddi
  - Most commonly **form in the bile ducts** (are *primary common bile duct stones*)
  - Tx: almost all patients with primary stones need a biliary drainage procedure – **sphincteroplasty** (90% successful)
- Cholesterol stones and black stones found in the CBD are considered *secondary common bile duct stones*.
- **Choledocholithiasis lab tests**
  - **GGT** – highest sensitivity (highest NPV)
  - **Alkaline phosphatase** – highest specificity (highest PPV)

CHOLECYSTITIS

- Due to obstruction of the **cystic duct** by a gallstone
- Results in gallbladder wall distention and wall inflammation
- Symptoms: RUQ pain (constant), referred pain to the right shoulder and scapula, nausea and vomiting, loss of appetite
  - Attacks frequently occur after a fatty meal; pain is persistent (unlike biliary colic).
- Murphy's sign – patient resists deep inspiration with deep palpation to the RUQ secondary to pain
- **Alkaline phosphatase** and **WBCs** are frequently elevated.
- **Suppurative cholecystitis** associated with frank purulence in the gallbladder → can be associated with sepsis and shock
- Most common organisms in cholecystitis – *E. coli (#1)*, *Klebsiella*, *Enterococcus*
- **Stone risk factors** – age > 40, female, obesity, pregnancy, rapid weight loss, vagotomy, TPN (pigmented stones), ileal resection
- **Ultrasound** - 95% sensitive for picking up stones → hyperechoic focus, posterior shadowing, movement of focus with changes in position
  - Best initial evaluation test for **jaundice** or **RUQ pain**
  - Findings suggestive of **acute cholecystitis** – gallstones, gallbladder wall thickening (> 4 mm), pericholecystic fluid
  - Dilated CBD (> 6 mm) suggests CBD stone and obstruction.
- **HIDA scan** – technetium taken up by liver and excreted in the biliary tract
- **CCK-CS test** (cholecystokinin cholescintigraphy)
  - *Most sensitive test for cholecystitis* (also uses HIDA above)
  - Indications for **cholecystectomy** after CCK-CS test:
    - If **gallbladder not seen** (the cystic duct likely has a stone in it; chronic cholecystitis)
    - Takes > **60 minutes to empty** (biliary dyskinesia)
    - **Ejection fraction** < **40%** (biliary dyskinesia)
- Indications for **emergent** ERCP (signs that a common bile duct stone is present) – jaundice, clinical cholangitis, dilated CBD *without* gallstone pancreatitis, or imaging shows CBD stone
- Indications for **preop** ERCP (any of following needs to be persistently high for > 24 hours to justify) – **AST** or **ALT** (> 200) *without* gallstone pancreatitis or **bilirubin** (> 3)
  - Consider **MRCP** for gallstone pancreatitis (*avoid* ERCP – no improvement in outcomes and stone will likely pass).
  - **< 5%** of patients undergoing cholecystectomy will have a retained CBD stone → 95% of these are cleared with ERCP
  - Consider **CBD exploration** with **intraop cholangiogram** (IOC) if ERCP *not* available (IV glucagon and normal saline flush if stones found).

- **Tx for cholecystitis** – cholecystectomy; cholecystostomy tube can be placed in patients who are very ill and cannot tolerate surgery.
    - No benefit to "cooling patient off" with antibiotics prior to surgery
    - Patients undergoing cholecystostomy tube placement need **interval cholecystectomy** when recovered from illness (high cholecystitis recurrence rate when tube removed).
- **ERCP** – best treatment for late common bile duct stone
    - Sphincterotomy allows for removal of stone.
    - Risks: bleeding, pancreatitis, perforation
- **Biliary colic** – transient cystic duct obstruction caused by passage of a gallstone
    - Resolves within 4–6 hours
    - If U/S shows gallstones, elective cholecystectomy is indicated.
- **Air in the biliary system** most commonly occurs with previous ERCP and sphincterotomy.
    - Can also occur with cholangitis or erosion of the biliary system into the duodenum (ie gallstone ileus)
- **Bacterial infection of bile** – dissemination from **portal system** is the most common route (<u>not</u> retrograde through sphincter of Oddi)
- **Highest incidence of positive bile cultures** occurs with **postoperative strictures** (usually *E. coli*, often polymicrobial).
- **Pregnancy** and **symptomatic cholelithiasis** – laparoscopic cholecystectomy (in 2nd trimester if possible)
    - Lower spontaneous abortion rate compared to nonoperative Tx
    - Open port placement (Hassan), low pneumoperitoneum, roll patient to left (off IVC)
- **Cirrhosis** and **acute cholecystitis** – patients with **Child's A or B** cirrhosis should undergo <u>laparoscopic cholecystectomy</u>; **Child's C** better off with <u>medical management</u> (antibiotics)
- **Choledocholithiasis after Roux-en-Y gastric bypass**
    - Issue is you can't easily access biliary system for ERCP.
    - If **gallbladder** still present – cholecystectomy and intraop CBD exploration
    - If **gallbladder** *not* present – double balloon ERCP or laparoscopic G tube placement in distal stomach remnant and perform ERCP through G tube

ACALCULOUS CHOLECYSTITIS

- Thickened wall, RUQ pain, ↑ WBCs, <u>no</u> stones
- Occurs most commonly after severe burns, prolonged TPN, trauma, or major surgery
- Primary pathology is **bile stasis** (narcotics, fasting), leading to distention and ischemia.
- Also have ↑ **viscosity** secondary to **dehydration, ileus, transfusions**
- Ultrasound shows **sludge**, gallbladder wall thickening, pericholecystic fluid, and ***no stones***.
- HIDA scan is positive.
- Tx: cholecystectomy; percutaneous drainage if patient too unstable

EMPHYSEMATOUS GALLBLADDER DISEASE

- Gas in the gallbladder wall – can see on plain film
- ↑ in diabetics; usually secondary to ***Clostridium perfringens***
- Symptoms: severe, rapid-onset abdominal pain, nausea, vomiting, and sepsis
- Perforation more common in these patients
- Tx: **emergent cholecystectomy**; percutaneous drainage if patient is too unstable

GALLSTONE ILEUS

- **Fistula** between **gallbladder** and **duodenum** that releases stone, causing small bowel obstruction; usually in elderly
    - Can see **pneumobilia** (air in the biliary system) on plain film
- **Terminal ileum** – most common site of obstruction

- Primary Tx: **Remove stone** through enterotomy proximal to obstruction.
  - Generally do _not_ perform cholecystectomy and fistula resection at time of operation as complication rate is high and recurrence is low.

COMMON BILE DUCT INJURIES

- Most commonly occur after laparoscopic cholecystectomy
- MCC – excess cephalad retraction of the gallbladder fundus
- Need **IOC** for suspected intraop CBD injury (ie stricture or leak; Trendelenburg, adjust catheter if not initially filling CBD); if CBD doesn't fill, need to open to investigate
- **Intraoperative CBD injury** – if < 50% the circumference of the common bile duct, can probably perform primary repair; in all other cases, will likely need hepaticojejunostomy (or choledochojejunostomy); _do not try to attach to duodenum – won't reach_
- Persistent **nausea and vomiting** or **jaundice** following **laparoscopic cholecystectomy** → get **U/S** to look for fluid collection
  - If **fluid collection is present**, may be bile leak → percutaneous drain into the collection
    - If fluid is bilious, get ERCP → sphincterotomy and stent if due to cystic duct remnant leak, small injuries to the hepatic or common bile duct, or a leak from a duct of Luschka
    - Larger lesions (ie complete duct transection) will require hepaticojejunostomy or choledochojejunostomy (see below for timing).
  - If **fluid collection not present** and the hepatic ducts are dilated, likely have a completely transected common bile duct (PTC tube initially, then hepaticojejunostomy or choledochojejunostomy)
    - For lesions that cause <u>early symptoms (≤ 7 days)</u> – **hepaticojejunostomy**
    - For lesions that cause <u>late symptoms (> 7 days)</u> – **hepaticojejunostomy** 6–8 weeks after injury (tissue too friable for surgery after 7 days)
- **Sepsis** following **laparoscopic cholecystectomy** → fluid resuscitation and stabilize
  - May be due to complete transection of the CBD and cholangitis → get U/S to look for dilated intrahepatic ducts or fluid collections (pathway same as above)
- **Anastomotic leaks** following transplantation or hepaticojejunostomy → usually handled with percutaneous drainage of fluid collection followed by **ERCP with temporary stent** (leak will heal)

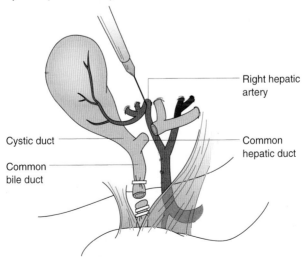

Classic laparoscopic bile duct injury. The common bile duct is mistaken for the cystic duct and transected. A variable extent of the extrahepatic biliary tree is resected with the gallbladder. The right hepatic artery, in background, is also often injured.

BILE DUCT STRICTURES

- **Ischemia** following **laparoscopic cholecystectomy** – most important cause of late postoperative biliary strictures
- Other causes – **chronic pancreatitis, gallbladder CA, bile duct CA**
- Symptoms: **jaundice**, sepsis, cholangitis
- Bile duct strictures without a history of pancreatitis or biliary surgery is CA until proven otherwise.
- Dx: **MRCP** (magnetic resonance cholangiopancreatography) defines anatomy, looks for mass → if CA not ruled out with MRCP, need ERCP with brush biopsies
- Tx: if due to **ischemia** or **chronic pancreatitis** → *choledochojejunostomy* (best long-term solution)
  - If due to CA, follow appropriate workup.

HEMOBILIA

- Fistula between **bile duct** and **hepatic arterial system** (most commonly)
- Patients classically present with hematemesis (UGI bleed), jaundice, and RUQ pain.
- Most commonly occurs with **percutaneous instrumentation** (eg PTC tube) or **trauma** to liver
- Dx: **EGD** (*first test*) will show blood coming out of the ampulla of Vater; angiogram
- Tx: **angioembolization**; operation if that fails

GALLBLADDER ADENOCARCINOMA

- Rare although most common CA of the biliary tract
- Often discovered incidentally after cholecystectomy
- 4× more common than bile duct CA; most have **stones** (#1 risk factor)
  - Other RFs – polyps ≥ 10 mm, inflammation, porcelain gallbladder, typhoid, primary sclerosing cholangitis, inflammatory bowel disease **porcelain gallbladder** – 3% risk of gallbladder CA; cholecystectomy indicated for **symptomatic** patients or who are **young/fit**
- **Liver** – most common site of metastasis
- Dx: MRCP
- 1st spreads to **segments IV** and **V** relatively early (*gallbladder has no submucosa*)
- 1st nodes are the **cystic duct nodes** (right side).
- Symptoms: **jaundice** 1st (bile duct invasion with obstruction) then **RUQ pain**
- Tx:
  - If muscle *not* involved (not beyond mucosa or lamina propria; **T1a**) – **cholecystectomy** alone sufficient
  - If in **muscle** (muscularis propria, **T1b**) but not beyond – also need **wedge resection** of **segments IVb** and **V**
  - If **beyond muscle** and **still resectable** – also need **formal resection of segments IVb and V**
  - Also need **portal regional lymphadenectomy** if in the **muscle** or beyond
  - Do *not* need to excise port sites if previous laparoscopic cholecystectomy and going back in for liver resection
- Overall 5-year survival – 20%

BILE DUCT CANCER (CHOLANGIOCARCINOMA)

- Occurs in elderly; males
- Risk factors: *C. sinensis* infection (liver fluke), ulcerative colitis, choledochal cysts, primary sclerosing cholangitis, chronic bile duct infection, HBV, HCV, inflammation
- Symptoms: <u>early</u> – **painless jaundice**; <u>late</u> – **weight loss**, pruritus
- Persistent ↑ in **bilirubin** and **alkaline phosphatase**

- Dx: **MRCP** (defines anatomy, looks for mass)
  - Can make diagnosis based on MRI and symptoms (_no biopsy necessary_)
- Invades contiguous structures early
- Discovery of a **focal bile duct stenosis** in patients without a history of biliary surgery or pancreatitis is highly suggestive of bile duct CA.
- **Diagnostic laparoscopy** prior to resection to rule out disseminated disease
- Consider surgery if no distant metastases and tumor is resectable:
  - **Intrahepatic** tumor – should have _no_ lymph node involvement **past porta hepatis**
  - **Extrahepatic** tumor – should _not_ involve SMA or celiac nodes
- Tx:
  - **Intrahepatic** – resection with negative margin (usually lobectomy; can be segmental or wedge resection)
  - **Extrahepatic** (also need **regional lymphadenectomy**; resection with negative margin):
    - **Upper** ⅓ (Klatskin tumors)
      - Most common type, worst prognosis, usually unresectable
      - Contralateral hemi-liver arterial/portal vein/biliary systems must be **tumor free.**
      - Tx: can try lobectomy; usually end up with hepaticojejunostomy
    - **Middle** ⅓ – hepaticojejunostomy
    - **Lower** ⅓ – Whipple
- Palliative stenting for unresectable disease
- Liver TXP _not_ an option for cholangiocarcinoma
- Overall 5-year survival rate – 10%

CHOLEDOCHAL CYSTS

- Female gender; Asians; 90% are extrahepatic; 15% CA risk (cholangiocarcinoma)
- Older patients have episodic pain, fever, jaundice, cholangitis.
- Infants can have symptoms similar to biliary atresia.
- Most are type I – fusiform or saccular dilatation of extrahepatic ducts (very dilated)
- Caused by **abnormal reflux of pancreatic enzymes** during uterine development
- (See Pediatric chapter for surgical management.)

PRIMARY SCLEROSING CHOLANGITIS

- Men in 4th–5th decade
- Can be associated with ulcerative colitis, pancreatitis, diabetes
- Symptoms: jaundice, fatigue, pruritus (from bile acids), weight loss, RUQ pain
- Have **multiple strictures** throughout the hepatic ducts
- Leads to **portal HTN** and **hepatic failure** (progressive fibrosis of intrahepatic and extrahepatic ducts)
- Does _not_ get better after colon resection for ulcerative colitis
- Complications – cirrhosis, cholangiocarcinoma
- Tx: **liver TXP** needed long term for most; PTC tube drainage, choledochojejunostomy or balloon dilatation of dominant strictures may provide some symptomatic relief.
  - **Cholestyramine** – can ↓ pruritus symptoms (↓ bile acids)
  - **UDCA** (ursodeoxycholic acid) – can ↓ symptoms (↓ bile acids) and improve liver enzymes

PRIMARY BILIARY CIRRHOSIS

- Women; medium-sized hepatic ducts
- Cholestasis → cirrhosis → portal hypertension
- Symptoms: jaundice, fatigue, pruritus, xanthomas
- Have **antimitochondrial antibodies**
- Tx: **liver TXP**; UDCA and cholestyramine for symptoms

CHOLANGITIS

- Usually caused by **obstruction of the bile duct** (most commonly due to gallstones)
- Can also be caused by **indwelling tubes** (eg PTC tube)
- **Charcot's triad** – RUQ pain, fever, jaundice
- **Reynolds' pentad** – Charcot's triad plus mental status changes and shock (suggests sepsis)
- **E. coli** (#1) and **Klebsiella** – most common organisms
- **Colovenous reflux** occurs at > 200 mm Hg pressure → **systemic bacteremia**
- Dx: ↑ AST/ALT, bilirubin, alkaline phosphatase, and WBCs
  - U/S – dilated CBD (> 6 mm, > 10 mm after cholecystectomy) if due to obstruction of the biliary system
- Stricture and hepatic abscess are late complications of cholangitis.
- Renal failure – #1 serious complication; related to **sepsis**
- Other causes – biliary strictures, neoplasm, choledochal cysts, duodenal diverticula
- Tx: *fluid resuscitation* and *antibiotics* initially
  - **Emergent ERCP** with **sphincterotomy** and **stone extraction**; if ERCP fails, place PTC tube to decompress the biliary system.
  - Generally needs cholecystectomy prior to discharge (prevents further episodes)
  - If the patient has cholangitis due to infected PTC tube, **change the PTC tube**.
- Mortality: 5%–10%

SHOCK FOLLOWING LAPAROSCOPIC CHOLECYSTECTOMY

- **Early** (1st 24 hours) – hemorrhagic shock from clip that fell off cystic artery
- **Late** (after 1st 24 hours) – septic shock from accidental clip on CBD with subsequent cholangitis

GALL BLADDER POLYPS

- Majority are **cholesterol polyps** (benign); other – hyperplastic (benign), adenoma (CA risk)
- Management based on size
  - **6–9** mm – need **annual U/S**; need **cholecystectomy** for **high-risk criteria** (see below)
  - **10–18** mm – **laparoscopic cholecystectomy**
  - **> 18** mm – treated like **gallbladder CA**
- **High-risk criteria** (need **cholecystectomy** *regardless* of size) – concurrent gallstones, symptomatic, fast-growing, sessile (wide base), long pedicle, age > 50, abnormal gallbladder wall, and infundibular polyp

OTHER CONDITIONS

- **Adenomyomatosis** – thickened nodule of mucosa and muscle associated with Rokitansky–Aschoff sinus
  - Not premalignant; does not cause stones, can cause RUQ pain
  - Tx: cholecystectomy
- **Granular cell myoblastoma** – benign neuroectoderm tumor of gallbladder
  - Can occur in biliary tract with signs of cholecystitis
  - Tx: cholecystectomy
- **Cholesterolosis** – speckled cholesterol deposits on the gallbladder wall
- **Delta bilirubin** – bound to albumin covalently, half-life of 18 days; may take a while to clear after long-standing jaundice
- **Mirizzi syndrome** – compression of the common hepatic duct by 1) a stone in the gallbladder infundibulum or 2) inflammation arising from the gallbladder or cystic duct extending to the contiguous hepatic duct, causing common hepatic duct stricture; Tx: cholecystectomy; may need hepaticojejunostomy for hepatic duct stricture
- **Ceftriaxone** – can cause gallbladder sludging and cholestatic jaundice
- **Indications for asymptomatic cholecystectomy** – in patients undergoing liver TXP or gastric bypass procedure (if stones are present)

33 Pancreas

ANATOMY AND PHYSIOLOGY

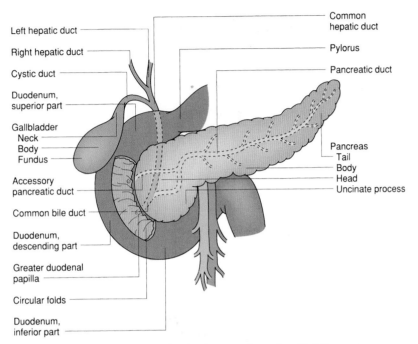

Relation of the pancreas to the duodenum and extrahepatic biliary system.

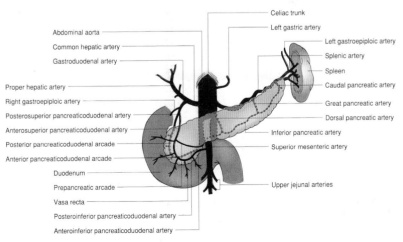

Arterial supply to the pancreas.

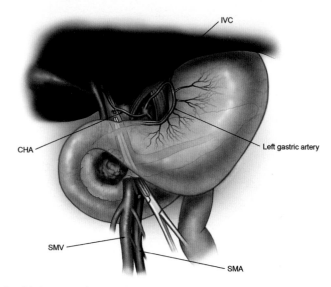

Relationship between the superior mesenteric vein and superior mesenteric artery.

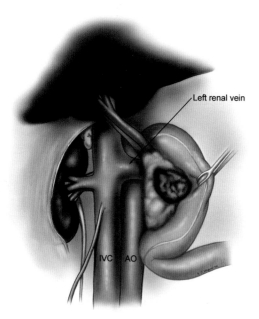

Kocher maneuver and relationship between the aorta and inferior vena cava.

- **Head** (including uncinate), **neck, body**, and **tail**
- **Uncinate process** – rests on aorta, behind SMV
- **SMV** and **SMA** – lay behind neck of pancreas
- **Portal vein** – forms behind the neck (SMV and splenic vein)
- **Blood supply**
  - **Head** – **superior** (off GDA) and **inferior** (off SMA) **pancreaticoduodenal arteries** (anterior and posterior branches for each)
  - **Body** – great, inferior, and dorsal pancreatic arteries (all off **splenic artery**)
  - **Tail** – splenic, gastroepiploic, and caudal pancreatic arteries
- **Venous drainage** into the **portal system**
- **Lymphatics** – celiac and SMA nodes
- **Ductal cells** – secrete **HCO_3^- solution** (have carbonic anhydrase)
- **Acinar cells** – secrete **digestive enzymes**
- **Exocrine function of the pancreas** – amylase, lipase, trypsinogen, chymotrypsinogen, carboxypeptidase; HCO_3^-
  - **Amylase** – <u>only pancreatic enzyme secreted in active form</u>; hydrolyzes alpha 1–4 linkages of glucose chains
- **Endocrine function of the pancreas** (islet cells)
  - **Alpha cells** – glucagon
  - **Beta cells** (at center of islets) – insulin
  - **Delta cells** – somatostatin
  - **PP or F cells** – pancreatic polypeptide
  - **Islet cells** – also produce vasoactive intestinal peptide (VIP), serotonin
- **Islet cells** receive **majority of blood supply** related to size.
  - After islets, blood goes to acinar cells.
- **Enterokinase** – released by the duodenum, activates trypsinogen to trypsin
  - Trypsin activates other pancreatic enzymes including trypsinogen.
- **Hormonal control of pancreatic excretion**
  - **Secretin** – ↑ HCO_3^- mostly
  - **CCK** – ↑ pancreatic enzymes mostly
  - **Acetylcholine** – ↑ HCO^- and enzymes
  - **Somatostatin** and **glucagons** – ↓ exocrine function
  - **CCK** and **secretin** – most released by cells in the duodenum
- **Ventral pancreatic bud**
  - Connected to duct of Wirsung; migrates posteriorly, to the right, and clockwise to fuse with the dorsal bud
  - Forms uncinate and inferior portion of the head
- **Dorsal pancreatic bud** – body, tail, and superior aspect of the pancreatic head; has duct of Santorini
- **Duct of Wirsung** – major pancreatic duct that merges with CBD before entering duodenum
- **Duct of Santorini** – small accessory pancreatic duct that drains directly into duodenum
- **Sphincter of Oddi** – **CCK** and **glucagon** relax the sphincter

ANNULAR PANCREAS

- 2nd portion of duodenum trapped in pancreatic band; can see double bubble on abdominal x-ray; get **duodenal obstruction** (N/V, abdominal pain)
- Associated with Down syndrome; forms from the <u>ventral pancreatic bud</u> from failure of clockwise rotation
- Tx: **duodenojejunostomy** or **duodenoduodenostomy**; possible sphincteroplasty
  - Pancreas <u>not</u> resected

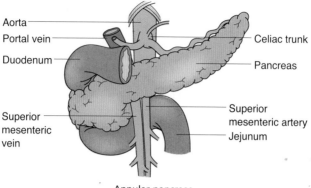

Annular pancreas.

PANCREAS DIVISUM

- Failed fusion of the pancreatic ducts; can result in pancreatitis from duct of Santorini (accessory duct) stenosis
- Most are asymptomatic; some get pancreatitis.
- Dx: ERCP – **minor papilla** will show long and large duct of Santorini; **major papilla** will show short duct of Wirsung
- Tx: **ERCP with sphincteroplasty**; open sphincteroplasty if that fails

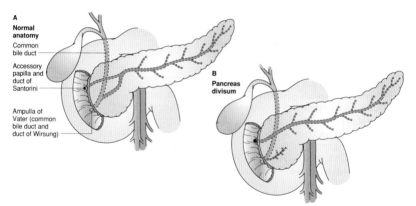

(A) Normal pancreatic ductal anatomy. **(B)** Pancreas divisum. There is no communication between the duct of Wirsung and the duct of Santorini. The duct of Wirsung is short or absent. Most of the pancreas is drained by the duct of Santorini through the accessory papilla. This anatomy is found in about 10%–15% of normal individuals.

HETEROTOPIC PANCREAS

- Most commonly found in **duodenum**
- Usually asymptomatic
- Surgical resection if symptomatic

ACUTE PANCREATITIS

- **Gallstones** and **ETOH** most common etiologies in the United States
  - Other etiologies – ERCP, trauma, hyperlipidemia, hypercalcemia, viral infection, medications (azathioprine, furosemide, steroids, cimetidine)

- **Gallstones** – can obstruct the ampulla of Vater, causing impaired extrusion of zymogen granules and activation of degradation enzymes → leads to pancreatic auto-digestion
- **ETOH** – can cause autoactivation of pancreatic enzymes while still in the pancreas
- Symptoms: **epigastric pain** radiating to the back; **nausea, vomiting, anorexia**
  - Can also get **jaundice**, left **pleural effusion**, **ascites**, or **sentinel loop** (dilated small bowel near the pancreas as a result of the inflammation)
- Mortality rate 10%; hemorrhagic pancreatitis mortality 50%
- MCC death – **sepsis**
- Pancreatitis without obvious cause → need to worry about malignancy
- **Ranson's criteria**
  - On admission → age > 55, WBC > 16, glucose > 200, AST > 250, LDH > 350
  - After 48 hours: Hct ↓ 10%, BUN ↑ of 5, Ca < 8, PaO2 < 60, base deficit > 4, fluid sequestration > 6 L
  - 8 Ranson criteria met → mortality rate near 100%
- Labs: ↑ **amylase**, **lipase**, and **WBCs**
- **Ultrasound** – needed to check for gallstones and possible CBD stone
- **Abdominal CT** – to check for complications (**necrotic pancreas** will <u>not</u> uptake contrast)
- Tx: **NPO**, NG tube, and aggressive **fluid resuscitation**
  - **ERCP** is <u>not</u> needed in patients with **gallstone pancreatitis** (stone usually passes on its own; no improvement in outcomes).
    - Consider ERCP for **clinical cholangitis, bilirubin > 3**, or **stone seen on imaging**.
  - **Antibiotics** (***Imipenem*** – **best**) for severe pancreatitis, failure to improve, suspected infected pancreatitis (eg fever, significantly elevated WBCs), or CT-guided aspiration showing organisms
  - Nasogastric or nasoduodenal **tube feeds** should be started **within 24–48 hours** of severe pancreatitis (reduces mortality compared to TPN).
  - Patients with gallstone pancreatitis should undergo **cholecystectomy** when recovered from pancreatitis (same hospital admission).
    - *Exception* – moderate to severe gallstone pancreatitis with fluid collections/ pseudocysts → **wait 6 weeks** before interval cholecystectomy to allow fluid collections to resolve and pseudocysts to mature
  - Morphine should be avoided as it can contract the sphincter of Oddi and worsen attack.
- **15% get pancreatic necrosis** – leave sterile necrosis <u>alone</u>
  - **Infected necrosis** (fever, sepsis, positive blood cultures; may need to sample necrotic pancreatic fluid with CT-guided aspiration to get diagnosis)
  - **Gas** in necrotic pancreas = infected necrosis or abscess
- **Infected pancreatic necrosis Tx** (*above plus*):
  1. ICU care, antibiotics, and early nutrition
  2. Continued **ongoing sepsis** – percutaneous or endoscopic drainage (transgastric)
  3. Continued **ongoing sepsis** – upsize drain
  4. If **> 3 weeks** therapy and **ongoing sepsis** – debridement (endoscopic transgastric vs minimally invasive video-assisted retroperitoneal)
- **Bleeding** (hemorrhagic pancreatitis)
  - **Grey Turner sign** – flank ecchymosis
  - **Cullen's sign** – periumbilical ecchymosis
  - **Fox's sign** – inguinal ecchymosis
- **Infection** – leading cause of death with pancreatitis; usually GNRs
- **Obesity** – most important risk factor for necrotizing pancreatitis
- **ARDS** – related to release of phospholipases
- **Coagulopathy** – related to release of proteases
- **Pancreatic fat necrosis** – related to release of phospholipases
- **Mild ↑ amylase** and **lipase** can be seen with cholecystitis, perforated ulcer, sialoadenitis, small bowel obstruction (SBO), and intestinal infarction.

PANCREATIC PSEUDOCYSTS

- Most common in patients with **chronic pancreatitis**; can also occur after acute pancreatitis or pancreatic trauma (generally presenting around 6 weeks after the initial event)
  - Cysts <u>not</u> associated with pancreatitis – **need to R/O CA** (eg mucinous cystadenocarcinoma)
- Symptoms: vague abdominal discomfort, early satiety, weight loss, bowel obstruction from compression
- Often occurs in the **head** of the pancreas; is a non-epithelialized sac of pancreatic fluid
- Most **resolve spontaneously** (especially if < 5 cm).
- Fluid has **high amylase.**
- Tx: *expectant management for 3 months* – (*most resolve on their own*; also allows pseudocyst to mature if cystogastrostomy is required)
  - May need to place these patients on **TPN** if unable to eat
  - Need **ERCP** *before* surgery/intervention to define ductal anatomy and see if pseudocyst connects with ductal system (MRCP may be alternative)
  - **Surgery/intervention** *only* for:
    - **Continued symptoms** (Tx: **cystogastrostomy** [open or laparoscopic] or **endoscopic transluminal drainage** [into stomach])
    - Pseudocysts that are **growing** (Tx: **resection** to rule out CA)
- **Complications of pancreatic pseudocyst** – infection of cyst, portal or splenic vein thrombosis
- **Incidental cysts** <u>not</u> associated with pancreatitis/trauma should be *resected* (worry about **intraductal papillary-mucinous neoplasms** [IPMNs] or **mucinous cystadenocarcinoma**) <u>unless</u> the cyst is purely serous and non-complex.
- **Non-complex, purely serous cystadenomas** have an extremely low malignancy risk (≤ 1%) and can be followed.

PANCREATIC FISTULAS

- Most **close spontaneously** (especially if low output < 200 cc/day).
- Are usually associated with pancreatic surgery
- Tx: Allow drainage, NPO, TPN, **octreotide**.
  - If failure to resolve with medical management, can try **ERCP**, **sphincterotomy**, and **pancreatic stent** placement (Fistula will usually close, then remove stent.)
  - Unusual to have to operate on these patients

PANCREATITIS-ASSOCIATED PLEURAL EFFUSION (OR ASCITES)

- Caused by retroperitoneal leakage of pancreatic fluid from the pancreatic duct or a pseudocyst (is <u>not</u> a pancreatic–pleural fistula); majority close on their own.
- Tx: **thoracentesis** (or paracentesis) followed by conservative Tx (**NPO, TPN, and octreotide**)
  - **Amylase** will be elevated in the fluid (> 1,000).

CHRONIC PANCREATITIS

- Corresponds to irreversible **parenchymal fibrosis**
- **ETOH** most common cause; **idiopathic** 2nd most common; other – biliary tract disease, autoimmune
- Increased risk of **pancreatic CA**
- **Pain** most common problem; anorexia, weight loss, malabsorption, steatorrhea
- <u>Endocrine</u> function usually **preserved** (Islet cell preserved); <u>exocrine</u> function **decreased**
- Can cause **malabsorption of fat-soluble vitamins** (Tx: pancrelipase; decreases steatorrhea)

- Dx: **Abdominal CT** (*best test*) will show **shrunken pancreas** (atrophy) with **calcifications** and fibrosis.
  - **Ultrasound** – shows pancreatic ducts > 4 mm, cysts, and atrophy
  - **ERCP** – very sensitive at diagnosing chronic pancreatitis
  - Advanced disease – **chain of lakes** → alternating segments of dilation and stenosis in pancreatic duct
- Tx: supportive, including **pain control** and nutritional support (**pancrelipase**)
- **Surgical indications** – pain that interferes with quality of life, nutrition abnormalities, addiction to narcotics, failure to rule out CA, biliary obstruction
- **Surgical options**
  - **Puestow procedure** – <u>lateral</u> pancreaticojejunostomy; for enlarged ducts > **6 mm** and pancreatic head free of disease (most patients improve) → open along main pancreatic duct and drain into jejunum

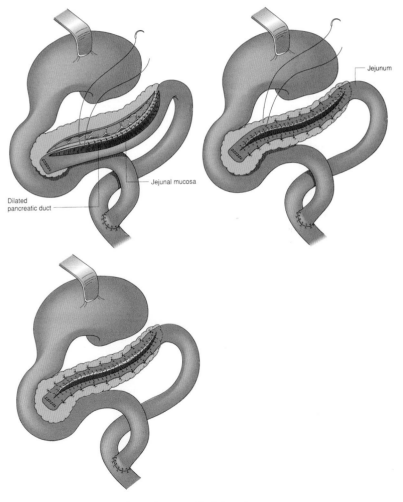

Jejunum

Jejunal mucosa

Dilated pancreatic duct

Lateral pancreaticojejunostomy.

- **Distal pancreatic resection** – for normal or small ducts and only distal portion of the gland is affected
- **Beger** (duodenal preserving **pancreatic head resection** with <u>end-to-side</u> pancreaticojejunostomy) – for normal or small ducts with isolated pancreatic head enlargement
- **Frey** (pancreatic head "core-out" procedure [*not* head resection] with <u>lateral</u> pancreaticojejunostomy) → for diffuse disease with enlarged ducts
- **Minimal change chronic pancreatitis** (patients having pain) – **bilateral thoracoscopic splanchnicectomy** or **celiac ganglionectomy** may be used for **pain control**
- **Common bile duct** (CBD) **stricture** from chronic pancreatitis – causes CBD dilation
  - Dx: MRCP
  - Tx: **hepaticojejunostomy or choledochojejunostomy** for pain, jaundice, progressive cirrhosis, or cholangitis (Make sure the stricture is not pancreatic CA.)
- **Splenic vein thrombosis** – <u>chronic pancreatitis</u> most common cause
  - Can get bleeding from isolated **gastric varices** that form as collaterals
  - Tx: **splenectomy** for isolated bleeding gastric varices

PANCREATIC INSUFFICIENCY

- Usually the result of long-standing pancreatitis or occurs after total pancreatectomy (Over 90% of the function must be lost.)
- Generally refers to exocrine function
- Symptoms: **malabsorption** and **steatorrhea**
- Dx: **fecal fat testing**
- Tx: high-carbohydrate, high-protein, **low-fat diet**; add **pancreatic enzymes** (Pancrease)

JAUNDICE WORKUP

- **Ultrasound 1st**
  - **Positive CBD stones**, **no mass** → ERCP (allows extraction of stones)
  - **No CBD stones**, **no mass** → MRCP
  - **Positive mass** → MRCP

PANCREATIC CYSTIC NEOPLASMS

- Often asymptomatic and picked up incidentally
- Dx: **MRCP** (*best*) – defines ductal anatomy and delineates lesion well
  - **EUS** – for aspiration of fluid (send for mucins, CEA, amylase, and cytology) →
    - **CEA: > 192 ng/mL** – suggests **mucinous** cyst; **< 192** suggests **serous** cyst
    - **High amylase** (> 250 U/L) – suggests **ductal communication** (IPMN or pseudocyst)
- **Serous cystadenoma**
  - Very low malignancy rate (≤ 1% lifetime)
  - Dx: low CEA, no mucin, well circumscribed, not complex
  - Tx: **observe**; resection only if symptomatic or growing
- **Mucinous cystadenoma**
  - Higher malignancy potential (15% malignant at time of resection)
  - Dx: high CEA, mucins, thick walled with internal septations
  - Tx: **resection**
- **Intraductal papillary mucinous neoplasm** (IPMN)
  - Divided into **main duct** and **branch duct** types
  - 30% have extrapancreatic malignancies (MC – **colorectal**; others esophageal, gastric).
  - Are cystic lesions
  - **Main duct IPMN** (also includes mixed duct)
    - 70% malignant at time of resection
    - Can be seen on **endoscopy** – "fish-mouth" ampullary papilla with mucin coming out is pathognomonic
    - Tx: surgical resection

- **Branch duct IPMN**
  - 5% malignant transformation rate over 5 years (much lower than main duct)
  - 40% are multifocal.
  - Surgery **recommended** for tumors **> 3 cm** or **high-risk features**.
  - **High-risk features**: thickened wall, mural nodules, lymphadenopathy, main pancreatic duct (MPD) > 10 mm, quick enlargement of MPD with distal atrophy, suspicious cytology, young patient with cyst > 2 cm (life-long risk of malignancy)
  - At surgery can encounter **multiple cysts** – just resect area with cysts having high-risk features (_Avoid_ total pancreatectomy.)
  - If elderly and frail may want to _avoid_ surgery (only 1%/year malignant transformation rate)

PANCREATIC ADENOCARCINOMA

- Male predominance; usually 6th–7th decades of life
- Pancreatic adenocarcinoma refers to pancreatic **ductal** (99%) or **acinar** (1%) CA.
- Pancreatic adenocarcinoma represents > 90% of all pancreatic CA.
- Symptoms: **weight loss** (most common symptom), **jaundice**, **pain** (epigastric or back)
- Risk factors – **tobacco #1**, heavy ETOH use, chronic pancreatitis, high BMI
- **CA 19-9** – serum marker for pancreatic CA
- 95% have **p16 mutation** (tumor suppressor, binds **cyclin** complexes)
- Lymphatic spread 1st
- **70%** are in the **head**.
- **Unresectable disease**
  - Invasion of retroperitoneum
  - Unreconstructable portal vein or SMV involvement
  - > 180-degree contact with SMA or celiac artery
  - Metastases to peritoneum, omentum, **liver** (MC site of metastasis), or other distant sites
  - Metastases to celiac or SMA nodal system (nodal systems outside area of resection)
- Most cures in patients with **pancreatic head disease**.

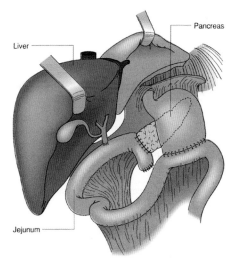

Reconstruction after standard pancreaticoduodenectomy (Whipple; the gallbladder is usually resected with the procedure).

- Labs: typically show ↑ conjugated **bilirubin** and **alkaline phosphatase**
- These patients usually do <u>not</u> get pancreatitis.
- Patients with a **resectable mass** (and no signs of metastatic disease) in the pancreas do **<u>not</u>** need a biopsy because you are taking it out regardless. If the patient appears to have metastatic disease or is undergoing neoadjuvant therapy, a biopsy (CT guided or endoscopic U/S) is warranted to direct therapy.
- **Workup:**
  - **MRCP** good at differentiating dilated ducts secondary to chronic pancreatitis versus CA
    - **Signs of CA on MRCP** – duct with irregular narrowing, displacement, destruction; can also detect vessel involvement
  - **Pancreatic protocol CT** – may show the lesion and double-duct sign for pancreatic head tumors (dilation of both the pancreatic duct and CBD)
  - **EUS** – can help define lymph node and vascular involvement
  - **PET/CT** – used if worried about metastatic disease
- **Staging laparoscopy** – look for **peritoneal metastases**
- **Preop biliary drainage**
  - Increases wound infection; <u>no</u> effect on survival
  - Consider for coagulopathy or pruritis; possibly for jaundiced patients getting neoadjuvant chemo
  - **Self-expanding metal** biliary stents have the best **patency** and **less migration**.
- Resectable **pancreatic head tumors** – pancreaticoduodenectomy (Whipple)
- Resectable **distal tumors** – distal pancreatectomy and splenectomy
- **Suspicious nodes** intraop <u>outside</u> area of resection – just biopsy (not lymphadenectomy)
- For **unresectable disease**, consider **palliation** with **biliary stents** (for biliary obstruction), **duodenal stents** (for duodenal obstruction), and **celiac plexus ablation** (for pain).
- Complications from Whipple – **delayed gastric emptying** #1 (Tx – metoclopramide), **fistula** (Tx: conservative therapy), **leak** (place drains and Tx like a fistula), **marginal ulceration** (Tx: PPI)
- **Bleeding** after Whipple or other pancreatic surgery – go to **angio for** *embolization* (The tissue planes are very friable early after surgery, and bleeding is hard to control operatively.)
- **All patients** get chemo postop – **FOLFIRINOX**
  - **FOL**inic acid, **F**luorouracil, **IRIN**otecan, **OX**aliplatnin
  - Neoadjuvant chemo +/− XRT if borderline resectable
- Prognosis for non-metastatic disease related to nodal invasion and ability to get a clear margin
- Overall 5-year survival – 10% (with resection for cure – 20%)

NON-FUNCTIONAL PANCREATIC NEUROENDOCRINE TUMORS

- **Non-functional** is the most common **PNET** (35%).
- 75% are **malignant**.
- Tend to be discovered **late** due to asymptomatic clinical course although often have **metastases** (MC – liver) at time of diagnosis
- Tend to have a more **indolent and protracted course** compared with pancreatic adenocarcinoma
- MC in **head of pancreas**
- Tx: **formal resection**: Metastatic disease precludes resection.
- **5FU** and **streptozocin** may be effective.

FUNCTIONAL PANCREATIC NEUROENDOCRINE TUMORS

- **Octreotide** – effective for symptoms with insulinoma, gastrinoma, glucagonoma, and VIPoma
- Most common in **pancreatic head** – gastrinoma, somatostatinoma

- All tumors can respond to debulking.
- **Liver** metastatic spread – 1st for all
- **Cholecystectomy** – indicated for **glucagonoma** and **VIPoma** to avoid **gallstones** with prolonged octreotide Tx for potentially metastatic disease; also needed for **somatostatinoma** (Metastases may continue to release somatostatin.)
- **MEN-**1 patients treated similarly to sporadic with exception of gastrinoma (see below)
- **Insulinoma**
  - Most common **functional PNET**
  - Symptoms: **Whipple's triad** – fasting **hypoglycemia** ($<$ 55), **symptoms** of hypoglycemia (confusion, LOC, seizures, ↑ HR, combativeness, diaphoresis), and **relief with glucose**
  - **90%** are **benign**; **evenly distributed** throughout pancreas
  - Dx (*after 72-hour fast*):
    - **Insulin** $>$ 36 pmol/L
    - **C peptide** $>$ 0.6 mg/mL ($>$ 0.2 nmol/L)
    - **Proinsulin** $>$ 5 pg/mL ($>$ 20 pmol/L)
    - **Insulin/C peptide ratio** $<$ 1 (*convert C peptide to pmol/L*)
    - **Beta-hydroxybutyrate** $<$ 2.7 mmol/L
    - *Absence* of sulfonylureas
  - If C peptide and proinsulin *not* elevated → suspect **Munchausen's syndrome**
  - Localization – **triple phase CT scan** (or MRI) and **EUS**
    - If not localized with above – need **selective intra-arterial calcium injection with hepatic venous sampling** for insulin
    - Somatostatin scintigraphy *not* effective for insulinoma
  - Tx: enucleate if $<$ 2 cm; formal resection if $>$ 2 cm
    - For metastatic disease → **5FU** and **streptozocin**; octreotide
    - **Diazoxide** for symptoms
- **Gastrinoma** (Zollinger–Ellison syndrome [ZES])
  - Most common PNET in **MEN-1 patients**
  - 50% **multiple**
  - 75% **malignant**
  - 75% **spontaneous** and 25% **MEN-1**
  - 75% in **gastrinoma triangle** – common bile duct, neck of pancreas, third portion of the duodenum
  - Symptoms: **refractory** or **complicated peptic ulcer disease** (despite aggressive PPI and *H. pylori* eradication Tx), **diarrhea** (improved with PPI), abdominal pain, weight loss
  - Can have multiple ulcers or ulcers that extend beyond 1st portion of the duodenum

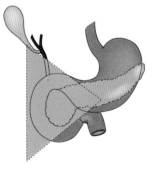

Most gastrinomas are found within the gastrinoma triangle.

- Elevated **serum gastrin** (> 200 pg/mL) _combined_ with **stomach basal acid output** > 15 mEq/hr _or_ **gastric pH < 2** (trying to make sure high gastrin level is not due to PPI/H$_2$ blockers)
  - Fasting gastrin levels > 1,000 is diagnostic.
- **Secretin stimulation test** (used if still not sure after above) – ZES patients (paradoxical effect): ↑ **gastrin** (> 200); normal patients: ↓ gastrin
- **Localization studies** – triphasic CT scan (or MRI), EUS
  - **Somatostatin receptor scintigraphy** (SRS) – _single best study for localizing tumor_
- **Sporadic gastrinoma** Tx: **enucleation** if < 2 cm; **formal resection** if > 2 cm; include **periduodenal lymph node dissection**; excise any other suspicious nodes.
  - Unable to localize → exploration with palpation, intraop U/S, and intraop upper endoscopy (with transillumination) to help localize; perform **duodenotomy** and look inside duodenum for tumor (15% of microgastrinomas there)
  - **Duodenal tumor** – resection with primary closure (need periduodenal lymph node dissection); may need Whipple if extensive; be sure to check pancreas for primary
  - **Debulking** – can improve symptoms; PPI helps palliate metastatic disease
- **MEN-1 gastrinoma Tx**: aims at **medical therapy** unless tumor > 2 cm
  - Due to multiplicity of small gastrinoma and rare surgical cure without extensive resection (ie total pancreatectomy)
- **Glucagonoma**
  - Symptoms (4 D's): **Diabetes**, **Dermatitis** (**rash** – necrolytic migratory erythema), **Depression**, **DVT**, weight loss
  - Most **malignant** (90%); most in **distal pancreas**
  - Diagnosis: fasting glucagon level and glucose intolerance
  - Localization: triphasic CT scan (or MRI), EUS, SRS
  - Tx: **formal resection** with regional lymph node dissection for all (_high malignancy rate_)
  - Perform **cholecystectomy** with resection.
  - Zinc, amino acids, or fatty acids may treat skin rash.
- **VIPoma** (Verner–Morrison syndrome)
  - Symptoms: **watery diarrhea, hypokalemia**, and **achlorhydria** (WDHA)
  - Hypokalemia from diarrhea
  - Most **malignant**; most in **distal pancreas**, 10% extrapancreatic (adrenal gland, retroperitoneal, mediastinum)
  - Dx: exclude other causes of diarrhea; ↑ VIP levels
  - Localization: triphasic CT scan (or MRI), EUS, SRS
  - Tx: **formal resection** with regional lymph node dissection for all (_high malignancy rate_)
  - Perform **cholecystectomy** with resection.
- **Somatostatinoma**
  - **Very rare**
  - Symptoms: **diabetes, gallstones, steatorrhea**
  - Diagnosis: fasting somatostatin level
  - Most **malignant**; most in **head of pancreas**
  - Localization: triphasic CT scan (or MRI), EUS, SRS
  - Perform **cholecystectomy** with resection.
  - Tx: **formal resection** with regional lymph node dissection for all (_high malignancy rate_)

34 Spleen

ANATOMY AND PHYSIOLOGY

- **Short gastrics** and **splenic artery** are end arteries.
  - **Gastrosplenic** ligament – contains **short gastric arteries**
  - **Splenorenal** ligament – contains **splenic vessels** and tail of pancreas
- Splenic vein is posterior and inferior to the splenic artery.
- Spleen serves as an **antigen-processing center** for macrophages.
- Is the largest producer of **IgM** (most common antibody in the spleen)
- **85% red pulp** – acts as a filter for aged or damaged RBCs
  - **Pitting** – removal of abnormalities in RBC membrane
    - <u>Howell–Jolly bodies</u> – nuclear remnants
    - <u>Heinz bodies</u> – hemoglobin
  - **Culling** – removal of less deformable RBCs
- **15% white pulp** – immunologic function; contains lymphocytes and macrophages
  - Spleen is body's largest concentration of lymphoid tissue.
    - Lymphoid follicles – B cells
    - Periarterial lymphatics – T cells
  - Major site of **bacterial clearance that lacks preexisting antibodies**
  - Site of removal of **poorly opsonized bacteria**, **particles**, and **cellular debris**
  - Antigen processing occurs with interaction between **dendritic cells/macrophages** and **helper T cells**.

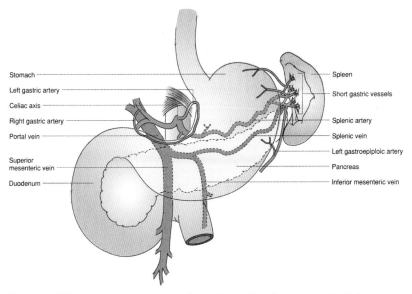

The arterial blood flow to the spleen is derived from the splenic artery, the left gastro-epiploic artery, and the short gastric arteries (vasa brevia). The venous drainage into this portal vein is also shown.

- **Tuftsin** – an opsonin; facilitates phagocytosis → produced in spleen
- **Properdin** – activates alternate complement pathway → produced in spleen
- **Hematopoiesis** – occurs in spleen before birth and in conditions such as myeloid dysplasia
- Spleen serves as a **reservoir for platelets**.
- **Accessory spleen** (20%) – most commonly found at *splenic hilum*
  - Dx: scintigraphy with ^{99}Tc-nanocolloid
- **Wandering spleen** – congenital lack of ligaments holding spleen in place
  - Spleen can end up in unusual parts of the abdomen (eg RLQ).
  - Can also twist around splenic artery (splenic torsion) causing infarction
  - Tx: **splenopexy**; splenectomy if infarcted
- **Indication for splenectomy** – idiopathic thrombocytopenic purpura (ITP) far greater than for thrombotic thrombocytopenic purpura (TTP)
- ITP most common nontraumatic condition requiring splenectomy

IDIOPATHIC THROMBOCYTOPENIC PURPURA (ITP)

- This can occur from many etiologies – drugs, viruses, etc.
- Caused by **anti-platelet antibodies (IgG to GpIIb/IIIa and Gp Ia/IIa)** – bind platelets; results in **decreased platelets**
- Petechiae, gingival bleeding, bruising, soft tissue ecchymosis
- **Spleen is normal.**
- In children < 10 years, ITP usually resolves spontaneously (*avoid* splenectomy in children).
- Tx: *steroids* (primary therapy); **IV-IG** (gammaglobulin) if steroid resistant
- Splenectomy indicated for those who <u>fail medical therapy</u> or who are <u>steroid dependent</u> (avoids long-term steroid use)
  - Removes IgG production and prevents platelets consumption
  - 80% respond after splenectomy.
  - Patients with a good response to steroids usually have a good response to splenectomy.
- Give platelets *after* ligation of the splenic artery if needed for intraop bleeding (prevents consumption of transfused platelets).

THROMBOTIC THROMBOCYTOPENIC PURPURA (TTP)

- Associated with medical reactions, infections, inflammation, autoimmune disease
- Due to ADAMTS13 defect (metalloproteinase that normally cleaves vWF)
- Causes **loss of platelet inhibition** – leads to platelet aggregation, thrombosis, and infarction; **profound thrombocytopenia**
- Purpura, fever, mental status changes, renal dysfunction, hematuria, hemolytic anemia
- 80% respond to medical therapy.
- Tx: *plasmapheresis* (primary); immunosuppression
- Death most commonly due to **intracerebral hemorrhage** or acute renal failure
- Splenectomy *rarely* indicated

POSTSPLENECTOMY SEPSIS SYNDROME (PSSS)

- 0.1% risk after splenectomy; ↑ risk in **children**
- Organisms – *S. pneumoniae* (#1), *H. influenzae, N. meningitidis*
- Secondary to specific lack of immunity (decreased **IgM**) to capsulated bacteria
- Highest in patients with splenectomy for **hemolytic disorders** (eg beta thalassemia) or **malignancy**
- Children also have ↑ risk of **acquiring** and of **mortality** after developing PSSS.
- Try to wait until at least **6 years old** before performing splenectomy → allows antibody formation; child can get fully immunized
- Most episodes occur within 2 years of splenectomy.

- Children < 10 years should be given prophylactic antibiotics for 6 months (daily Augmentin).
- **Vaccines needed _before_ splenectomy** – _Pneumococcus, Meningococcus, H. influenzae_
- Give vaccines at least 14 days before elective surgery or 14 days after emergency surgery.
- Inform parents to take child to the ED for any signs of infection so IV antibiotics can be started immediately.

Definition of Hypersplenism

Decrease in circulating cell count of erythrocytes and/or platelets and/or leukocytes
and
Normal compensatory hematopoietic responses present in bone marrow
and
Correction of cytopenia by splenectomy
with or without
Splenomegaly

HEMOLYTIC ANEMIAS: MEMBRANE PROTEIN DEFECTS

- **Spherocytosis**
  - **Most common congenital hemolytic anemia requiring splenectomy**
  - **Spectrin** deficit (**membrane protein**, autosomal dominant) leads to less deformable RBCs and splenic culling/sequestration (**hypersplenism**).
  - Causes anemia, splenomegaly, jaundice, pigmented stones
  - Try to perform splenectomy after age 6 in symptomatic patients (give immunizations 1st).
  - Tx: **splenectomy** and **cholecystectomy**
  - Splenectomy curative
- **Elliptocytosis**
  - Symptoms and mechanism similar to spherocytosis; less common
  - Spectrin and protein 4.1 deficit (**membrane protein**)

HEMOLYTIC ANEMIAS: NON–MEMBRANE PROTEIN DEFECTS

- **Pyruvate kinase deficiency**
  - Results in congenital hemolytic anemia
  - Caused by **altered glucose metabolism**
  - RBC survival is enhanced and transfusion requirements are decreased by splenectomy.
  - Is the most common congenital hemolytic anemia not involving a membrane protein that requires splenectomy
- **G6PD deficiency**
  - Precipitated by infection, certain drugs, fava beans
  - Splenectomy usually not required
- **Warm antibody–type acquired immune hemolytic anemia**
  - MC autoimmune hemolytic disease
  - Indication for splenectomy if refractory
- **Sickle cell anemia** – HgbA replaced with HgbS
  - Spleen usually autoinfarcts and splenectomy not required
- **Beta thalassemia**
  - Most common thalassemia; due to persistent HgbF
  - Major – both chains affected; minor – 1 chain, asymptomatic
  - Symptoms: pallor, retarded body growth, head enlargement
  - **Splenectomy** (if patient has splenomegaly) may decrease hemolysis and transfusion requirement.
  - Most die in teens secondary to hemosiderosis.
  - Medical Tx: blood transfusions and iron chelators (deferoxamine, deferiprone)

HODGKIN'S DISEASE

- A – asymptomatic
- B – symptomatic (night sweats, fever, weight loss) → unfavorable prognosis
- Stage I – 1 area or 2 contiguous areas on the same side of diaphragm
- Stage II – 2 non-contiguous areas on the same side of diaphragm
- Stage III – involved on each side of diaphragm
- Stage IV – liver, bone, lung, or any other non-lymphoid tissue except spleen
- See **Reed–Sternberg cells.**
- **Lymphocyte predominant** – best prognosis
- **Lymphocyte depleted** – worst prognosis
- **Nodular sclerosing** – most common
- **Lymphoma workup** – need 1) core needle biopsy of lymph node, 2) bone marrow biopsy, and 3) gallium MRI or PET scan of the liver and spleen
- Tx: chemo
- **MCC of chylous ascites** – *lymphoma*

NON-HODGKIN'S LYMPHOMA

- Worse prognosis than Hodgkin's; 90% are **B-cell** lymphomas.
- Generally systemic disease by the time the diagnosis is made
- Tx: chemo

OTHER CONDITIONS

- **Hairy cell leukemia** – Tx: rarely need splenectomy
- **Spontaneous splenic rupture** – mononucleosis, malaria, sepsis, sarcoid, leukemia, polycythemia vera
- **Splenosis** – splenic implants; usually related to trauma
- **Hyposplenism** – see Howell–Jolly bodies (*most reliable finding*)
  - If you don't see Howell–Jolly bodies and other signs of hyposplenism (see below) after splenectomy, suggest **accessory spleen.**
- **Pancreatitis** – most common cause of splenic artery or splenic vein thrombosis
- **Postsplenectomy changes** – ↑ RBCs, ↑ WBCs, ↑ platelets; if platelets $> 1 \times 10^6$, give ASA
- **Hemangioma** – #1 splenic tumor overall; #1 benign splenic tumor; Tx: splenectomy if symptomatic
- **Non-Hodgkin's lymphoma** – #1 malignant splenic tumor; MCC of splenomegaly
  - Rarely need splenectomy for **pan-cytopenia**
- **Angiosarcoma** – #1 malignant non-blood cell splenic tumor; RFs – arsenic, vinyl chloride, thorium dioxide, very aggressive with high mortality: Tx: **splenectomy** if resectable
- **Sarcoidosis of spleen** – anemia, ↓ platelets; Tx: splenectomy for symptomatic splenomegaly
- **Felty's syndrome** – rheumatoid arthritis, hepatomegaly, splenomegaly, and pancytopenia
  - Tx: methotrexate; treatment for RA usually helps.
  - Splenectomy for symptomatic splenomegaly
- **Splenic abscess** – usually from IVDA or endocarditis; sickle cell disease
  - Usually *Streptococcus*
  - **Unilocular** with a **thick wall** in a **stable** patient – U/S- or CT-guided percutaneous drainage
  - **Multilocular** or **thin-walled** or **unstable** patient – splenectomy
- **Simple splenic cysts** (congenital; is a primary cyst [true cyst] with epithelial lining)
  - Also called splenic **epithelial cysts** or splenic **epidermoid cysts**
  - **CT scan** – homogenous, well-defined hypodense lesion with nonenhancing rim

- <u>CT scan</u> and <u>serology</u> used to rule out parasitic (eg echinococcus) or malignant cysts
- **Infection** and **rupture risk** increased for cysts > 5 cm
- Tx: **Leave alone** unless **symptomatic** or **> 5 cm**; surgery is usually cyst excision, fenestration, or partial splenectomy (send cyst wall to pathology).
- **Posttraumatic splenic cyst** (is a <u>secondary</u> cyst [false cyst], <u>no</u> epithelial lining) – similar surgical indications as above
- **Echinococcal splenic cyst** – splenectomy
- **Splenic injury** (capsular tear) can occur with **stomach/colon** surgery.
- **Tail of the pancreas** – can be injured with splenectomy causing pancreatic leak and fluid collection; can cause fullness/pain
  - **CT scan** – shows low attenuation fluid collection in lesser sac/postsplenectomy space
  - **Tx**: percutaneous drain (<u>not</u> repeat surgery)

Results of Splenectomy/Hyposplenic Condition
ERYTHROCYTES
Howell–Jolly bodies (nuclear fragments)
Heinz bodies (hemoglobin deposits)
Pappenheimer bodies (iron deposits)
Target cells
Spur cells (acanthocytes)
PLATELETS
Transient thrombocytosis
LEUKOCYTES
Transient leukocytosis
Persistent lymphocytosis
Persistent monocytosis

35 Small Bowel

ANATOMY AND PHYSIOLOGY

- **Small intestine** – nutrient and water absorption
- **Large intestine** – water absorption
- **Duodenum**
  - **Bulb** (1st portion) – 90% of ulcers here
  - **Descending** (2nd) – contains ampulla of Vater (duct of Wirsung) and duct of Santorini
  - **Transverse** (3rd)
  - **Ascending** (4th)
  - Descending and transverse portions are **retroperitoneal**.
  - 3rd and 4th portions – transition point at the acute angle between the aorta (posterior) and **SMA** (anterior)
  - Vascular supply is **superior** (off gastroduodenal artery) and **inferior** (off SMA) **pancreaticoduodenal arteries**.
    - Both have anterior and posterior branches.
    - Many communications between these arteries

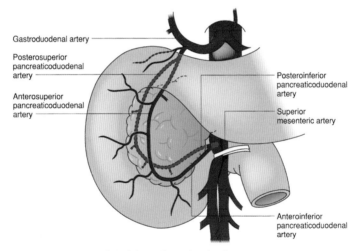

Arterial supply to the duodenum.

- **Jejunum**
  - 100 cm long; long vasa recta, circular muscle folds
  - Is the **maximum site of all absorption** except for B_{12} (terminal ileum), bile acids (ileum – nonconjugated; terminal ileum – conjugated), iron (duodenum), and folate (terminal ileum)
  - 95% of NaCl absorbed and 90% of water absorbed in jejunum
  - Vascular supply – SMA
- **Ileum** – 150 cm long; short vasa recta, flat
  - Vascular supply – SMA
- **Glutamine** is primary nutrient for small bowel.
- **Intestinal brush border** – maltase, sucrase, limit dextrinase, lactase
- **Normal sizes** – small bowel/transverse colon/cecum → **3/6/9 cm**

- SMA eventually branches into the **ileocolic artery**.
- **Cell types**
  - **Absorptive cells**
  - **Goblet cells** (mucin secretion)
  - **Paneth cells** (secretory granules, enzymes)
  - **Enterochromaffin cells** (APUD, 5-hydroxytryptamine release, carcinoid precursor)
  - **Brunner's glands** (alkaline solution)
  - **Peyer's patches** (lymphoid tissue); increased in the ileum
  - **M cells** – antigen-presenting cells in intestinal wall
- **IgA** – released into gut; also in mother's milk
- **Fe** – small bowel has both heme and Fe transporters
- **Migrating motor complex** (gut motility)
  - Phase I – rest
  - Phase II – acceleration and gallbladder contraction
  - Phase III – peristalsis
  - Phase IV – deceleration
  - **Motilin** is most important hormone in migrating motor complex (acts on **phase III peristalsis**).
- **Bile salts** (acids)
  - **95% of bile salts are reabsorbed.**
    - 50% passive absorption (nonconjugated bile salts) – 45% ileum, 5% colon
    - 50% active resorption (conjugated bile salts) in **terminal ileum** (Na/K ATPase); conjugated bile salts are absorbed only in the terminal ileum.
  - Gallstones form after terminal ileum resection from malabsorption of bile salts (get cholesterol stones).

SHORT-GUT SYNDROME

- Diagnosis is made on symptoms, not length of bowel.
- Symptoms: steatorrhea, weight loss, nutritional deficiency
- Lose fat, B_{12}, electrolytes, water
- **Sudan red stain** – checks for fecal fat
- **Schilling test** – checks for B_{12} absorption (radiolabeled B_{12} in urine)
- Probably need at least 75 cm to survive off TPN; 50 cm with competent ileocecal valve
- Tx: **Restrict fat**, **PPI** to reduce acid, **Lomotil** (diphenoxylate and atropine).

CAUSES OF STEATORRHEA

- **Gastric hypersecretion of acid** → ↓ pH → ↑ intestinal motility; interferes with fat absorption
- **Interruption of bile salt resorption** (eg terminal ileum resection) interferes with micelle formation and fat absorption.
- **Decreased pancreatic enzymes** (eg chronic pancreatitis)
- Steatorrhea causes malnutrition with **weight loss** as well as deficiency in **fat-soluble vitamins** (A, D, E, K) and **essential fatty acids**.

NONHEALING FISTULA

- **"FRIENDSS"** – mnemonic for nonhealing fistula causes: **f**oreign body, **r**adiation, **i**nflammatory bowel disease, **e**pithelialization, **n**eoplasm, **d**istal obstruction, **s**epsis/infection, **s**teroids
- High-output fistulas are more likely with proximal bowel (duodenum or proximal jejunum) and are less likely to close with conservative management.
- Colonic fistulas are more likely to close than those in small bowel.
- Patients with **persistent fever** or **sepsis** – need to check for **abscess** (fistulogram, abdominal CT, upper GI with small bowel follow-through)
- Can cause fluid/electrolyte loss, nutritional depletion, and skin erosion of abdominal wall

- Most fistulas are **iatrogenic** and treated conservatively 1st → NPO, TPN, skin protection (stoma appliance), octreotide
- Majority close spontaneously without surgery.
- Surgical options: Resect bowel segment containing fistula and perform primary anastomosis.

BOWEL OBSTRUCTION

- **Without previous surgery** (most common)
  - Small bowel – <u>hernia</u>
  - Large bowel – <u>cancer</u>
- **With previous surgery** (most common)
  - Small bowel – <u>adhesions</u>
  - Large bowel – <u>cancer</u>

Symptoms and Signs of Bowel Obstruction

Symptom or Sign	Proximal Small Bowel (Open Loop)	Distal Small Bowel (Open Loop)	Small Bowel (Closed Loop)	Colon and Rectum
Pain	Intermittent, intense, colicky; often relieved by vomiting	Intermittent to constant	Progressive, intermittent constant; rapidly worsens	Continuous
Vomiting	Large volumes; bilious and frequent	Low volume and frequency; progressively feculent with time	May be prominent (reflex)	Intermittent, not prominent; feculent when present
Tenderness	Epigastric or periumbilical; quite mild unless strangulation is present	Diffuse and progressive	Diffuse, progressive	Diffuse
Distention	Absent	Moderate to marked	Often absent	Marked
Obstipation	May not be present	Present	May not be present	Present

- Symptoms: nausea and vomiting, crampy abdominal pain, failure to pass gas or stool
- Abdominal x-ray: air–fluid level, distended loops of small bowel, distal decompression

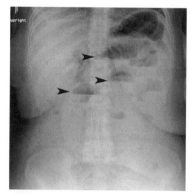

Plain upright abdominal film of a patient with small intestinal obstruction. Note the air–fluid levels in the stomach and multiple dilated loops of small intestine (*black arrows*) and absence of air in the colon or rectum.

- 3rd spacing of fluid into bowel lumen occurs – need **aggressive fluid resuscitation**
- Air with bowel obstruction – from **swallowed nitrogen**
- Tx: bowel rest, NG tube, IV fluids → cures 80% of partial SBO, 40% of complete SBO
- Surgical indications: **progressing pain**, **peritoneal signs**, **fever**, **increasing WBCs** (all signs of strangulation or perforation), or **failure to resolve**
- Obstruction from hernias should all be operated on to eliminate the hernia (either emergently if incarcerated or electively if reducible).

GALLSTONE ILEUS

- Small bowel obstruction from **gallstone** usually in the **terminal ileum**
- Classically see **air in the biliary tree** in a patient with small bowel obstruction
- Caused by a **fistula** between the **gallbladder** and **second portion of duodenum**
- Tx: Remove stone from terminal ileum.
  - Can leave gallbladder and fistula if patient too sick
  - If not too sick, perform cholecystectomy and close duodenum.

MECKEL'S DIVERTICULUM

- 2 ft from ileocecal valve; 2% of population; usually presents in 1st 2 years of life with bleeding; is a true diverticulum
- Caused by failure of closure of the **omphalomesenteric duct**
- Accounts for 50% of all **painless lower GI bleeds in children < 2 years**
- **Pancreas tissue** – most common tissue found in Meckel's (can cause **diverticulitis**)
- **Gastric mucosa** – most likely to be symptomatic (**bleeding** most common)
- **Obstruction** – most common presentation in adults
- **Incidental** → usually not removed unless gastric mucosa suspected (diverticulum feels thick) or has a very narrow neck
- Dx: can get a **Meckel's scan** (^{99}Tc) if having trouble localizing (mucosa lights up)
- Tx: **diverticulectomy** for uncomplicated diverticulitis or bleeding
  - Need **segmental resection** for **complicated** diverticulitis (eg perforation), **neck > ⅓ the diameter** of the normal bowel lumen, or if **diverticulitis involves the base**

DUODENAL DIVERTICULA

- Need to rule out gallbladder-duodenal fistula
- **Observe** unless perforated, bleeding, causing obstruction, or highly symptomatic.
- Frequency of diverticula: duodenal > jejunal > ileal
- Tx: **segmental resection** if significantly symptomatic and outside the 2nd portion of the duodenum
  - If **juxta-ampullary** usually can't get resection and need **choledochojejunostomy** for <u>biliary</u> or **ERCP with stent** for <u>pancreatitis</u> symptoms (*avoid* Whipple here)

CROHN'S DISEASE

- Inflammatory bowel disease causing intermittent **abdominal pain**, **diarrhea**, and **weight loss**; can also cause **bowel obstructions** and **fistulas**
- Bimodal distribution at presentation: 20–30s, 50–60s; ↑ in Ashkenazi Jews
- Extraintestinal manifestations – arthritis, arthralgias, pyoderma gangrenosum (erythema nodosum), ocular diseases (uveitis), growth failure, megaloblastic anemia from folate and vitamin B$_{12}$ malabsorption in terminal ileum
- Can occur anywhere from mouth to anus; usually **spares rectum**
- **Terminal ileum** – most commonly involved bowel segment
- **Anal/perianal disease** – 1st presentation in 5% (MC: large skin tags – *do not resect*)

- **Most common sites for initial presentation**
  - **Terminal ileum** and cecum – 40%
  - Colon only – 35%
  - Small bowel only – 20%
  - Perianal – 5%
- Dx: Colonoscopy with biopsies and enteroclysis can help make the diagnosis.

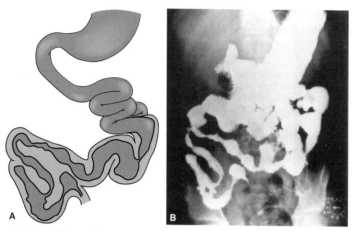

Typical radiographic appearance of extensive jejunoileal Crohn's disease.

- **Pathology** – transmural involvement, segmental disease (skip lesions), cobblestoning, narrow deep ulcers, creeping fat
- Medical Tx: **mesalamine** and **loperamide** for maintenance; **steroids** for acute flares
  - **Remicade** (infliximab; TNF-α inhibitor) – for fistulas or steroid-resistant disease
  - **Flagyl** – good for fistulas and perianal disease
  - Add **Cipro** and **Flagyl** for acute flares if worried about infection or toxic megacolon/colitis.
  - <u>No</u> agents affect the natural course of disease.
  - **TPN** – may induce remission and fistula closure with small bowel Crohn's disease
- **90%** eventually need an **operation**.
- **Complications related to Crohn's** – unlike ulcerative colitis, surgery is <u>not</u> curative
  - **Obstruction** – from **inflammation**; often partial; can be initially treated conservatively
  - **Strictures** – from **scarring**; consider stricturoplasty vs resection (see below)
    - Can try balloon dilatation if reachable by endoscopy
  - **Abscess** – usually treated with percutaneous drainage
  - **Free perforation** – unusual but can occur (2%); need resection
  - **Toxic megacolon/colitis** – unusual but can occur; surgery if refractory
  - **Hemorrhage** – unusual in Crohn's but can occur
  - **Blind loop obstruction** – need resection
  - **Fissures** – *no lateral internal sphincteroplasty in patients with Crohn's disease*
  - **Enterocutaneous fistula** – can usually be treated conservatively
  - **Perineal fistula** – rule out abscess; use draining setons; let heal on its own
  - **Anorectovaginal fistulas** – may need <u>rectal advancement flap</u>; possible colostomy
- Do <u>not</u> need clear margins; just get 2 cm away from gross disease with surgery.
- Try to **preserve bowel** as much as possible; patients will often need multiple resections over their lifetime (short gut syndrome becomes a problem).

- Patients with **diffuse severe disease of colon** – proctocolectomy and ileostomy the procedures of choice (*no pouches or ilio-anal anastomosis with Crohn's*)
- **Incidental finding of inflammatory bowel disease** in patient with presumed appendicitis who has normal appendix – Tx: **remove appendix** if cecum not involved (avoids future confounding diagnosis)
- **Stricturoplasty**
  - Simplest – longitudinal incision through stricture, close transversely (good for strictures **< 10 cm** in length)
  - Consider if patient has multiple bowel strictures to save small bowel length.
  - Probably not good for patient's 1st operation as it leaves disease behind
  - Isolated short segment stricture – resection preferred
  - Need biopsy of strictured segment to rule out CA
  - Contraindications to stricturoplasty – fistula, perforation, inflammation, malnutrition, CA
  - 10% leakage/abscess/fistula rate with stricturoplasty (all of which can usually be treated conservatively)
- 50% recurrence rate requiring surgery for Crohn's disease after resection
- **Crohn's pancolitis** – same **colon CA risk** as UC however colon CA sites are **evenly distributed throughout the colon** (unlike UC which has rectosigmoid predominance)
- Complications from **removal of terminal ileum**
  - ↓ **B_{12} uptake** can result in **megaloblastic anemia**.
  - ↓ **bile salt uptake** causes osmotic **diarrhea** (bile salts) and **steatorrhea** (fat) in colon.
  - ↓ **oxalate binding to calcium secondary to** ↑ **intraluminal fat** (fat binds Ca) → oxalate then gets absorbed in colon → released in urine → **Ca oxalate kidney stones** (hyperoxaluria)
  - **Gallstones** can form after terminal ileum resection from malabsorption of bile salts.

CARCINOID

- **Serotonin** is produced by **Kulchitsky cells** (enterochromaffin cell or argentaffin cell).
  - Part of amine precursor uptake decarboxylase system (**APUD**)
  - **5-HIAA** is a breakdown product of serotonin – can measure this in urine
- **Carcinoid syndrome** – caused by bulky **liver metastases**
  - Intermittent **flushing** (kallikrein) and **diarrhea** (serotonin) – hallmark symptoms
  - Can also get **asthma-type symptoms** (bradykinin) and **right heart valve lesions**
  - If patient has carcinoid syndrome with small bowel carcinoid primary, it **indicates metastasis to liver** (liver usually clears serotonin).
  - If resection of liver metastases is performed, perform cholecystectomy in case of future embolization.
  - **Octreotide scan** – best for *localizing* tumor not seen on CT scan
  - **Chromogranin A level** – highest sensitivity for *detecting* a carcinoid tumor
- **Appendix carcinoid** – most common site for carcinoid tumor (50% of carcinoids arise here; ileum and rectum next most common)
- **Small bowel carcinoid** – patients at ↑ risk for **multiple primaries** and **second unrelated malignancies**
- **Carcinoid Tx:**
  - **Carcinoid in appendix** – **< 2 cm** → appendectomy; **≥ 2 cm or involving base** → right hemicolectomy
  - **Chemotherapy – streptozocin** and **5FU**; usually just for **unresectable disease**
  - **Octreotide** – useful for carcinoid syndrome palliation
  - **Bronchospasm** – Tx: **albuterol inhalers**
  - **Flushing** – Tx: **α-blockers** (phenothiazine)
  - **False 5-HIAA** – fruits

INTUSSUSCEPTION IN ADULTS

- Can occur from small bowel or cecal tumors
- Most common presentation is obstruction.
- Worrisome in adults as it often has a **malignant lead point** (ie cecal CA)
- Tx: resection

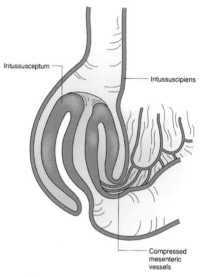

Anatomy of intussusception. The intussusceptum is the segment of bowel that invaginates into the intussuscipiens.

BENIGN SMALL BOWEL TUMORS

- **Adenomas** – most found in duodenum; present with bleeding, obstruction
  - Need resection when identified (often done with endoscope)
- **Peutz–Jeghers syndrome** (STK11 gene mutation; autosomal dominant)
  - Benign **hamartomas** throughout GI tract (small and large bowel)
  - Mucocutaneous melanotic **skin pigmentation**
  - Patients have ↑ **extraintestinal malignancies** (most common – **breast CA**).
  - Small risk (< 3%) of GI malignancies; **_no prophylactic colectomy_**

MALIGNANT SMALL BOWEL TUMORS (RARE)

- **Adenocarcinoma** (rare) – most common malignant small bowel tumor
  - High proportion is in the **duodenum**.
  - Symptoms: obstruction, jaundice
  - Can also arise from the ampulla of Vater (Sx's – jaundice, anemia, guaiac-positive stools)
  - Tx: resection and adenectomy; **Whipple** if in **2nd portion of duodenum**
- **Duodenal CA risk factors**: FAP, Gardner's, polyps, adenomas, von Recklinghausen's
- **Leiomyosarcoma**
  - Usually in **jejunum** and **ileum**; most extraluminal
  - Hard to differentiate compared with leiomyoma (> 5 mitoses/50 HPF, atypia, necrosis)
  - Make sure it is not a GIST (check for C-Kit).
  - Tx: resection; <u>no</u> adenectomy required

- **Lymphoma**
  - Usually in **ileum**; associated with Wegener's, SLE, AIDS, Crohn's, celiac sprue
  - Usually **NHL B cell** type
  - Posttransplantation – ↑ **risk of bleeding** and **perforation**
  - Dx: abdominal CT, node sampling
  - Tx: **wide en bloc resection** (include nodes) unless 1st or 2nd portion of the duodenum (chemo-XRT, <u>no</u> Whipple)
  - 40% 5-year survival rate

STOMAS

- **Parastomal hernias** – highest incidence with colostomies; generally well tolerated and do not need repair unless symptomatic
- *Candida* – most common stomal infection
- **Diversion colitis** (Hartmann's pouch) – secondary to lack of short-chain fatty acids
  - Tx: short-chain fatty acid enemas
- **Ischemia** – most common cause of stenosis of stoma
  - Tx: dilation if mild
- **Crohn's disease** – most common cause of fistula near stoma site
- **Abscesses** – underneath stoma site, often caused by irrigation device
- **Gallstones** (loss of bile salts) and **uric acid kidney stones** (loss of HCO_3^-) – increased in patients with ileostomy

APPENDICITIS

- **Appendicitis** – 1st: anorexia; 2nd: abdominal pain (periumbilical); 3rd: vomiting
- Pain gradually migrates to the RLQ as peritonitis sets in.
- Most commonly occurs in patients 20–35 years
- Patients can have normal WBC count.
- **CT scan** – <u>diameter > 7 mm</u> or <u>wall thickness > 2 mm</u> (looks like a bull's eye), fat stranding, no contrast in appendiceal lumen; try to give rectal contrast
- **Midpoint of anti-mesenteric border** – area most likely to **perforate**
- **Lymphoid hyperplasia** – most common cause in children; can follow a viral illness
- **Fecalith** – most common cause in adults
- Luminal obstruction is followed by distention of the appendix, venous congestion and thrombosis, ischemia, gangrene necrosis, and finally rupture.
- **Nonoperative situation** – CT scan shows walled-off perforated appendix (usually in **elderly**)
  - Tx: **percutaneous drainage** and **interval appendectomy** at later date as long as symptoms are improving
  - Consider follow-up barium enema or colonoscopy to rule out perforated cecal colon CA.
- **Children** and **elderly** have higher propensity to rupture secondary to <u>delayed diagnosis</u>.
  - Children often have **higher fever** and more **vomiting and diarrhea**.
  - **Elderly** – signs and symptoms can be minimal; may need right hemicolectomy if cancer suspected
- **Appendicitis is infrequent in infants.**
- **Perforation** – patient generally more ill; can have evidence of sepsis
- **Appendicitis during pregnancy**
  - **Most common cause** of **acute abdominal pain** in the **1st trimester**
  - More likely to **occur** in the **2nd trimester** but is not the most common cause of abdominal pain
  - More likely to **perforate** in the **3rd trimester** – confused with contractions
  - **Need to make the incision where the patient is having pain** – the appendix is *displaced superiorly (cephalad)*

- May have symptoms of RUQ pain in the 3rd trimester
- 35% fetal mortality with rupture
- Women with suspected appendicitis need beta-HCG drawn and abdominal ultrasound to rule out OB/GYN causes of abdominal pain.

OTHER APPENDIX

- **Appendix mucocele** – can be benign or malignant mucinous tumor (signet ring cells); needs resection (**should open** for these so you don't spill tumor contents)
  - Need right hemicolectomy if malignant
  - Can get **pseudomyxoma peritonei** with rupture (spread of tumor implants throughout the peritoneum)
  - **MCC of death** – **small bowel obstruction** from peritoneal tumor spread
- **Regional ileitis** – can mimic appendicitis; 10% go on to Crohn's disease
- **Gastroenteritis** – nausea, vomiting, diarrhea
- **Presumed appendicitis** but find ruptured ovarian cyst, thrombosed ovarian vein, or regional enteritis not involving cecum → **still perform appendectomy** (prevents future confounding diagnosis)

ILEUS

- Causes include surgery (most common), electrolyte abnormalities ($\downarrow$ K), peritonitis, ischemia, trauma, drugs.
- **Ileus** – dilatation is uniform throughout the stomach, small bowel, colon, and rectum *without* decompression; no passage of gas; absent bowel sounds
- **Obstruction** – there is <u>bowel decompression</u> distal to the obstruction

TYPHOID ENTERITIS (SALMONELLA)

- Children; get RLQ pain, diarrhea, fever, headaches, maculopapular rash, leukopenia; rare bleeding/perforation
- Large mesenteric lymph nodes
- Tx: **Bactrim**

36 Colorectal

ANATOMY AND PHYSIOLOGY

- Colon secretes **K** and reabsorbs **Na and water** (mostly in right colon and cecum).
- **4 layers** – mucosa (columnar epithelium) → submucosa → muscularis propria → serosa
  - **Muscularis mucosa** – small interwoven inner muscle layer just below mucosa but above basement membrane
  - **Muscularis propria** – circular layer of muscle
- Ascending, descending, and sigmoid colon are all **retroperitoneal**.
  - Peritoneum covers anterior upper and middle ⅓ of the rectum.
- **Plicae semilunares** – transverse bands that form haustra
- **Taenia coli** – 3 bands that run longitudinally along colon. At rectosigmoid junction, the taeniae become broad and completely encircle the bowel.
- **Rectum** – extends from where taenia splay to anorectal ring (12–15 cm in length)
- **Anal canal** – extends from anorectal ring (puborectalis) to anal verge (squamous mucosa and perianal skin junction)
- **Anal margin** – from squamous mucocutaneous junction to 5 cm out radially

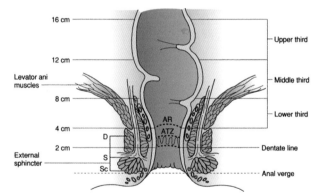

Anorectal anatomy with important landmarks. Approximate measurements are relative to the anal verge. AR, anorectal ring; ATZ, anal transition zone; D, deep; S, superficial; Sc, subcutaneous.

- **Vascular supply**
  - **Ascending** and ⅔ **of transverse colon** supplied by **SMA** (ileocolic, right and middle colic arteries)
  - ⅓ **transverse, descending colon**, **sigmoid colon**, and **upper portion of the rectum** supplied by **IMA** (left colic, sigmoid branches, superior rectal artery)
  - **Marginal artery** – runs along colon margin, connecting SMA to IMA (provides collateral flow)
  - **Arc of Riolan** (meandering mesenteric artery) – short direct collateral connection between SMA and IMA
  - 80% of blood flow goes to mucosa and submucosa.
- **Venous drainage** follows arterial except IMV, which goes to the splenic vein.
  - Splenic vein joins the SMV to form the portal vein behind the pancreas.
- **Superior rectal artery** – branch of **IMA**

- **Middle rectal artery** – branch of **internal iliac** (the lateral stalks during low anterior resection [LAR] or abdominoperineal resection [APR] contain the middle rectal arteries)
- **Inferior rectal artery** – branch of <u>internal pudendal</u> (which is a branch of **internal iliac**)
- <u>Superior</u> rectal vein drain into the IMV and eventually the <u>portal vein</u>.
- <u>Middle</u> and <u>inferior</u> rectal veins drain into the internal iliac veins and eventually the <u>IVC</u>.
- **Superior** and **middle rectum** – drain to IMA nodal lymphatics
- **Lower rectum** – drains primarily to IMA nodes, also to internal iliac nodes

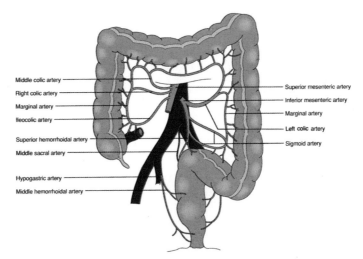

Arterial blood supply of the colon. The superior mesenteric artery (SMA) and inferior mesenteric artery (IMA) are the major blood supplies to the colon.

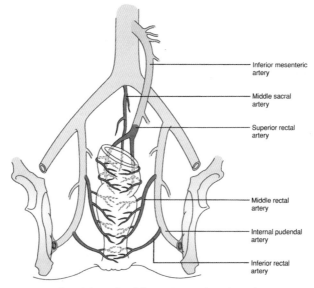

Arterial supply of the rectum and anal canal.

- Bowel wall contains mucosal and submucosal lymphatics.
- **Watershed areas**
  - Splenic flexure (Griffith's point) – SMA and IMA junction
  - Rectum (Sudeck's point) – superior rectal and middle rectal junction
  - **Hypotension** or low-flow state causes ischemia in these areas.
  - Colon more sensitive to ischemia than small bowel secondary to ↓ collaterals
- **External sphincter** (puborectalis muscle) – under CNS (voluntary) control
  - Inferior rectal branch of **internal pudendal nerve**
  - Is the continuation of the **levator ani muscle** (striated muscle)
- **Internal sphincter** – involuntary control
  - **Pelvic splanchnic nerves**
  - Is the continuation of the **muscularis propria** (smooth muscle)
  - Is normally contracted
- **Meissner's plexus** – inner nerve plexus
- **Auerbach's plexus** – outer nerve plexus
- **Pelvic splanchnic nerves** – parasympathetic
- **From anal verge** – anal canal 0–5 cm, rectum 5–15 cm, rectosigmoid junction 15–18 cm
- **Levator ani** – marks the transition between anal canal and rectum
- **Crypts of Lieberkühn** – mucin-secreting goblet cells
- **Colonic inertia** – slow transit time; patients may need subtotal colectomy
- **Short-chain fatty acids** (Butyrate) – main nutrient of colonocytes
- **Stump pouchitis** (diversion or disuse proctitis) – Tx: short-chain fatty acid enema
- **Infectious pouchitis** – Tx: metronidazole (Flagyl)
- **Denonvilliers' fascia** (anterior) – rectovesicular and rectoprostatic fascia in men; rectovaginal fascia in women
- **Waldeyer's fascia** (posterior) – rectosacral fascia

POLYPS

- **Hyperplastic polyps** – most common polyp; no cancer risk
- **Tubular adenoma** – most common (75%) intestinal neoplastic polyp
  - These are generally pedunculated.
- **Villous adenoma** – most likely to produce symptoms
  - These are generally sessile and larger than tubular adenomas.
  - 50% of villous adenomas have **cancer**.
- **> 2 cm**, **sessile**, or **villous** lesions have ↑ cancer risk.
- Polyps have left-side predominance.
- Most **pedunculated polyps** can be removed endoscopically.
- If not able to get all of the polyp (which usually occurs with **sessile polyps**) → need **segmental resection**
- **High-grade dysplasia** – basement membrane is intact (carcinoma in situ)
- **Intramucosal cancer** – into muscularis mucosa (carcinoma in situ → still has not gone through basement membrane)
- **Invasive cancer** – into submucosa (T1)
- **Screening** – **45–75** for **normal risk**, **40–75** (or 10 years before youngest case) for **intermediate risk** (1 first-degree relative with colon CA or 2 second-degree relatives with colon CA)
- **Screening options**:
  1) **colonoscopy** every 10 years _or_;
  2) **CT colonography** every 5 years _or_;
  3) **flexible sigmoidoscopy** every 5 years _or_;
  4) **mt-sDNA** stool tests every 3 years _or_;
  5) **highly sensitive** fecal immunochemical **(FIT)** or guaiac **(gFOBT)** stool tests every year
  - **False-positive guaiac** – beef, vitamin C, iron, cimetidine
  - <u>No</u> colonoscopy with recent MI, splenomegaly, pregnancy (if fluoroscopy planned)

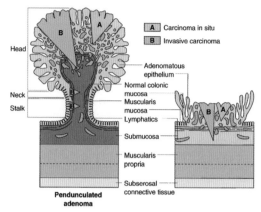

Pedunculated adenoma

Diagrammatic representation of cancer-containing polyps. Pedunculated adenoma is described on the left and a sessile adenoma on the right. In carcinoma in situ, malignant cells are confined to the mucosa. These lesions are adequately treated by endoscopic polypectomy. Polypectomy is adequate treatment for invasive carcinoma only if the margin is sufficient (2 mm), the carcinoma is not poorly differentiated, and no evidence of venous or lymphatic invasion is found.

- **Polypectomy shows T1 lesion** – polypectomy is adequate if margins are clear (2 mm), is well moderately differentiated, has no vascular/lymphatic/nerve invasion, and ability to remove polyp in 1 piece; otherwise, need formal colon resection
- **Extensive low rectal villous adenomas with atypia** – Tx: transanal excision (can try mucosectomy) as much of the polyp as possible
  - **No APR unless cancer is present.**
- **Pathology shows T1 lesion after transanal excision of villous rectal polyp** → transanal excision is adequate if < 4 cm, < ⅓ of bowel lumen diameter, margins are clear (2 mm), it is well moderately differentiated, and it has no vascular/lymphatic/nerve invasion
- **Pathology shows T2 lesion after transanal excision of villous rectal polyp** → patient needs APR or LAR
- **Repeat colonoscopy** interval after polyp removal:
  - Hyperplastic polyps (normal screening)   10 years
  - **1–2** tubular adenomas (well-moderate differentiation)   5 years
  - **3–10** or advanced adenoma (> 1 cm, high grade, dysplasia, or villous)   3 years
  - **> 10** (consider syndrome)   1 year
  - Large sessile adenoma (confirms complete resection, get biopsy)   3 months

COLORECTAL CANCER

- **2nd leading cause of CA death**
- Symptoms: **anemia**, **constipation** (narrow caliber stools), and lower GI **bleeding**
- Red meat and **fat** → O_2 radicals are thought to have a role
- Colon CA has had an association with *Clostridium septicum* infection.
- **Colon CA** – main gene mutations are **APC, DCC, p53**, and **k-ras**
- **Sigmoid colon** – most common site of primary
- **Disease spread**
  - Spreads to **nodes** first
  - **Nodal status** – most important prognostic factor
    - Need tumor deposit ≥ **0.2 mm** to be considered positive

- **Liver** – #1 site of metastases; lung – #2 site of metastases
  - Portal vein → **liver metastases**; iliac vein → **lung metastases**
  - **Liver metastases** – if resectable and leaves adequate liver function, patients have 35% 5-year survival (5-YS) rate
  - **Lung metastases** – 25% 5-YS rate in selected patients after resection
  - Potentially resectable **isolated liver** or **lung metastases** should be **resected** (preop chemo [+ XRT for rectal CA], re-stage, resect).
- 5% get drop metastases to **ovaries**.
- **Rectal CA** – can metastasize to **spine directly via Batson's plexus** (venous)
- **Colon CA** typically does not go to bone.
- Colorectal CA growing into **adjacent organs** can be resected **en bloc** with a portion of the adjacent organ (eg partial bladder resection, Whipple for colon CA growing into pancreatic head).
- **Lymphocytic penetration** – patients have an improved prognosis
- **Mucoepidermoid** – worst prognosis
- **Workup:**
  - Need **total colonoscopy** to rule out **synchronous lesions**
  - **CT chest/abdomen/pelvis** – look for metastatic disease
  - **Rigid proctoscopy** – for rectal tumors to assess level of tumor
  - **Endorectal ultrasound** (ERUS) – for rectal tumors; good at assessing depth of invasion (sphincter involvement), recurrence, and lymphadenopathy; best test for T and N status
  - **Rectal MRI** – good at assessing **circumferential margin** (distance between tumor and mesorectum; prognostic indicator)
  - **CEA**
- **Goals of resection**
  - **En bloc resection** – ensure adequate margins (ideally **5–7 cm**)
    - Include mesocolon and regional adenectomy.
    - Take Waldeyer's and Denonvilliers' fascia (**mesorectal fascia**) for rectal tumors.
  - Want at least **12 nodes** for adequate lymphadenectomy
    - **Higher number of nodes taken** equates with **improved survival** for colon CA (not clear for rectal CA).
  - Usually want at least **2-cm margins**
    - **1-cm margins** can be accepted in low rectal tumors if it means LAR vs APR.
  - **Most right-sided colon CAs** can be treated with primary anastomosis without ostomy.
  - **Rectal pain with rectal CA** – patient needs APR
- **Intraoperative ultrasound** (U/S) – best method of picking up intrahepatic metastases
  - Conventional U/S resolution: 10 mm
  - Abdominal CT: 5-10 mm
  - Abdominal MRI: 5-10 mm (better resolution than CT)
  - Intraoperative U/S: 3-5 mm
- **Low anterior resection** (LAR) – removes **sigmoid colon** and varying amount of **rectum**
- **Abdominoperineal resection** (APR)
  - Permanent colostomy; anal canal is excised along with the rectum.
  - Can have impotence and bladder dysfunction (injured pudendal nerves)
  - Indicated for malignant lesions only (not benign tumors) that are not amenable to LAR
  - Need at least a **1-cm margin** (1 cm from levator ani muscles) for LAR, otherwise will need APR
  - Risk of local recurrence higher with rectal CA than with colon CA in general
- **Preoperative chemo-XRT** – produces complete response in some patients with rectal CA; preserves sphincter function in some

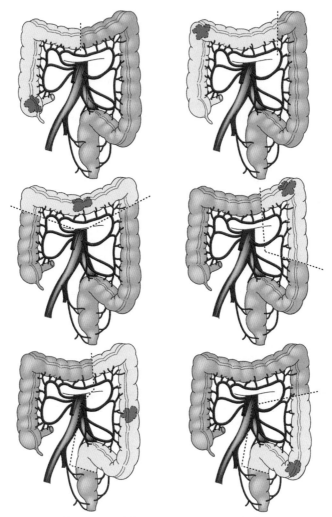

Segmental resections for cancers of the colon and upper third of the rectum. Note the blood supply taken with each form of resection.

- **Low rectal T1** (limited to submucosa) – can be excised transanally if < 4 cm, < ⅓ of bowel lumen diameter, has negative margins (need **2 mm**), is well moderately differentiated, and there is no nerve/vascular/nodal invasion; otherwise, patient needs APR or LAR.
- **Low rectal T2** or higher (muscularis propria or greater) – Tx: APR or LAR
- **Chemotherapy**
  - **Stage III colon CA** (nodes positive) → **postop chemo**, no XRT
  - **Stage IV colon CA** that is potentially resectable (distant metastases) → **preop chemo**, re-stage, and **postop chemo**, no XRT
  - Unresectable colon CA – **chemo** only

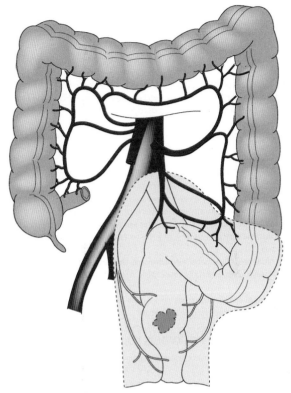

Extent of surgery in abdominoperineal resection.

TNM STAGING SYSTEM FOR COLORECTAL CANCER

- **T1**: into submucosa. **T2**: into muscularis propria. **T3**: into subserosa or through muscularis propria if no serosa is present. **T4a**: through serosa into free peritoneal cavity **T4b**: into adjacent organs/structures if no serosa is present
- **N0**: nodes negative. **N1**: 1–3 nodes positive, **N2a**: 4–6 nodes positive, **N2b**: ≥ 7 nodes positive, **N3**: central nodes positive
- **M1**: distant metastases

Stage	TNM Status
0	Tis, N0, M0
I	T1–2, N0, M0
IIA	T3, N0, M0
IIB	T4, N0, M0
IIIA	T1–2, N1, M0
IIIB	T3–4, N1, M0
IIIC	Any T, N2, M0
IV	Any T, Any N, M1

- **Stage II** and **III rectal CA** → **preop chemo-XRT** (neoadjuvant) and **postop chemo**
- **Stage IV rectal CA** that is potentially resectable → **preop chemo-XRT**, re-stage, and **postop chemo**
- Unresectable rectal CA → **chemo-XRT** _only_
- For unresectable colon/rectal CA – surgery only for bleeding, perforation, or obstruction
  - **Stent** preferred for obstruction; resection vs colostomy if that fails
- **Chemo regimen** – **5FU**, _leucovorin_, and _oxaliplatin_ (_FOLFOX_) for **6 months** postop (or **3 months preop** and **3 months postop**)
- XRT
  - ↓ local recurrence and ↑ survival when _combined_ with **chemotherapy**
  - **XRT damage** – _rectum_ most common site of injury → vasculitis, thrombosis, ulcers, strictures, bleeding
  - **Preop chemo-XRT** may help shrink **rectal tumors**, allowing down-staging of the tumor and possibly allowing LAR versus APR.
  - **XRT regimen** – 5,000 cGY over 6 weeks (5FU acts as radiosensitizer)
- **20% have a recurrence** (usually occurs within 1 year).
  - 5% get **another primary** – _main reason for_ **surveillance colonoscopy after 1 year**
- **Follow-up colonoscopy at 1 year** – mainly to check for **new primary colon CA** (metachronous)
- **Complete clinical response after neoadjuvant therapy** – still need **resection** (of primary area and any previous potentially resectable metastases) as complete pathologic response is rare
- **Isolated peritoneal carcinomatosis** (no other distant metastases); Tx: **cytoreductive surgery** and heated **intraperitoneal chemo**

FAMILIAL ADENOMATOUS POLYPOSIS (FAP)

- Autosomal dominant; all have cancer by age 40
- **APC gene** – chromosome 5
- 20% of FAP syndromes are spontaneous
- Polyps <u>not</u> present at birth; are present in **puberty**
- Start yearly screening colonoscopy at **age 10**.
- Get **1,000s of polyps** (carpet the colon).
- Do <u>not</u> need colonoscopy for surveillance in patients with suspected FAP → just need flexible sigmoidoscopy to check for polyps
- All need **total colectomy prophylactically** at **age 20**.
- **Also get duodenal polyps** → need to check duodenum with endoscopy every 1–2 years
- **Surgery** – **proctocolectomy**, **rectal mucosectomy**, and **ileoanal pouch** (J-pouch)
  - Need lifetime surveillance of residual rectal mucosa
  - **Total proctocolectomy with end ileostomy** is also an option.
  - Following colectomy, most common cause of death in FAP patients is **periampullary tumors of duodenum**.
- **Gardner's syndrome** – patients get colon CA (associated with APC gene) and intra-abdominal desmoid tumors/osteomas
- **Turcot's syndrome** – patients get colon CA (associated with APC gene) and brain tumors

LYNCH SYNDROMES (HEREDITARY NONPOLYPOSIS COLON CANCER)

- 5% of population, autosomal dominant
- Associated with **DNA mismatch repair gene**
- Predilection for right-sided and multiple cancers
- **Lynch I** – just colon CA risk
- **Lynch II** – patients _also_ have ↑ risk of ovarian, endometrial, bladder, and stomach cancer
- **Amsterdam criteria** for **Lynch syndrome** – "3, 2, 1" → at least **3** first-degree relatives, over **2** generations, **1** with cancer before age 50

- Need surveillance colonoscopy every 1–2 years starting at age 25 or 10 years before primary relative got cancer (also need surveillance program for the other CA types in the family)
- 50% get metachronous lesions within 10 years; often have multiple primaries
- Need **total proctocolectomy** with first cancer operation

SIGMOID VOLVULUS

- More common with high-fiber diets (Iran, Iraq) and in elderly
- Risk factors – debilitated, psychiatric patients, neurologic dysfunction, laxative abuse
- Symptoms: pain, distention, and obstipation (can't pass stool/gas)
- Causes closed-loop obstruction – **sigmoid colon twists on itself**
- AXR – bent inner tube sign with apex pointing to RUQ; colon distension
- Gastrografin enema may show bird's beak sign (tapered colon).
- Dx: need **abdominal CT scan with contrast** (to confirm diagnosis and check colon wall viability)
- Do not attempt decompression with **gangrenous bowel, diffuse peritoneal signs**, or **full thickness injury** (eg dusky colon with ulceration) → go to OR for **sigmoidectomy and end-colostomy**
- Tx: **Decompress with colonoscopy** (80% reduce, 50% will recur), place rectal decompression tube (1–3 days), give bowel prep, and perform **sigmoidectomy with primary anastomosis** during same admission.

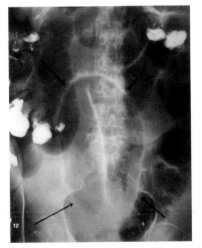

Plain supine abdominal film of a patient with sigmoid volvulus. The centrally located sigmoid loop is outlined by trapped air. The proximal small intestine is dilated as well, suggesting that the volvulus has been present for sufficient time to cause accumulation of air and fluid proximally.

CECAL VOLVULUS

- Less common than sigmoid volvulus; occurs in 20s–30s
- AXR – can appear as an SBO; can have "coffee bean" sign with dilated cecum in the RLQ with apex pointing to LUQ

- Endoscopic decompression is _not_ recommended.
- Tx: **OR → right hemicolectomy** with primary anastomosis (_best_); can try **cecopexy** if colon is viable and patient is frail; _avoid_ cecostomy

ULCERATIVE COLITIS

- Symptoms: **bloody diarrhea, abdominal pain, fever**, and **weight loss**
- Chronic inflammation involves the **mucosa** and **submucosa**.
- Strictures and fistulae unusual with ulcerative colitis
- **Spares anus** – unlike Crohn's disease
- Usually starts distally in **rectum**, extends **proximally**, and is **contiguous** (no skip areas like Crohn's)
- **Bleeding** is universal and has mucosal friability with pseudopolyps, collar button ulcers, and crypt abscesses.
- Always need to rule out infectious etiology
- Backwash ileitis can occur with proximal disease.

Clinicopathologic Features of Ulcerative Colitis versus Crohn Disease

Manifestation	Ulcerative Colitis	Crohn Disease
Transmural inflammation	Seldom	Common
Granulomas	Seldom	> 50%
Fissuring	Rare	Common
Fibrosis	Rare	Common
Submucosal inflammation	Rare	Common
Crypt abscesses	Common	Uncommon
Small-bowel involvement	Rare (backwash ileitis)	Common
Anatomic location	Continuous	Skip
Rectal involvement	Common	May be spared
Bleeding	Common	Absent
Fistulas	Rare	Common
Perianal disease	Rare	Common
Ulcers	Rare	Common
Surrounding mucosa	Pseudopolyps	Relatively normal
Cobblestoning of mucosa	None	Long-standing disease
Mucosal friability	Common	Uncommon
Vascular pattern	Absent	Normal
Fat wrapping	Rare	Common

- **Barium enema** – with chronic disease see loss of haustra, narrow caliber, short colon, and loss of redundancy
- **Medical Tx**: **mesalamine** and **loperamide** for maintenance therapy
  - **Steroids** for acute flares
  - Consider **infliximab** for steroid-resistant disease.
  - Add **Cipro** and **Flagyl** for acute flares if worried about infection or toxic megacolon/colitis.
- **Toxic colitis** and **toxic megacolon**
  - Toxic colitis: > 6 bloody stools/d, fever, ↑ HR, drop in Hgb, leukocytosis
  - Toxic megacolon (colon **> 6 cm**): above plus distension, abdominal pain, and tenderness
  - Initial Tx: **NG tube, fluids, steroids, bowel rest**, and **antibiotics** (ciprofloxacin and Flagyl) will treat 50% adequately; other 50% require surgery.
  - Follow clinical response and abdominal radiographs.
  - _Avoid_ barium enemas, narcotics, anti-diarrheal agents, and anti-cholinergics.

Indications for Surgery with Toxic Colitis and Toxic Megacolon

Absolute	Relative
Pneumoperitoneum (perforation)	Inability to promptly control sepsis
Diffuse peritonitis	Increasing megacolon
Localized peritonitis with increasing abdominal pain and/or colonic distension >10 cm	Failure to improve within 24–48 h
Uncontrolled sepsis	Increasing toxicity or other signs of clinical deterioration
Major hemorrhage	Continued transfusion requirements

- **Perforation** with **ulcerative colitis** – <u>transverse colon</u> more common
- **Perforation** with **Crohn's** – <u>distal ileum</u> most common
- **Surgical indications for ulcerative colitis**: medical intractability (*most common*), massive hemorrhage, refractory toxic megacolon/fulminant colitis (occurs in 15%), obstruction, stricture, multifocal or high-grade dysplasia, CA, systemic complications, failure to thrive (children), avoidance of chronic steroids, and long-standing disease (> 20 years) as prophylaxis against colon CA (some controversy here)
- **Emergent/urgent resections** – total proctocolectomy and bring up end ileostomy
  - Perform definitive hook-up later.
- **Elective resections**
  - **Ileal pouch and anal anastomosis** – total proctocolectomy, rectal mucosectomy, J-pouch, and ileoanal (low rectal) anastomosis; <u>*not used with Crohn's disease*</u>
  - Can protect bladder and sexual function
  - Need lifetime surveillance of residual rectal area
  - Must have good baseline continence prior to pouch
  - Many ileoanal anastomoses need resection secondary to cancer, dysplastic changes, refractory pouchitis, or pouch failure (incontinence).
  - Need temporary diverting ileostomy (6–8 weeks) while pouch heals
  - **Leak** (most common major morbidity) – can lead to sepsis (Tx: drainage, antibiotics)
  - **Infectious pouchitis** (fever, pelvic pain, increased stools) – Tx: **Cipro** and **Flagyl**; **budesonide enemas** if refractory
    - Suspect undiagnosed <u>Crohn's disease</u> if chronic.
  - **APR with ileostomy** – can also be performed
- **Cancer risk** is **1% per year** starting **8 years** after initial diagnosis for patients with **extensive colitis** (extending proximal to the splenic flexure).
  - Need colonoscopy every 1–2 years starting 8 years after diagnosis
  - Need 4 quadrant biopsies at 10 cm intervals for entire length of affected colon (also biopsy any suspicious areas)
  - **Cancer** in ulcerative colitis most common in **recto-sigmoid colon**; due to **chronic inflammation**
- **Extraintestinal manifestations of ulcerative colitis**
  - Most common extraintestinal manifestation requiring total colectomy – **failure to thrive in children**
  - Do **not** get better with colectomy → primary sclerosing cholangitis, ankylosing spondylitis
  - **Get better with colectomy** → most ocular problems (episcleritis), arthritis, and anemia
  - **50% get better** → skin problems (pyoderma gangrenosum, erythema nodosum)
  - **HLA B27** – sacroiliitis, ankylosing spondylitis, ulcerative colitis
  - Can get **thromboembolic disease**
  - **Pyoderma gangrenosum** – Tx: steroids

CARCINOID OF THE COLON AND RECTUM

- Represents 15% of all carcinoids; infrequent cause of carcinoid syndrome
- Metastases related to size of tumor
- ⅔ of colon carcinoids have either local or systemic spread.
- **Low rectal carcinoids**
    - **< 2 cm** → wide local excision with negative margins
    - **> 2 cm or invasion of muscularis propria** → APR
- **Colon or high rectal carcinoids**
    - **< 1 cm** – polypectomy
    - **> 1 cm** – formal resection

COLONIC OBSTRUCTION

- **Colon perforation with obstruction** – most likely to occur in **cecum**
    - Law of LaPlace: tension = pressure × diameter
- **Closed-loop obstructions** – can be worrisome; can have rapid progression and perforation with minimal distention
    - Competent ileocecal valve can lead to closed-loop obstruction.
- **Colonic obstruction** – #1 cancer; #2 diverticulitis
- **Pneumatosis intestinalis** – air on the bowel wall, associated with ischemia and dissection of air through areas of bowel wall
- **Air in the portal system** – usually indicates significant infection or necrosis of the large or small bowel; often an ominous sign

OGILVIE'S SYNDROME

- Pseudo-obstruction of colon
- Associated with: opiate use, bedridden or older patients, recent surgery, infection, trauma, electrolyte imbalances (low K, Mg, or Ca)
- Get a **massively dilated colon**, which can **perforate**.
- High risk of **perforation** for **cecum > 12 cm** or duration **> 6 days**
- **Initial Tx**: fluid resuscitation, replace electrolytes (especially K and Mg), discontinue drugs that slow the gut (eg morphine), NG tube, bowel rest, stop anti-cholinergics (eg Benadryl).
    - 2nd-line Tx: **neostigmine** (indicated for **cecum > 12 cm, no improvement after 3 days**, or **duration > 4 days**); can cause **bradycardia** (need to give in a monitored area; Tx: **Atropine**)
    - 3rd-line Tx: **colonoscope decompression** (indicated if neostigmine fails)
    - Surgical indications: perforation, gangrenous colitis, or no improvement after 6 days
        - If **perforation** (diffuse peritonitis) or suspected **gangrenous/toxic colitis** – extent of resection depends on intraop findings (right hemi-colectomy vs subtotal colectomy)
        - If **simple failure of conservative Tx** (duration **> 6 days**; without perforation/ gangrene/toxic colitis) – tube cecostomy vs resection

AMOEBIC COLITIS

- **Entamoeba histolytica**; from contaminated food and water with feces that contain cysts
- **Primary infection** – occurs in colon; **secondary infection** – occurs in liver
- Risk factors – travel to Mexico, ETOH; fecal–oral transmission
- Symptoms: similar to ulcerative colitis (dysentery); chronic more common form (3–4 bowel movements/day, cramping, and fever)
- Dx: endoscopy → ulceration, trophozoites; 90% have anti-amebic antibodies
- Tx: **Flagyl**, diiodohydroxyquin

ACTINOMYCES

- Can present as a mass, abscess, fistula, or induration; suppurative and granulomatous
- Cecum most common location; can be confused with CA
- Pathology shows **yellow-white sulfur granules**.
- Tx: **penicillin** or tetracycline, drainage of any abscess

DIVERTICULA

- Herniation of mucosa through the colon wall at sites where arteries enter the muscular wall
- Circular muscle thickens adjacent to diverticulum with luminal narrowing.
- Caused by **straining** (↑ intraluminal pressure)
- Most diverticula occur on **left side** (80%) in the sigmoid colon (not rectum).
  - **Bleeding** is more likely with <u>right-sided diverticula</u> (50% of bleeds occur on right).
  - **Diverticulitis** is more likely to present on the <u>left side</u>.
- Present in 35% of the population

LOWER GI BLEEDING

- Stool guaiac can stay positive up to 3 weeks after bleed.
- **Hematemesis** – bleeding anywhere from nose to ligament of Treitz
- **Melena** – passage of tarry stools; need as little as 50 cc
- **Jaundice** – from hemoglobin absorption (broken down to bilirubin)
- **Azotemia after GI bleed** – caused by production of urea from bacterial action on intraluminal blood (↑ BUN; also get elevated total bilirubin)
- Lower GI bleeding can occur from angiodysplasia, diverticulosis, hemorrhoids, polyps, or cancer.
- If **significant bleed** – place 2 large-bore IVs, T and C for 6 units pRBCs (transfuse as necessary), serial Hcts, ICU care
- Rule out an **upper GI source** in patients with **melena** or **red blood per rectum** by placing an **NG tube**.
  - If **clear** fluid is aspirated, need upper endoscopy (Pylorus may be closed and duodenum may be the source.)
  - If **bilious** fluid is aspirated, an upper GI source has been ruled out.
  - If **bloody** fluid is aspirated, the diagnosis of upper GI bleeding is made.

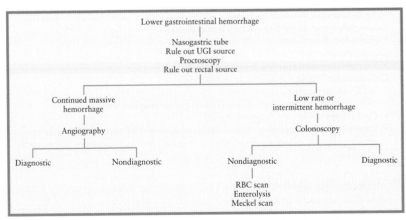

Diagnostic steps in the evaluation of acute lower gastrointestinal hemorrhage. RBC, red blood cell; UGI, upper gastrointestinal.

- Most bleeds stop **spontaneously**.
- Can try repeated attempts at **localization** if the patient **rebleeds** and is **stable**
- If patient becomes **unstable** or continues to have **significant transfusion requirement** – need surgery
  - **Segmental colectomy** if bleeding was **localized** on diagnostic studies
  - **Total abdominal colectomy** if bleeding site was **not located** on diagnostic studies
- **Arteriography** – bleeding must be $\geq$ 0.5 cc/min
- **Tagged RBC scan** – bleeding must be $\geq$ 0.1 cc/min
- **Video capsule study** – also an option

DIVERTICULITIS

- Result of **mucosal perforations** in the diverticulum with adjacent fecal contamination
- Denotes infection and inflammation of the colonic wall as well as surrounding tissue
- LLQ pain, tenderness, fever, $\uparrow$ WBCs
- Dx: CT scan is needed only if worried about **complicated disease**.
  - **Complicated disease** – perforation, abscess, obstruction, fistula, stricture (late)
  - Extraluminal gas and phlegmon (contained inflammation area) are _not_ considered complicated disease.
- **Signs of complication** – obstruction symptoms, fluctuant mass, peritoneal signs, temperature > 39, WBCs > 20; _all warrant_ **hospital admission**
- Most common complication – **abscess formation**
  - < 4 cm abscess – usually resolve with **antibiotics** _only_
  - $\geq$ 4 cm abscess – need **percutaneous drainage**
- **Uncomplicated diverticulitis** – Tx: **levofloxacin** and **Flagyl**; bowel rest for 3–4 days
  - **Mild** cases – can be treated as an outpatient
  - **Moderate to severe** cases and can't tolerate oral hydration – admit as inpatient, NPO, and IV fluid resuscitation
  - **Septic shock** or **diffuse peritonitis** – OR for **urgent resection** (sigmoid colectomy usual with colostomy and Hartman's pouch)
    - **Septic shock** patients may need **fluid resuscitation** before OR
- **Surgery** – for **significant complications** (eg total obstruction not resolved with medical Tx, perforation, abscess not amenable to percutaneous drainage) or **inability to exclude CA**
  - Need to resect all of the **sigmoid colon** down to the superior rectum (distal margin should be **normal rectum**); place colostomy with Hartman's pouch.
- Need **follow-up colonoscopy 6 weeks** after an episode of diverticulitis to rule out **colorectal cancer** and **inflammatory bowel disease**
- **Right-sided diverticulitis** – 80% discovered at the time of incision for appendectomy
  - Tx: right hemicolectomy
- **Colovesicular fistula** – fecaluria, pneumaturia
  - MCC – diverticulitis
  - Occurs in men; women are more likely to get **colovaginal fistula**.
  - **Cystoscopy** is the best diagnostic test.
  - Tx: close bladder opening, resect involved segment of colon, and perform reanastomosis, diverting ileostomy; interpose omentum between the bladder and colon.

DIVERTICULOSIS BLEEDING

- Most common cause of lower GI bleed
- Usually causes significant bleeding
- 75% stops spontaneously; recurs in 25%

- Caused by disrupted **vasa rectum**; creates **arterial bleeding**
- Dx: **NG tube** to rule out upper GI source
  - **Colonoscopy** usually as a 1st step → can be therapeutic (hemoclips best) and can localize bleeding should surgery be required
  - **Angio** 1st if **massive bleed** (hypotension, tachycardia) – want to localize area for surgery; may be able to treat at angio with highly selective coil embolization
  - **Go to operating room** if hypotensive and not responding to resuscitation → colectomy at site of bleeding if identified or total abdominal colectomy if bleeding source has not been localized
  - **Tagged RBC scan** for intermittent bleeds that are hard to localize (most sensitive test)
- Tx: **Colonoscopy** can ligate bleeder.
  - With arteriography, can use vasopressin (to temporize) or **highly selective coil embolization**; also demonstrates where the bleed is should surgery be required
  - May need segmental colectomy or possible total abdominal colectomy if bleeding is not localized and not controlled
- Patients with **recurrent diverticular bleeds** should have **resection** of the area.

ANGIODYSPLASIA BLEEDING

- ↑ on right side of colon
- Bleeds are usually less severe than diverticular bleeds but are more likely to recur (80%).
- Causes **venous bleeding**
- Soft signs of angiodysplasia on angiogram – **tufts**, **slow emptying**
- 20% of patients with angiodysplasia have **aortic stenosis** (usually gets better after valve replacement).

ISCHEMIC COLITIS

- Symptoms: abdominal pain, bright red bleeding
- Generally involves the **left colon**
- Can be caused by a low-flow state (eg recent MI, CHF), ligation of the IMA at surgery (eg AAA repair), embolus or thrombosis of the IMA, sepsis
- **Splenic flexure** and **upper rectum** most vulnerable to low-flow state
- **Griffith's point** (splenic flexure) – SMA and IMA junction
- **Sudeck's point** – superior rectal and middle rectal artery junction
- Dx: CT scan or colonoscopy (best test) → cyanotic edematous mucosa covered with exudates
  - Lower ⅔ of the rectum is spared → supplied by the middle and inferior rectal arteries (off internal iliacs)
  - If gangrenous colitis is suspected (peritonitis), <u>no</u> colonoscopy and go to OR → sigmoid resection or left hemicolectomy usual
  - **Black bowel** on colonoscopy, **sepsis**, or **perforation** → go to the OR for resection
- If not going to the OR – Tx: NPO, antibiotics, IVFs

PSEUDOMEMBRANOUS COLITIS (C. DIFFICILE COLITIS; ANAEROBIC GRAM-NEGATIVE ROD)

- Profuse, watery, green, mucoid diarrhea; pain and cramping; fever
- Can occur up to 3 weeks after antibiotics; increased in postop, elderly, and ICU patients
- Carrier state not eradicated; 15% recurrence
- Key finding – **PMN inflammation of mucosa** and **submucosa**
  - Pseudomembranes, plaques, and ring-like lesions
- Most common in the **distal colon**
- Dx: **antigen** (Ab's to GDH enzyme) and **B toxin** PCR tests (*best combination*)

- Tx: **oral vancomycin** first line for all cases (can also give vancomycin enemas)
  - **Fidaxomicin** (oral macrolide) for resistant strains
  - Consider IV or oral **Flagyl** if not able to take vancomycin.
  - Lactobacillus can also help; stop other antibiotics or change them; avoid anti-diarrheals.
- **Toxic colitis/megacolon** (eg patient requiring increasing **vasopressors**) can occur requiring emergency **subtotal colectomy** and **end-ileostomy** (may need **total abdominal colectomy** depending on disease extent; carries a higher mortality, less re-explorations).
  - Colon may look **normal** at surgery as infection is **mucosal/submucosal**.

NEUTROPENIC TYPHLITIS (ENTEROCOLITIS)

- Follows chemotherapy when WBCs are low (nadir)
- Can mimic surgical disease
- Can often see pneumatosis intestinalis (not a surgical indication here)
- Tx: **antibiotics**; patients will improve when WBCs ↑; surgery _only_ for free perforation

OTHER COLON DISEASES

- Other causes of colitis – *Salmonella*, *Shigella*, *Campylobacter*, CMV, *Yersinia* (can mimic appendicitis in children), other viral infections, *Giardia*
- **Yersinia** – can mimic appendicitis; comes from contaminated food (feces/urine)
  - Tx: tetracycline or Bactrim
- **Megacolon** – propensity for volvulus; enlargement is proximal to non-peristalsing bowel
  - **Hirschsprung's disease** – rectosigmoid most common. Dx: rectal biopsy
  - **Trypanosoma cruzi** – most common acquired cause, secondary to destruction of nerves

INTRODUCTION

Arterial supply to the anus – inferior rectal artery
Venous drainage – above the dentate is **internal hemorrhoid plexus** and below the dentate is **external hemorrhoid plexus**

HEMORRHOIDS

- Caused by **straining**
- Left lateral, right anterior, and right posterior hemorrhoidal plexuses
- **External hemorrhoids** usually cause **pain** when they thrombose (somatic innervation).
  - Can also cause swelling, bleeding, and itching
  - Are **distal** to the dentate line, covered by sensate squamous epithelium
- **Internal hemorrhoids** usually **prolapse** and **bleed** (autonomic innervation).
  - **Primary** – slides below dentate with strain (internal only)
  - **Secondary** – prolapse that reduces spontaneously
  - **Tertiary** – prolapse that has to be manually reduced
  - **Quaternary** – not able to reduce
- Tx: **fiber** and **stool softeners** (_avoid_ straining); sitz baths; drink fluids
- **Thrombosed external hemorrhoid** → lance open (if > 72 hours) or elliptical excision (if < 72 hours) to relieve pain
- **Surgical indications**: recurrence, thrombosis multiple times, large external component
- _External_ hemorrhoids can be resected with **elliptical excision**.
- Can **band primary** and **secondary** _internal_ hemorrhoids
  - Do _not_ band _external_ hemorrhoids (painful).
- **Surgery** for **tertiary** and **quaternary** _internal_ hemorrhoids – 3 quadrant resection
  - Need to resect down to the **internal anal sphincter** (do _not_ go through it)
  - Postop – sitz baths, stool softener, high-fiber diet, drink fluids
- Complications of banding/surgery – bleeding, ulcer, pain, infection (rare Fournier's gangrene)

RECTAL PROLAPSE

- Starts 6–7 cm from anal verge
- See full-thickness rectal wall with concentric rings protruding on exam.
- Secondary to pudendal neuropathy and laxity of the anal sphincters
- ↑ with female gender, straining, chronic diarrhea, previous pregnancy, and redundant sigmoid colons; psychiatric meds, elderly
- Prolapse involves all layers of the rectum.
- **Medical Tx**: high-fiber diet
- **Surgical Tx**:
  - **Perineal rectosigmoid resection** (Altemeier) transanally if patient is older and frail
    - Less morbidity however higher recurrence
  - **Transabdominal posterior suture rectopexy** (rectal fixation; _key to repair_) if good condition patient
    - Lower morbidity with laparoscopic approach vs open
    - Consider resection (sigmoidectomy or LAR) if the patient also has constipation (can decrease symptoms).

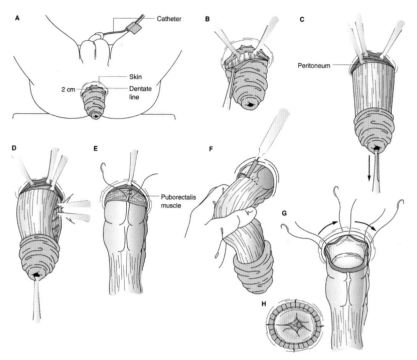

Perineal rectosigmoidectomy. The patient is placed in the lithotomy position with both legs in gynecologic stirrups. **(A and B)** A circular incision is made on the prolapsed rectum 2 cm proximal to the dentate line. **(C)** The peritoneal attachment is dissected from the anterior rectal wall, thus opening into the peritoneal cavity. **(D)** The mesorectum or meso-sigmoid is clamped and divided laterally and posteriorly. **(E)** The previously opened peritoneum is sutured to the anterior wall of the rectum or sigmoid colon as high as possible. This is followed by approximation of the puborectalis (optional). **(F)** The anterior wall of the protruding rectum is cut 1 cm distal to the anal verge. **(G)** Stay sutures of 3-0 synthetic absorbable material are placed in four quadrants. **(H)** Anastomosis with running stitches.

CONDYLOMATA ACUMINATA

- Cauliflower mass; papillomavirus (HPV)
- Tx: laser surgery

ANAL FISSURE

- Pain and bleeding after defecation; chronic ones will see a **sentinel pile**.
- Straining bowel movements, constipation
- Caused by a split in the anoderm
- 90% in **posterior midline**
- First-line medical Tx: **sitz baths**, **bulk** (psyllium), **lidocaine jelly**, **stool softeners**, **nitroglycerin** cream (S/E – headaches), **diltiazem** ointment (*90% heal with medical Tx*)
  - Second-line medical Tx: **botulinum toxin** (+/− results); incontinence after botulinum injection is a <u>*contraindication*</u> to sphincterotomy.
- Surgical Tx: **lateral subcutaneous internal sphincterotomy**
  - Better long-term results than medical Tx
  - **Fecal incontinence** is the most serious complication of surgery (small risk).

- *Contraindications* to surgery – Crohn's disease, ulcerative colitis, women of child-bearing age, prior obstetrical injury, history of incontinence, sphincter dysfunction
- **Anorectal flap** – inferior healing rates compared to sphincterotomy; less risk of incontinence
- **Lateral or recurrent fissures** – worry about IBD, anal CA, syphilis

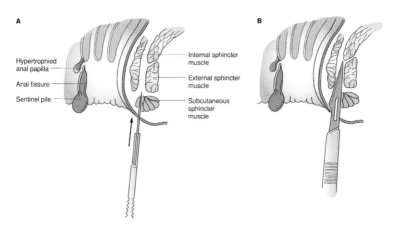

Lateral internal sphincterotomy (closed technique). **(A)** Triad of fissure, sentinel pile, and hypertrophied anal papilla. With an anal speculum used for exposure of the lateral quadrant, a no. 11 scalpel blade stabs into the subcutaneous tissue from the anal verge to the dentate line, with the knife in the horizontal position. **(B)** The knife is turned 90 degrees, and the internal sphincter muscle is cut while the anal canal is stretched open.

ANORECTAL ABSCESS

- Can cause severe pain and fever
- **Perianal**, *superficial*, **intersphincteric** (between internal/external sphincters) and **ischiorectal** (between rectal wall and pubic tubercle) **abscesses** all treated with **external** incision and drainage through the **skin** (all are *below* the levator muscles).
  - **Intersphincteric and ischiorectal abscesses** can form horseshoe abscess (extension to **postanal space** between anococcygeal ligament and levator muscles).
- **Supralevator** and *deep* **intersphincteric abscesses** need **internal** incision and drainage with **transanal** approach.
- **Antibiotics** given for systemic signs of infection, cellulitis, DM, immunosuppressed, or prosthetic hardware
- Rule out anal cancer with biopsy.
- 30% eventually develop a **fistula-in-ano**.

FISTULA-IN-ANO

- Fecal soiling, occasional perianal discomfort
- Do <u>not</u> need to excise the tract
- Often occurs after anorectal abscess
- **Goodsall's rule**
  - Anterior fistulas connect with anus/rectum in a straight line.
  - Posterior fistulas go toward a midline internal opening in the anus/rectum.
- Tx:
  - If **simple, superficial** and ***not* involving the external anal sphincter** – **fistulotomy** (open tract up, curettage out, let it heal by secondary intention)

- **Less than lower ¼** of external anal sphincter involved → **fistulotomy** (generally safe; avoid if previous incontinence issues; contraindications same as fissure surgery above)
- **Greater than lower ¼** of the external anal sphincter involved → **draining seton stitch** as _first_ procedure (induces fibrosis of the tract); _second_ procedure options:
  - **LIFT** (ligation of intersphincteric fistula tract) – intersphincteric incision, ligate fistula close to internal opening, scrape out track, ligate distal opening at external anal sphincter; possibly decreased incontinence rates compared to advancement flap
  - **Anorectal advancement flap**
  - _Avoid_ fistula plugs and fibrin glue.
- Most worrisome complication is **risk of incontinence** – you want to avoid damage to the external anal sphincter so fistulotomy is not used for fistulas above the lower ¼ of the external anal sphincter
- Rule out necrotic and draining tumor with biopsies.

RECTOVAGINAL FISTULAS

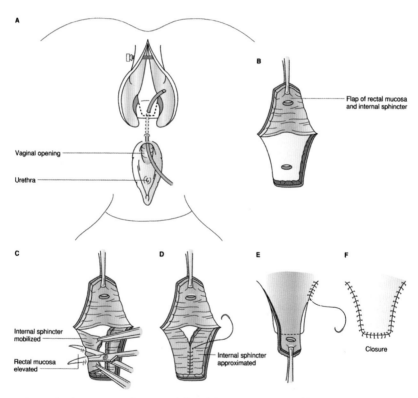

Endorectal advancement of anorectal flap. **(A)** Exposure is gained by an anal speculum, and the fistula is identified. Outline of endorectal flap, extending proximally to 7 cm from the anal verge. **(B)** The full-thickness flap is created to include the internal sphincter muscle. **(C)** Lateral mobilization is made on each side in the submucosal plane. **(D)** Anorectal wall on each side is approximated. **(E and F)** The endorectal flap is pulled down to cover the wound and sutured. The fistula is excised. The aperture in the vagina is not sutured but is left open for drainage.

- **Simple** – low to mid-vagina; MCC – obstetrical trauma
  - Tx: transanal **rectal mucosa advancement flap**
  - Many obstetrical fistulas heal spontaneously.
- **Complex** – high in vagina; MCC – diverticulitis
  - Tx: **abdominal** or combined **abdominal and perineal approach** usual; resection and reanastomosis of rectum, close hole in vagina, interpose omentum, temporary ileostomy

ANAL INCONTINENCE

- **Neurogenic** (gaping hole) – no good treatment
- **Abdominoperineal descent** – chronic damage to levator ani muscle and pudendal nerves (obesity, multiparous women) and anus falls below levators; Tx: high-fiber diet, limit to 1 bowel movement a day; hard to treat
- **Obstetrical trauma** – Tx: **anterior anal sphincteroplasty**

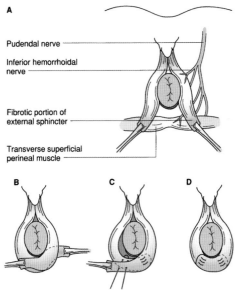

Overlapping anal sphincteroplasty.

PILONIDAL CYSTS

- Sinus or abscess formation over the sacrococcygeal junction; ↑ in men
- Tx: drainage and packing; follow-up surgical resection of cyst

AIDS ANORECTAL PROBLEMS

- **Kaposi's sarcoma** – see nodule with ulceration; most common cancer in patients with AIDS
- **CMV** – see shallow ulcers; similar presentation as appendicitis. Tx: ganciclovir
- **HSV** – #1 rectal ulcer
- **B cell lymphoma** – can look like abscess or ulcer
- Need biopsies of these ulcers to rule out cancer and figure out above

ANAL CANCER

- Association with **HPV** (16 and 18), **HIV**, **XRT**, and **immunosuppression**
- Anal canal – above dentate line
- Anal margin – below dentate line
- **Anal intra-epithelial neoplasm** (AIN) is a precursor for anal squamous cell CA (SCCA).
  - AIN I, II, and III (low-, moderate-, and high-grade dysplasia, respectively)
  - **Low rate of conversion** to SCCA overall (higher for **immunosuppressed**)
  - Tx: topical imiquimod (5%), topical 5FU (5%), ablation Tx (eg laser, Bovie), photodynamic Tx, surveillance with biopsy every 4–6 months
- **Anal canal lesions** (*above dentate line*)
  - **Squamous cell CA** (eg epidermoid CA, mucoepidermoid CA, cloacogenic CA, basaloid CA)
    - **Symptoms**: pruritus, bleeding, and palpable mass; may have palpable inguinal nodes
    - Tx: **Nigro protocol** (*chemo-XRT with **5FU** and **mitomycin**; 3000 cGy XRT*), **not** surgery
    - Cures 80%
    - APR for treatment failures or recurrent cancer
  - **Adenocarcinoma**
    - Tx: **APR** usual; WLE if < 4 cm, < ½ circumference, limited to submucosa (T1 tumors, 2–3 mm margin needed), well differentiated, and no vascular/lymphatic/nerve invasion
    - Postoperative chemo/XRT same as rectal CA
  - **Melanoma**
    - 3rd most common site for melanoma (skin and eyes #1 and #2)
    - ⅓ has spread to mesenteric lymph nodes.
    - Hematogenous spread to the liver and the lung is early and accounts for most deaths.
    - Symptomatic disease is often associated with significant metastatic disease.
    - Most common symptom – **rectal bleeding**
    - Most tumors are lightly pigmented or not pigmented at all.
    - Tx: **APR** usual; margin dictated by depth of lesion standard for melanoma
- **Anal margin lesions** (*below dentate line*) – have better prognosis than anal canal lesions
  - **Squamous cell CA**
    - Ulcerating, slow growing; men with better prognosis
    - Metastases – go to **inguinal nodes**
    - **WLE** for lesions < 5 cm (need 0.5 cm margin)
    - **Chemo-XRT** (**5FU** and **cisplatin**) primary Tx for lesions > 5 cm, if involving sphincter or if positive nodes (trying to preserve the sphincter here and avoid APR)
    - Need inguinal node dissection if clinically positive
  - **Basal cell CA** – central ulcer, raised edges, rare metastases
    - Tx: WLE usually sufficient, only need 3-mm margins; rare need for APR unless sphincter involved

NODAL METASTASES

- **Superior and middle rectum** – IMA nodes
- **Lower rectum** – primarily IMA nodes, also to internal iliac nodes
- **Anal canal** – internal iliac nodes
- **Anal margin** – inguinal nodes

ANATOMY

- **External abdominal oblique fascia** – forms the <u>inguinal ligament</u> (shelving edge and roof) at inferior portion of the inguinal canal
- **Internal abdominal oblique** – forms <u>cremasteric muscles</u>
- **Transversalis muscle** – along with the conjoined tendon, forms inguinal canal <u>floor</u>
- **Conjoined tendon** – composed of the aponeurosis of the internal abdominal oblique and transversalis fascia
- **Inguinal ligament** – from external abdominal oblique fascia, runs from anterior superior iliac spine to the pubis; anterior to the femoral vessels
  - **Lacunar ligament** – where inguinal ligament splays out to insert into the pubis; the pectineal ligament is an extension of lacunar ligament
- **Pectineal ligament** (Cooper's ligament) – <u>posterior</u> to femoral vessels; lies against bone
- **Iliopubic tract** – <u>anterior</u> to femoral vessels; runs from anterior superior iliac spine to pubis
- **Spermatic cord structures** – testicular artery, pampiniform plexus, cremasteric muscle, vas deferens, ilioinguinal nerve, genital branch of the genitofemoral nerve (all can be injured with open inguinal hernia repair)
  - **Vas deferens** – runs medial to cord structures
- **Hesselbach's triangle** – rectus muscle, inferior inguinal ligament, and inferior epigastrics
  - **Direct hernias** are inferior/medial to epigastric vessels (in Hesselbach's triangle).
  - **Indirect hernias** are superior/lateral to epigastric vessels.

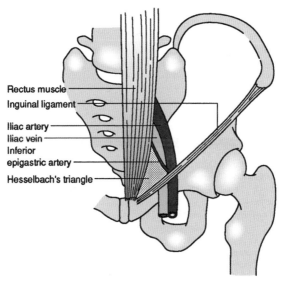

Rectus muscle
Inguinal ligament
Iliac artery
Iliac vein
Inferior epigastric artery
Hesselbach's triangle

The inguinal (Hesselbach's) triangle.

INGUINAL HERNIAS

- **Indirect hernias** – most common; <u>congenital</u> from persistently **patent processus vaginalis**
- **Direct hernias** – from <u>weakness</u> in inguinal canal floor; lower risk of incarceration
  - Rare in females, **higher recurrence** than indirect
  - Risk factors: age, obesity, heavy lifting, coughing (COPD, smoking), chronic constipation, straining (BPH), ascites, pregnancy, peritoneal dialysis, poor nutrition
- **Pantaloon hernia** – direct and indirect components
- **Incarcerated hernia** (<u>not</u> able to reduce) – can lead to obstruction and bowel strangulation; should be repaired emergently
- **Strangulation** (compromised blood supply) – severe tenderness and pain; skin changes; dusky bowel intraop
  - If bowel **infarcted** (black) – need to resect
  - Need tissue hernia repair or biologic mesh with bowel resection
- **Sliding hernias** – retroperitoneal organ makes up part of the hernia sac
  - **Females** – ovaries or fallopian tubes most common
  - **Males** – cecum or sigmoid most common
  - Bladder can also be involved.
  - Careful when opening sac to not injure involved organ
- **Females with ovary in canal**
  - Ligate the round ligament (found in the inguinal canal in women).
  - Return ovary to peritoneum.
  - Perform biopsy if looks abnormal.

INGUINAL HERNIA REPAIR

- Goal is to achieve **tension-free repair**.
- Usually **remove hernia sac** in adults with open repair.
- **Lichtenstein repair** – mesh sewn between conjoined tendon and inguinal ligament
  - **Lower recurrence** with use of **mesh** (less tension)
- **Bassini repair** – direct approximation of conjoined tendon to free edge of inguinal ligament (shelving edge, inferior)
- **Cooper's ligament repair** – direct approximation of the conjoined tendon to Cooper's ligament (pectineal ligament, inferior)
  - Needs a relaxing incision in the external abdominal oblique fascia
  - Can use this for femoral hernia repair
- **Laparoscopic hernia repair** – usually indicated for bilateral or recurrent inguinal hernias
  - TEP – total extraperitoneal repair (peritoneum and abdomen are <u>not</u> entered)
  - TAPP – transabdominal preperitoneal repair (need to **close peritoneum** after mesh placement to prevent adhesions)
  - Mesh is used to cover indirect, direct, and femoral areas (covers **myopectineal orifice**).
  - **Pectineal ligament** (Cooper's ligament) near pubic bone origin serves as **mesh anchor**.
  - **Areas of injury**
    - **Triangle of doom** – vas deferens (medial), spermatic vessels (lateral), peritoneal fold (inferior); contains iliac artery and vein; also genital branch of the genitofemoral nerve; located inferior to iliopubic tract
    - **Triangle of pain** (just lateral to triangle of doom) – iliopubic tract (superior), spermatic vessels (medial), peritoneal fold (lateral); contains femoral nerve, lateral femoral (cutaneous) nerve, and femoral branch of the genitofemoral nerve
    - **Avoiding the triangles** – <u>*avoid*</u> placing tacks that are lateral to vas deferens and inferior to the iliopubic tract

- **Inferior epigastric artery** (vein) – runs along abdominal wall (can be injured with abdominal wall tacks – just skip over it when placing tacks)
- **Vas deferens** and **spermatic vessels** – can be injured when placing tacks in pectineal ligament (avoid when placing tacks)
- **Corona mortis** – can be found at lacunar ligament near mesh anchor site
  - Is a collateral between obturator and external iliac artery (can just ligate)
- **Urinary retention** – most common early complication following hernia repair
- **Wound infection** – 1% (most common cause of hernia **recurrence**)
  - Infected mesh (purulent drainage) requires **excision**
- **Recurrence rate** – 2%
- **Testicular atrophy** – usually secondary to dissection of the distal component of the hernia sac causing vessel disruption
  - Thrombosis of **spermatic cord veins**
  - Usually occurs with indirect hernias
- **Ilioinguinal nerve injury** – loss of cremasteric reflex; numbness on ipsilateral penis, scrotum, and thigh
  - Most commonly **injured nerve** with open inguinal hernia repair
  - Nerve is usually injured at **external ring** when opening **external abdominal oblique fascia**; nerve runs on top of cord (anterior).
- **Genitofemoral nerve injury** – **genital branch** can be injured with open inguinal repair
  - From dissection of cord structures
  - Genital branch – cremaster (motor) and scrotum (sensory)
  - Femoral branch – upper lateral thigh (sensory)
- **Pain after open hernia repair** – most commonly compression of **ilioinguinal nerve**
  - Tx: Local infiltration can be diagnostic and therapeutic (near anterior superior iliac spine).
- **Lateral femoral cutaneous nerve** – lateral thigh sensation
  - Most commonly injured nerve with laparoscopic hernia repair (lateral thigh numbness)
  - From placing tack too laterally and below iliopubic tract (triangle of pain)
- **Cord lipomas** – should be removed
- **Attempted open inguinal hernia repair** in woman and cannot find hernia sac – likely has femoral hernia (divide floor of inguinal canal to find femoral hernia)
- **External iliac artery and vein** – can be injured with open repair if sutures are too deep into inguinal ligament floor (Tx: remove suture and hold pressure)
- **Unable to dissect hernia sac from scrotum** – confirm it is not a sliding hernia, then ligate sac proximally (return to abdomen) and leave distal sac in scrotum (keep distal sac open to avoid hydrocele)

FEMORAL HERNIA

- Most common in **women** and **elderly**
- Femoral canal boundaries – Cooper's ligament (pectineal, posterior), inguinal ligament (anterior), femoral vein (lateral), and lacunar ligament (medial)
- **Femoral hernia** is medial to the femoral vein and lateral to lymphatics/lacunar ligament (in empty space).
- High risk of incarceration → may need to **divide the inguinal ligament** to reduce the bowel
- Hernia passes under the inguinal ligament.
- Characteristic **bulge on the anterior–medial thigh** below the ligament
- Hernia is usually repaired through an inguinal approach with Cooper's ligament repair (open floor of inguinal canal, conjoint tendon sutured to pectineal ligament to close space).

OTHER HERNIAS

- **Umbilical hernia**
  - Usually congenital; usually contains **omentum** (other – bowel)
  - ↑ incidence in African Americans; often close on their own in children
  - Risk of incarceration in adults, not children
  - **Children** – delay repair until age **5 years** (**primary repair** in children, not laparoscopic)
  - **Adults** – primary repair if < 1 cm; consider laparoscopic if larger
  - **Pregnancy** – majority small; _rarely_ need surgery during pregnancy unless incarcerated
  - If **large** and **significantly symptomatic** (eg pain, intermittent obstructive symptoms) can offer surgery in 2nd trimester
- **Spigelian hernia**
  - Lateral border of rectus muscle, adjacent to the **linea semilunaris**
  - Almost always **inferior** to the semicircularis (arcuate line)
  - Is **intramuscular**, between the muscle fibers of the internal abdominal oblique muscle and insertion of the external abdominal oblique aponeurosis into the rectus sheath
- **Obturator hernia** (anterior pelvis)
  - Can present as tender medial thigh mass or as small bowel obstruction
  - **Howship–Romberg sign** – inner thigh pain with internal rotation
  - Elderly women, previous pregnancy, bowel gas below superior pubic ramus
  - Tx: operative reduction, may need mesh; check other side for similar defect.
- **Sciatic hernia** (posterior pelvis)
  - Herniation through the greater sciatic foramen; high rate of strangulation
- **Incisional/ventral hernia**
  - Highest recurrence rate of all hernias: defect in the midline rectus sheath
  - **Inadequate closure** is the most common cause (use 5 × 5 mm bites to avoid).
  - Risk factors – wound infection, coughing (smoking, COPD), obesity
  - Encourage **smoking cessation** prior to repair.
  - Repairs aim to approximate rectus muscles or place mesh to cover defect.
  - Tx: **macroporous mesh** used in various configurations
    - **Underlay** usual (posterior to rectus muscle; is intraperitoneal)
    - **Onlay** (anterior to rectus muscle)
    - **Sublay** is also posterior to rectus muscle although anterior to peritoneum (avoids **adhesions** to mesh).
    - High recurrence with **inlay** (between rectus muscles; _avoid_)
    - Use biologic mesh if contaminated.

COMPONENT SEPARATION TECHNIQUE

- Layers of abdominal wall are separated to **reduce tension** when closing large ventral hernias.
- Use of additional **mesh** to techniques below reduces complications although may not be able to use due to **contamination**.
- Not clear if this offers better results compared to simple mesh techniques
- **Anterior technique** – external abdominal oblique fascia is incised and the muscle is mobilized; internal abdominal oblique and transversalis are advanced toward midline; rectus muscle is re-approximated.
- **Posterior technique** – transversalis fascia is divided and the muscle is mobilized; external abdominal oblique and internal abdominal oblique are advanced toward midline; rectus muscle is re-approximated.

RECTUS SHEATH

- Anterior – complete
- Posterior – absent below semicircularis (arcuate line; just below umbilicus)

- The posterior aponeurosis of the internal abdominal oblique and transversalis moves anterior just below the umbilicus.
- Blood supply – **superior** and **inferior epigastric** arteries
- **Rectus sheath hematomas**
  - Most common after trauma; epigastric vessel injury
  - Painful abdominal wall mass
  - Mass more prominent and painful with flexion of the rectus muscle (Fothergill's sign)
  - Tx: nonoperative usual; **angio-embolization** if expanding (surgical ligation of epigastric vessels if that fails)

DESMOID TUMORS

- Women, benign but locally invasive; ↑ recurrences
- Gardner's syndrome
- Painless mass
- Tx: wide local excision if possible; if involving significant small bowel mesentery, excision may not be indicated → often not completely resectable
  - Medical Tx: **sulindac** and **tamoxifen**

RETROPERITONEAL FIBROSIS

- Can occur with hypersensitivity to methysergide
- **IVP** most sensitive test (constricted ureters)
- Symptoms usually related to **trapped ureters** and **lymphatic obstruction**
- Tx: **steroids**, nephrostomy if infection is present, and surgery if renal function becomes compromised (free up ureters and wrap in **omentum**)

MESENTERIC TUMORS

- Of the primary tumors, most are cystic.
  - **Malignant tumors** – closer to the **root** of the mesentery
  - **Benign tumors** – more **peripheral**
- Malignant – **liposarcoma** (#1), leiomyosarcoma
- Dx: abdominal CT
- Tx: resection

RETROPERITONEAL TUMORS

- 15% in children, others in 5th-6th decade
- Malignant > benign
- Most common malignant retroperitoneal tumor – #1 **lymphoma**, #2 liposarcoma
- Symptoms: vague abdominal and back pain
- **Retroperitoneal sarcomas**
  - < 25% resectable; local recurrence in 40%; 10% 5-year survival rate
  - Have pseudocapsule but cannot shell out → would leave residual tumor
  - Metastases go to the lung.

OMENTAL TUMORS

- Most common omental solid tumor is **metastatic disease**.
- Omentectomy for metastatic cancer has a role for some cancers (eg ovarian CA).
- Omental cysts are usually asymptomatic, can undergo torsion.
- Primary solid omental tumors are rare; ⅓ are malignant.
  - <u>No</u> biopsy → can bleed
  - Tx: resection

PERITONEAL MEMBRANE
- Blood is absorbed through fenestrated lymphatic channels in the peritoneum.
- Most drugs are not removed with peritoneal dialysis.
- NH_3, Ca, Fe, and lead are removed.
- Movement of fluid into the peritoneal cavity can occur with hypertonic intraperitoneal saline load (mechanism of peritoneal dialysis); can cause hypotension

CO_2 PNEUMOPERITONEUM
- Normal is 10–15.
- Cardiopulmonary dysfunction can occur with intra-abdominal pressure > 20.
- *Increased*: mean arterial pressure, pulmonary artery pressure, HR, systemic vascular resistance, central venous pressure, mean airway pressure, peak inspiratory pressure, and CO_2
- *Decreased*: pH, venous return (IVC compression), cardiac output, renal flow secondary to decreased cardiac output
- Hypovolemia lowers pressure necessary to cause compromise.
- PEEP worsens effects of pneumoperitoneum.
- CO_2 can cause some $\downarrow$ in myocardial contractility.
- **CO_2 embolus** (sudden transient rise in $ETCO_2$, followed by a drop, then hypotension) – Tx: head down, turn patient to the left; can try to aspirate CO_2 through central line; prolonged CPR

SURGICAL TECHNOLOGY
- **Harmonic scalpel**
  - Cost-effective for medium vessels (short gastrics)
  - Disrupts protein H-bonds, causes coagulation
- **Ultrasound**
  - **B-mode** used most commonly (B = brightness; assesses relative density of structures)
  - **Shadowing** – dark area posterior to object indicates mass
  - **Enhancement** – brighter area posterior to object indicates fluid-filled cyst
  - **Lower frequencies** – deep structures
  - **Higher frequencies** – superficial structures
  - **Duplex** – adds Doppler; color visual description of blood flow (direction, stenosis, velocity)
- **Argon beam** – energy transferred across argon gas
  - Depth of necrosis related to power setting (2 mm); causes superficial coagulation
  - Is non-contact – good for hemostasis of the liver and spleen; smokeless
- **Laser** – return of electrons to ground state releases energy as heat → coagulates and vaporizes
  - Used for condylomata acuminata (wear mask)
- **Nd:YAG laser** – good for deep tissue penetration; good for bronchial lesions
  - 1–2 mm cuts, 3–10 mm vaporizes, and 1–2 cm coagulates
- **Gore-Tex** (PTFE) – cannot get fibroblast ingrowth
- **Dacron** (polypropylene) – allows fibroblast ingrowth
- **Incidence of vascular or bowel injury with Veress needle or trocar** – 0.1%

ANATOMY AND PHYSIOLOGY

- **Gerota's fascia** – around kidney
- **Anterior to posterior** – renal vein, renal artery, and renal pelvis
  - **Right renal artery** crosses posterior to the IVC.
  - **Left renal vein** is anterior to the aorta.
- **Ureters** cross **over iliac vessels**.
- **Left renal vein** – can be ligated from IVC secondary to increased collaterals (left adrenal vein, left gonadal vein, and left ascending lumbar vein); right renal vein lacks collaterals
  - **Left renal vein** usually crosses anterior aorta.
- **Epididymis** – connects to vas deferens
- **Seminal vesicles** are connected to the **vas deferens**.
- **Spermatic cord structures** – testicular artery, pampiniform plexus, vas deferens, cremasteric muscle, ilioinguinal nerve, genital branch of the genitofemoral nerve
- **Erection** – parasympathetic
- **Ejaculation** – sympathetic
- **Hypotension** – most common cause of acute renal insufficiency following surgery

KIDNEY STONES

- **Symptoms**: severe, colicky, flank (back) pain; restlessness; nausea and vomiting
- **Urinalysis** – blood or stones
- **Abdominal CT** – can demonstrate stones and associated hydronephrosis
- **Calcium oxalate** stones – most common (75%); radiopaque; ↑ in patients with **terminal ileum resection** due to ↑ oxalate absorption in colon
- **Struvite** stones (magnesium ammonium phosphate; radiopaque) – occur with infections (*Proteus mirabilis*) that are <u>urease</u> producing; cause <u>staghorn calculi</u> (fill renal pelvis)
- **Uric acid** stones (radiolucent) – ↑ in patients with **ileostomies**, gout, and myeloproliferative disorders
- **Cysteine stones** (radiolucent) – associated with congenital disorders in the reabsorption of cysteine (cystinuria); prevention – tiopronin
- **Medical Tx**: IV fluids, analgesics, watchful waiting
- **Surgery indications** for kidney stones:
  - Intractable pain or infection
  - Progressive obstruction
  - Progressive renal damage
  - Solitary kidney
  - Stones with low probability of passing
- 90% of kidney stones opaque; > 6 mm not likely to pass
- Tx: **ESWL** (extra-corporeal shock wave lithotripsy; not used in pregnancy, with bleeding diathesis, or stones that are several centimeters in size); other options – ureteroscopy with stone extraction or placement of stent past obstruction, percutaneous nephrostomy tube, open nephrolithotomy

TESTICULAR CANCER

- **#1 cancer killer** in men 25–35
- Symptom: **painless hard mass**
- **Testicular mass** – patient needs an **orchiectomy** through an **inguinal incision** (<u>not</u> a trans-scrotal incision → do not want to disrupt lymphatics)
  - The testicle and attached mass constitute the biopsy specimen.

- Most testicular masses are **malignant**.
- **Ultrasound** can help with diagnosis.
- Chest and abdominal CT – to check for retroperitoneal and chest metastases
- **LDH** correlates with tumor bulk.
- Check **beta-HCG** and **AFP** level.
- 90% are **germ cell** – seminoma or nonseminoma
- **Undescended testicles** (cryptorchidism) – ↑ risk of testicular CA
  - Most likely to get seminoma
- **Seminoma**
  - #1 testicular tumor
  - 10% of seminomatous tumors have beta-HCG elevation.
  - Should <u>not</u> have AFP elevation (if elevated, need to treat like nonseminomatous)
  - **Seminoma** is **extremely sensitive to XRT**.
  - Tx: All stages get *orchiectomy* and *retroperitoneal XRT*.
    - Chemo reserved for **metastatic disease** or **bulky retroperitoneal disease** (cisplatin, bleomycin, VP-16)
    - Surgical resection of residual disease after above
- **Nonseminomatous testicular CA**
  - **Types** – embryonal, teratoma, choriocarcinoma, yolk sac
  - **Alpha-fetoprotein** and **beta-HCG** – 90% have these markers
  - Classically, tumors with ↑ teratoma components are more likely to metastasize to the retroperitoneum.
  - Tx: All stages get *orchiectomy* and *retroperitoneal node dissection*.
    - *Stage II or greater* – *also give chemo (cisplatin, bleomycin, VP-16)*
    - Surgical resection of residual disease after above

PROSTATE CANCER

- **Posterior lobe** – most common site
- **Bone** – most common site of metastases
  - **Osteoblastic**; x-ray demonstrates **hyperdense areas**.
- Many patients become impotent after resection; can get incontinence
- Can also get urethral strictures
- Dx: transrectal Bx, chest/abdomen/pelvic CT, PSA, alkaline phosphatase; possible bone scan
- **Intracapsular tumors** and no metastases (T1 and T2) → options:
  - XRT <u>or</u>
  - Radical prostatectomy + pelvic lymph node dissection (if life span > 10 years) <u>or</u>
  - Nothing (depending on age and health)
- **Extracapsular invasion** or **metastatic disease**
  - Tx: **XRT** and **androgen ablation** (leuprolide [GnRH agonist], flutamide [testosterone receptor blocker], or bilateral orchiectomy)
- **Stage IA disease found with TURP** – Tx: nothing
- **With prostatectomy**, PSA should go to 0 after 3 weeks → if not, get bone scan to check for metastases
- **A normal PSA is < 4** in a patient who has a prostate gland.
  - **PSA** can be ↑ with prostatitis, BPH, and chronic catheterization.
- ↑ **alkaline phosphatase** in a patient with prostate CA → worrisome for metastases or extracapsular disease

RENAL CELL CARCINOMA (RCC, HYPERNEPHROMA)

- #1 primary tumor of kidney (15% calcified)
- Risk factor: **smoking**
- **Flank pain, mass,** and **hematuria**

- Dx: CT scan – ⅓ have metastatic disease at the time of diagnosis → can perform **wedge resection** of **isolated lung** or **colon metastases**
- **Lung** – most common location for RCC metastases
- **Erythrocytosis** can occur secondary to ↑ erythropoietin (HTN).
- Tx: **radical nephrectomy** with regional nodes; XRT, chemotherapy
  - Radical nephrectomy takes kidney, <u>adrenal</u>, fat, Gerota's fascia, and regional nodes.
  - Predilection for growth in the IVC; can still resect even if going up IVC → can pull the tumor thrombus out of the IVC
  - Partial nephrectomies should be considered only for patients who would require dialysis after nephrectomy (tumors < 4 cm, creatinine ≥ 2.5).
  - Most common tumor in kidney – **metastasis from breast CA**
  - **RCC paraneoplastic syndromes** – renin, erythropoietin, PTHrp, ACTH, insulin
  - **Transitional cell CA of renal pelvis** – Tx: radical nephroureterectomy
  - **Oncocytomas** – benign
  - **Angiomyolipomas** – hamartomas; can occur with tuberous sclerosis; **benign**
  - **Von Hippel–Lindau syndrome** – multifocal and recurrent RCC, renal cysts, CNS tumors, and pheochromocytomas

BLADDER CANCER

- Usually **transitional cell CA**
- **Painless hematuria**
- Males; prognosis based on stage and grade
- Risk factors: smoking, aniline dyes, and cyclophosphamide
- Dx: cystoscopy
- Tx: **intravesical BCG** or **transurethral resection if muscle is not involved (T1)**
  - **If muscle wall is invaded** (T2 or greater) → cystectomy with ileal conduit, chemotherapy (MVAC: methotrexate, vinblastine, Adriamycin [doxorubicin], and cisplatin), and XRT
  - Metastatic disease – chemotherapy
- **Ileal conduit is standard reconstruction option** – avoid stasis as this predisposes to infection, stones (calcium resorption), and ureteral reflux
- **Reservoirs** or **neobladders** may also be options.
- **Squamous cell CA of bladder** – schistosomiasis infection

TESTICULAR TORSION

- Peaks in 15-year-olds; sudden onset of severe testicular pain
- Testis is swollen, tender, high riding, and may have a horizontal lie.
- Torsion is usually toward the midline.
- Tx: emergency **detorsion** and **bilateral orchiopexy**
  - If testicle not viable, resection and orchiopexy of contralateral testis

URETERAL TRAUMA

- If going to repair end-to-end →
  - Spatulate ends.
  - Use **absorbable suture** to avoid stone formation.
  - **Stent the ureter** to avoid stenosis.
  - **Place drains** to identify and potentially help treat leaks.
- Avoid stripping the soft tissue on the ureter, as it will compromise blood supply.

BENIGN PROSTATIC HYPERTROPHY (BPH)

- Arises in **transitional zone**
- **Symptoms**: nocturia, frequency, dysuria, weak stream, urinary retention

- **Initial therapy**
  - **Alpha blockers** – terazosin, doxazosin (relax smooth muscle)
  - **5-alpha-reductase inhibitors** – finasteride (inhibits the conversion of testosterone to dihydrotestosterone → inhibits prostate hypertrophy)
- **Surgery** (trans-urethral resection of prostate; TURP): for recurrent UTIs, gross hematuria, stones, renal insufficiency, or failure of medical therapy
  - **Post-TURP syndrome** – hyponatremia secondary to irrigation with water; can precipitate **seizures** from cerebral edema
  - Tx: careful correction of Na with diuresis
- Most patients with TURP have retrograde ejaculation.

NEUROGENIC BLADDER

- Most commonly secondary to spinal compression
- Patient urinates all the time.
- Nerve injury above T12
- Tx: surgery to improve bladder resistance

NEUROGENIC OBSTRUCTIVE UROPATHY

- Incomplete emptying
- Nerve injury below T12; can occur with APR
- Tx: intermittent catheterization

INCONTINENCE

- **Stress incontinence** (cough, sneeze)
  - Because of hypermobile urethra or loss of sphincter mechanism; women; multiple pregnancies and vaginal deliveries
  - Tx: Kegel exercises, alpha-adrenergic agents, surgery for urethral suspension or pubovaginal sling
- **Overflow incontinence**
  - Incomplete emptying of an enlarged bladder
  - Obstruction (BPH) leads to the distention and leakage.
  - Tx: tamsulosin (Flomax); TURP

OTHER UROLOGIC DISEASES

- **Ureteropelvic obstruction** – Tx: pyeloplasty
- **Vesicoureteral reflux** – prophylactic antibiotics and see if the child outgrows it; failure to suppress infections or complicated disease requires surgery
  - **Dx**: voiding cystourethrogram
  - **Surgical Tx**: reimplantation of ureter with long bladder portion
- **Ureteral duplication** – most common urinary tract abnormality; Tx: reimplantation if obstruction occurs
- **Ectopic ureter** – often seen with ureteral duplication; can connect to **urethra** (usually asymptomatic unless obstruction occurs; usually no Tx necessary) or **vagina** (need to reimplant in the bladder)
- **Ureterocele** – Tx: resect and reimplant if symptomatic
- **Posterior urethral valves** – most common reason for newborn boy not to urinate
  - Place urinary catheter to temporize (valves will not block catheter).
  - **Dx**: voiding cystourethrogram
  - Tx: resection of valves
- **Hypospadias** – ventral urethral opening; Tx: repair at 6 months with penile skin (use foreskin; _no circumcision in these patients_)
- **Epispadias** – dorsal urethral opening; Tx: surgery

- **Horseshoe kidney** – usually joined at lower poles
  - Complications: UTI, urolithiasis, and hydronephrosis
  - Tx: may need pyeloplasty
- **Polycystic kidney disease** – resection only if symptomatic
- **Failure of closure of urachus** – connection between umbilicus and bladder; occurs in patients with bladder outlet obstructive disease (wet umbilicus)
  - Tx: resection of sinus/cyst and closure of the bladder; relieve bladder outlet obstruction
- **Epididymitis** – sterile epididymitis can occur from ↑ abdominal straining
- **Infectious acute epididymitis** – sexually active; severe testicular pain of sudden onset; fever and pyuria; swollen and tender testis; cord is tender as well; get U/S to rule out testicular torsion; Tx: antibiotics
- **Acute bacterial prostatitis** – older men with fever, chills, dysuria, frequency, diffuse back pain, and tender prostate; Tx: antibiotics (avoid prostate compression, which could lead to sepsis)
- **Varicocele** – worrisome for <u>renal cell CA</u> (left gonadal vein inserts into left renal vein; obstruction by renal tumor causes varicocele); could also be caused by another retroperitoneal malignancy
- **Spermatocele** – fluid-filled cystic structure separate from and superior to the testis along the epididymis; Tx: surgical removal if symptomatic
- **Hydrocele in adult** – if acute, suspect tumor elsewhere (pelvic, abdominal); translucent
- **Pneumaturia** – most common cause is diverticulitis and subsequent formation of colovesical fistula; Dx – cystoscopy
- **WBC casts** – pyelonephritis, glomerulonephritis
- **RBC casts** – glomerulonephritis
- **Pyelonephritis** – fever, chills, flank pain, nausea, vomiting
  - Dx: CT or U/S to rule out obstruction
  - Tx: antibiotics and relief of any obstruction (eg ureteral stone) with stent, stone removal, or percutaneous nephrostomy tube
- **Interstitial nephritis** – fever, rash, arthralgias, eosinophils
- **Vasectomy** – 50% pregnancy rate after repair of vasectomy
- **Priapism** (erection lasting more than 4 hours) – Tx: aspiration of the corpus cavernosum with dilute epinephrine or phenylephrine
  - May need to create a communication through the glans with scalpel
  - Risk factors: sickle-cell anemia, hypercoagulable states, trauma, intracorporeal injections for impotence
- **SCC of penis** – penectomy with 2-cm margin
- **Indigo carmine** or **methylene blue** (intravenous) – used to check for urine leak
- **Phimosis found at time of laparotomy** – Tx: dorsal slit
- **Erythropoietin** – ↓ production in patients with renal failure

40 Gynecology

LIGAMENTS
- **Round ligament** – allows anteversion of the uterus
- **Broad ligament** – contains uterine vessels
- **Infundibular ligament** – contains ovarian artery, nerve, and vein
- **Cardinal ligament** – holds cervix and vagina

ULTRASOUND
- Very good at diagnosing disorders of the female genital tract

PREGNANCY
- Can see most pregnancies on ultrasound at **6 weeks**
- **Gestational sac** is seen with beta-HCG of 1,500.
- **Fetal pole** usually is seen with beta-HCG of 6,000.

ABORTIONS
- **Missed** – 1st-trimester bleeding, closed os, positive sac on ultrasound, and no heartbeat
- **Threatened** – 1st-trimester bleeding, positive heartbeat
- **Incomplete** – tissue protrudes through os
- **Ectopic pregnancy** (life threatening) – acute abdominal pain; positive beta-HCG, negative ultrasound for sac; can also have missed period, vaginal bleeding, hypotension
  - **Risk factors for ectopic pregnancy**: previous tubal manipulation, PID, previous ectopic pregnancy
  - **MC site** – ampullary portion of the fallopian tubes
  - Significant shock and hemorrhage can occur from an ectopic pregnancy.
  - **Stable** – methotrexate or salpingotomy
  - **Unstable** – salpingectomy

ENDOMETRIOSIS
- Symptoms: dysmenorrhea, infertility, dyspareunia
- Can involve the rectum and cause bleeding during menses → endoscopy shows **blue mass**
- **Ovaries** – most common site
- Tx: OCPs

PELVIC INFLAMMATORY DISEASE
- Has ↑ risk of infertility and ectopic pregnancy
- Symptoms: pain, nausea, vomiting, fever, vaginal discharge
  - Most commonly occurs in the first ½ of the menstrual cycle
- Risk factors: multiple sexual partners
- Dx: cervical motion tenderness, cervical cultures, positive Gram stain
- Tx: ceftriaxone, doxycycline
- **Complications**: persistent pain, infertility, ectopic pregnancy
- **HSV** – vesicles; **HPV** – condylomata
- **Syphilis** – positive dark-field microscopy, chancre
- **Gonococcus** – diplococci

MITTELSCHMERZ

- Rupture of graafian follicle
- Causes pain that can be confused with appendicitis
- Occurs 14 days after the 1st day of menses

VAGINAL CANCER

- #1 primary – squamous cell CA
- **DES** (diethylstilbestrol) – can cause clear cell CA of vagina
- **Botryoides** – rhabdosarcoma that occurs in young girls
- **XRT** – used for most cancers of vagina

VULVAR CANCER

- Elderly, nulliparous, obese; usually unilateral
- Majority **squamous cell CA**
- Tx: **< 2 cm** (stage I) – **WLE** and <u>ipsilateral</u> **inguinal node dissection** (2-cm margins)
  - **> 2 cm** (stage II or greater) – **radical vulvectomy** (bilateral labia) with <u>bilateral inguinal dissection</u>, postop **XRT** if close margins (< 1 cm)
  - Paget's VIN III or higher – **premalignant**
  - VIN – vulvar intra-epithelial neoplasia

OVARIAN CANCER

- **Leading cause of gynecologic death**
- Abdominal or pelvic pain; change in stool or urinary habits; vaginal bleeding
- ↓ **risk** – OCPs, bilateral tubal ligation
- ↑ **risk** – nulliparity, late menopause, early menarche
- **Types** – teratoma, granulosa-theca (estrogen secreting, precocious puberty); Sertoli-Leydig (androgens, masculinization); struma ovarii (thyroid tissues); choriocarcinoma (beta-HCG); mucinous; serous; and papillary
- **Clear cell type** – worst prognosis

Staging of Ovarian Cancer	
Stage	Location
I	One or both ovaries only
II	Limited to pelvis
III	Spread throughout abdomen
IV	Distant metastases

- **Bilateral ovary** involvement still **stage I**
- **MC initial site of regional spread** – other ovary
- **Debulking tumor** – can be effective; including omentectomy (helps intraperitoneal chemo and XRT)
- Tx: **total abdominal hysterectomy** and **bilateral oophorectomy** for all stages; *plus*:
  - Pelvic and para-aortic LN dissection
  - Omentectomy
  - 4 quadrant washes
  - Chemotherapy: cisplatin and paclitaxel (Taxol)
- **Krukenberg tumor** – stomach CA that has metastasized to ovary
  - Pathology classically shows **signet ring cells**.
- **Meige's syndrome** – pelvic ovarian fibroma that causes **ascites** and **hydrothorax**
  - Excision of tumor cures syndrome.

ENDOMETRIAL CANCER

- **Most common malignant tumor in female genital tract**
- **Risk factors** – nulliparity, late 1st pregnancy, obesity, tamoxifen, unopposed estrogen
- Vaginal bleeding in postmenopausal patient is endometrial CA until proved otherwise.
- Uterine polyps have very low chance of malignancy (0.1%).
- **Clear cell subtype** – worst prognosis
- **Abdominal approach** with surgery (not trans-vaginal)

Staging and Treatment		
Stage	Location	Treatment
I	Endometrium	Total abdominal hysterectomy and BSO or XRT
II	Cervix	Total abdominal hysterectomy and BSO or XRT
III	Vagina, peritoneum, and ovary	Total abdominal hysterectomy and BSO and XRT
IV	Bladder and rectum	Total abdominal hysterectomy and BSO and XRT

CERVICAL CANCER

- Goes to **obturator nodes 1st**
- Associated with **HPV 16** and **18**
- **Squamous cell CA** – most common

Staging of Cervical Cancer	
Stage	Location
I	Cervix
II	Upper ⅔ of vagina
III	Pelvis, side wall, and lower ⅓ of vagina; hydronephrosis
IV	Bladder and rectum

- Tx: **microscopic disease** without basement membrane invasion → **cone biopsy** (conization sufficient to remove disease; inner lining of the cervix is removed)
- **Stages I and IIa** – total abdominal hysterectomy (TAH)
- **Stages IIb to IV** – chemo-XRT (cisplatin and paclitaxel [Taxol])

OVARIAN CYSTS

- **Postmenopausal patient**
  - If **septated**, has ↑ **vascular flow** on Doppler, has **solid components**, or has **papillary projections** → oophorectomy with intraoperative frozen sections; TAH if ovarian CA
  - If none of the above are present, follow with ultrasound for 1 year → if persists or gets larger → oophorectomy with intraoperative frozen sections; TAH if ovarian CA
- **Premenopausal patient**
  - If **septated**, has ↑ **vascular flow** on Doppler, has **solid components**, or has **papillary projections** → oophorectomy with intraoperative frozen sections usual
    - Algorithm becomes very complicated after this, weighing how aggressive the cancer is (based on histology and stage at the time of operation) compared with whether the patient desires future pregnancy.
  - If none of the above are present → can follow with ultrasound; surgery if suspicious findings appear

ABNORMAL UTERINE BLEEDING

- < **40** years old – if **anovulation**. Tx: **clomiphene citrate**
  - If **leiomyomas** → Tx: **GnRH agonists** (leuprolide)
- > **40** years old – **cancer** or **menopause** → need biopsy

OTHER GYNECOLOGIC CONSIDERATIONS

- **Contraindications to estrogen therapy** – endometrial CA, thromboembolic disease, undiagnosed vaginal bleeding, breast CA
- **Uterine endometrial polyp** – can present as progressively heavier menses
- **Uterine fibroids** (leiomyomas) – under hormonal influence; recurrent abortions, infertility, bleeding
- **Most common vaginal tumor** – invasion from surrounding or distant structure
- **Hydatidiform mole** – malignancy risk with <u>partial mole</u>; complete mole is of paternal origin; Tx: chemo (methotrexate)
- **Toxic shock syndrome** – fever, erythema, diffuse desquamation, nausea, vomiting; associated with highly absorbent tampons
- **Ovarian torsion** – Tx: remove torsion and check for viability
- **Adnexal torsion with vascular necrosis** – Tx: adnexectomy
- **Ruptured tuboovarian abscess** – Tx: percutaneous drainage and antibiotics
- **Ovarian vein thrombosis** – Dx: CT scan; Tx: heparin
- **Postpartum pelvic thrombophlebitis** – can lead to ovarian vein, IVC, and hepatic vein thrombosis; get liver failure with ascites after pregnancy; Tx: **heparin** and **antibiotics**

INTRODUCTION

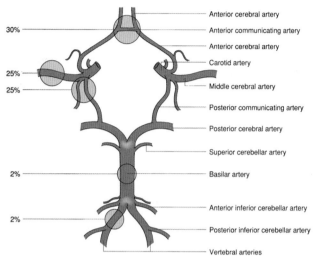

Locations of aneurysms of the circle of Willis and their relative occurrence.

CIRCLE OF WILLIS

- **Vertebral arteries** – come together to form a single **basilar artery**, which branches into 2 **posterior cerebral arteries**
- **Posterior communicating arteries** – connect **middle cerebral arteries** to **posterior cerebral arteries**
- **Anterior cerebral arteries** – branches off **middle cerebral arteries** and are connected to each other through the 1 **anterior communicating artery**

NERVE INJURY

- **Neurapraxia** – no axonal injury (temporary loss of function, foot falls asleep)
- **Axonotmesis** – disruption of **axon** with preservation of axon sheath, will improve
- **Neurotmesis** – disruption of **axon** and **myelin sheath** (whole nerve is disrupted), may need surgery for recovery
- Regeneration of nerves occurs at a rate of **1 mm/day**.
- **Nodes of Ranvier** – bare sections; allow salutatory conduction

ANTIDIURETIC HORMONE (ADH)

- Release controlled by **supraoptic nucleus of hypothalamus**, which descends into the posterior pituitary gland
- Released in response to high plasma osmolarity; ADH increases water absorption in collecting ducts.

STROKE

- CT scan to rule out **hemorrhage** (can't use tPA)
- Tx: tPA if within 3 hours of symptoms; endovascular stent retriever can be used for large emboli or failure of tPA if within 6 hours of stroke.

HEMORRHAGE

- **Arteriovenous malformations** – 50% present with hemorrhage; are congenital
  - Usually in patients < 30; sudden headache and loss of consciousness
  - Tx: resection if symptomatic
  - Can coil embolize these prior to resection
- **Cerebral aneurysms** – usually occur in patients > 40; most are congenital
  - Can present with bleeding, mass effect, seizures, or infarcts
  - Occur at branch points in artery, most off middle cerebral artery
  - Tx: Often place coils before clipping and resecting aneurysm.
- **Subdural hematoma** – caused by **torn bridging veins**
  - Has crescent shape on head CT and conforms to brain
  - Higher mortality than epidural hematoma
  - Tx: Operate for significant neurologic degeneration or mass effect (thickness > 10 mm or midline shift > 5 mm).

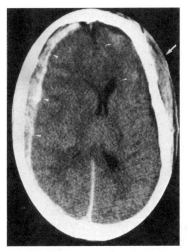

Acute subdural hematoma imaged by noncontrast computed tomography.

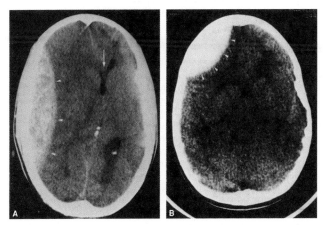

Two examples of acute epidural hematoma imaged by noncontrast computed tomography.

- **Epidural hematoma** – caused by injury to **middle meningeal artery**
  - Has lens shape on head CT and pushes brain away
  - Patients classically lose consciousness, have a lucid interval, and then lose consciousness again.
  - Tx: Operate for significant neurologic degeneration or mass effect (shift > 0.5 cm).
- **Subarachnoid hemorrhage** (nontraumatic)
  - Caused by cerebral aneurysms (50% middle cerebral artery) and AVMs
  - Symptoms: spontaneous stiff neck (nuchal rigidity), severe headache (worst headache of their life), photophobia, neurologic defects
  - Tx: Goal is to isolate the aneurysm from systemic circulation (clipping vascular supply), maximize cerebral perfusion to overcome vasospasm, and prevent rebleeding; use hypervolemia and calcium channel blockers to overcome vasospasm.
  - Go to OR **only if neurologically intact**.
  - Can get subarachnoid hemorrhages with trauma as well
- **Intracerebral hematomas** – temporal lobe most often affected
  - Those that are large and cause focal deficits should be drained.
- **Symptoms** of ↑ ICP – stupor, headache, nausea and vomiting, stiff neck
- **Signs** of ↑ ICP – hypertension, HR lability, slow respirations
  - **Intermittent bradycardia** is a sign of severely elevated ICP and impending herniation.
  - **Cushing's triad** – hypertension, bradycardia, slow respiratory rate

SPINAL CORD INJURY

- **Cord injury with deficit** → give **high-dose steroids (↓ swelling)**
- **Most sensitive test for spinal cord injury** – MRI
- **Spinal shock** – hypotension, **normal or slow heart rate**, and **warm extremities** (vasodilated)
  - Occurs with spinal cord injuries above T6 (loss of sympathetic tone)
  - Tx: fluids initially, may need phenylephrine drip (alpha agonist)
- **Complete cord transection** – bilateral areflexia, flaccidity, anesthesia, and paralysis below the level of the lesion
- **Anterior spinal artery syndrome** (anterior spinal cord syndrome) – occurs from compromise of the anterior spinal artery
  - **Causes** – aortic dissection, aneurysm, or atherosclerosis; ruptured disc; vertebral body burst fracture
  - **Bilateral loss of motor, pain,** and **temperature** sensation below the level of lesion
  - **Preservation of position–vibratory sensation** and **light touch**
  - About 10% recover to ambulation.
- **Hemisection** (Brown-Sequard syndrome) – incomplete cord transection (hemisection); most commonly due to penetrating injury
  - **Loss of ipsilateral motor** and **contralateral pain/temperature** below level of lesion
  - About 90% recover to ambulation.
- **Central cord syndrome** – most commonly occurs with hyperextension of the cervical spine (eg rear-end collision; often in elderly patients with preexisting cervical spondylosis)
  - Most common cervical spinal cord injury
  - **Bilateral loss motor, pain,** and **temperature** sensation in **upper extremities**; lower extremities spared
- **Cauda equina syndrome** – pain and weakness in lower extremities due to compression of lumbar nerve roots
- **SCIWORA** (spinal cord injury without radiographic abnormality) – usually seen in pediatric trauma (Dx: MRI)

- **Spinothalamic tract** (dorsal) – carries pain and temperature sensory neurons
- **Corticospinal tract** (ventral) – carries motor neurons
- **Rubrospinal tract** (ventral) – carries motor neurons
- **Dorsal nerve roots** – are generally afferent; carry sensory fibers
- **Ventral nerve roots** – are generally efferent; carry motor neuron fibers

BRAIN TUMORS

- Most are metastatic from other primary sites (eg breast, lung).
- Symptoms: **headache**, seizures, blurred vision, progressive neurologic deficit, and persistent vomiting
- High-dose **steroids** can help reduce intracranial pressure.
- Cushing reflex – HTN and bradycardia from increased intracranial pressure
- Adults – ⅔ supratentorial
- Children – ⅔ infratentorial (cerebellum; Sx's: ataxia, stumbling)
- **Gliomas** – most common primary brain tumor in adults and overall
  - **Glioma multiforme** – most common subtype, uniformly fatal
- **Meningioma** – benign; Tx: resection
- **Lung** – #1 metastasis to brain
- Most common brain tumor in children – **medulloblastoma**
- Most common metastatic brain tumor in children – **neuroblastoma**
- **Acoustic neuroma** – arises from the **8th cranial nerve** at **cerebellopontine angle**
  - Symptoms – hearing loss, unsteadiness, vertigo, nausea, and vomiting
  - Tx: surgery usual

SPINE TUMORS

- Overall, most are benign; #1 tumor overall **neurofibroma**
- **Intradural tumors** are more likely benign, and **extradural tumors** are more likely malignant.
- **Paraganglionoma** – check for metanephrines in urine

PEDIATRIC NEUROSURGERY

- **Intraventricular hemorrhage** (subependymal hemorrhage)
  - Seen in premature infants secondary to rupture of the fragile vessels in germinal matrix
  - Risk factors: ECMO, cyanotic congenital heart disease
  - Symptoms: bulging fontanelle, neurologic deficits, ↓ BP, and ↓ Hct
  - Tx: ventricular catheter for drainage and prevention of hydrocephalus
- **Myelomeningocele**
  - Neural cord defect – herniation of spinal cord and nerve roots through defect in vertebra
  - Most commonly occurs in the lumbar region

MISCELLANEOUS

- **Wernicke's area** – speech comprehension, temporal lobe
- **Broca's area** – speech motor, frontal lobe
- **Pituitary adenoma**, **undergoing XRT**, **patient now in shock**
  - Dx: pituitary apoplexy
  - Tx: steroids
- **Cervical nerves roots 3–5** innervate diaphragm (phrenic nerve).
- **Microglial cells** – act as brain macrophages

Cranial Nerves

Nerve	Name	Function	Muscle
I	Olfactory	Smell	
II	Optic	Sight	
III	Oculomotor		Motor to eye
IV	Trochlear		Superior oblique (eye)
V	Trigeminal: ophthalmic, maxillary, and mandibular branches	Sensory to face	Muscles of mastication
VI	Abducens		Lateral rectus (eye)
VII	Facial	Taste to anterior ⅔ of tongue	Motor to face
VIII	Vestibulocochlear	Hearing	
IX	Glossopharyngeal	Taste to posterior ⅓ of tongue	Swallowing muscles
X	Vagus	Many functions	
XI	Accessory		Trapezius Sternocleidomastoid
XII	Hypoglossal		Tongue

- **Brain abscess** – usually from adjacent otitis media or mastoiditis; fever; elevated ICP symptoms
  - Tx: need drainage if > 2.5 cm, otherwise just antibiotics
- **Reflex sympathetic dystrophy** (causalgia)
  - Develops several months after initial injury
  - Constant burning pain; aggravated by stimulation of area; area may be cold, cyanotic, and moist
  - Tx: sympathectomy

42 Orthopedics

BACKGROUND

- **Osteoblasts** –synthesize nonmineralized bone cortex
- **Osteoclasts** – reabsorb bone
  - Stages of bone healing – 1) inflammation, 2) soft callus formation, 3) mineralization of the callus, 4) remodeling of the callus
- Cartilage receives nutrients from synovial fluid (osmotic).
- **Salter-Harris** fractures **III**, **IV**, and **V** – cross the epiphyseal plate and can affect the growth plate of the bone (growth plate is in 2 pieces); need open reduction and internal fixation (**ORIF**)
- **Salter-Harris** fractures **I** and **II** – **closed reduction**
- **Greenstick fracture** – buckling of the cortex

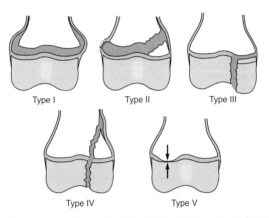

Type I   Type II   Type III

Type IV   Type V

Salter-Harris classification of epiphyseal injuries. Type I injury is an epiphysiolysis of the involved growth plate without associated fracture. Type II has an additional metaphyseal fracture fragment; type I and II injuries have a good prognosis and are usually treated with closed reduction and casting. Type III injury results in a fracture through the growth plate and epiphysis. Type IV fracture crosses the epiphysis, growth plate (physis), and metaphysis. Type III and IV injuries require careful open reduction and internal fixation if displaced. Type V injury involves a crush of the growth plate without a fracture and is usually detected late by asymmetric or premature closure of the growth plate.

- Fractures associated with **avascular necrosis** (AVN) – scaphoid, femoral neck, talus, hip dislocation
- Fractures associated with **nonunion** – clavicle, 5th metatarsal fracture (Jones' fracture)
- Fractures associated with **compartment syndrome** – supracondylar humerus, tibia, calcaneus
- **Biggest risk factor for nonunion** – smoking

LOWER EXTREMITY NERVES

- **Obturator nerve** – hip adduction
- **Superior gluteal nerve** – hip abduction
- **Inferior gluteal nerve** – hip extension
- **Femoral nerve** – knee extension

LUMBAR DISC HERNIATION

- Presents with back pain, sciatica
- Herniated **nucleus pulposus**
- Nerve root compression affects 1 nerve root below disc:
  - **L3 nerve** compression (L2–3 disc) – weak hip flexion
  - **L4 nerve** compression (most common; L3–4 disc) – weak knee extension (quadriceps), weak patellar reflex
  - **L5 nerve** compression (L4–5 disc) – weak dorsiflexion (footdrop)
    - ↓ sensation in big toe web space
  - **S1 nerve** compression (L5–S1 disc) – weak plantar flexion, weak Achilles reflex
    - ↓ sensation in lateral foot
- Dx: Patients with neurologic findings need **MRI**.
- Tx: NSAIDs, heat, and rest for majority; surgery for substantial/progressive neurologic deficit, refractory cases, severe sciatica, or disc fragments that have herniated into the cord (laminectomy)
- **Cauda equina syndrome** – distended bladder, flaccid rectal sphincter, perineal saddle anesthesia; Tx: emergency decompression

TERMINAL BRANCHES OF BRACHIAL PLEXUS

- **Ulnar nerve**
  - **Motor** – <u>intrinsic musculature of hand</u> (palmar interossei, palmaris brevis, adductor pollicis, and hypothenar eminence); finger abduction (spread fingers); wrist flexion
  - **Sensory** – all of 5th and ½ 4th fingers, back of hand
  - Injury results in **claw hand**.
- **Median nerve**
  - **Motor** – thumb apposition (anterior interosseous muscle, OK sign); finger flexors
  - **Sensory** – most of palm and 1st 3 and ½ 4th fingers on palmar side
  - Nerve is involved in **carpal tunnel syndrome**.
- **Radial nerve**
  - **Motor** – wrist extension, finger extension, thumb extension, and triceps; <u>no</u> hand muscles
  - **Sensory** – 1st 3 and ½ 4th fingers on dorsal side
- **Axillary nerve** – motor to deltoid (abduction)
- **Musculocutaneous nerve** – motor to biceps, brachialis, and coracobrachialis
- **Radial nerve roots** – on the superior portion of the brachial plexus
- **Ulnar nerve roots** – on the inferior portion of the brachial plexus

UPPER EXTREMITY

- **Clavicle fracture** – usually just treated with sling (risk of vascular impingement)
- **Shoulder dislocation**
  - **Anterior** (90%) risk of **axillary <u>nerve</u> injury**. Tx: closed reduction
  - **Posterior** (seizures, electrocution) risk of **axillary <u>artery</u> injury**. Tx: closed reduction
- **Acromioclavicular separation** – Tx: sling (risk of brachial plexus and subclavian vessel injury)
- **Scapula fracture** – sling unless glenoid fossa involved, then need internal fixation
- **Midshaft humeral fracture** – Tx: sling for almost all
- **Supracondylar humeral fracture** – adults → ORIF
  - **Children: nondisplaced** → <u>closed reduction</u>; **displaced** → ORIF
- **Monteggia fracture** – fall on outstretched hand; proximal ulnar fracture and radial head dislocation
  - Tx: ORIF
- **Colles fracture** – fall on outstretched hand, distal radius. Tx: closed reduction
- **Nursemaid's elbow** – subluxation of the radius at the elbow caused by pulling on an extended, pronated arm. Tx: closed reduction

- **Combined radial and ulnar fracture**
  - **Adults** – ORIF
  - **Children** – closed reduction
- **Scaphoid fracture** – snuffbox tenderness; can have negative x-ray
  - MC carpal bone fracture
  - Tx: all patients require cast to elbow, may need ORIF if displaced and angulated
  - High risk of **avascular necrosis** and **nonunion**
- **Metacarpal fracture** – typically 4th or 5th (when closed fist hits solid surface)
  - Tx: closed reduction with ulnar gutter splint; Kirschner wires if severely displaced
- **Volkmann's contracture**: supracondylar humerus fracture → occluded **anterior interosseous artery** → closed reduction of humerus → artery opens up → reperfusion injury, edema, and **forearm compartment syndrome** (flexor compartment most affected)
  - Symptoms: forearm pain with passive extension; weakness, tense forearm, hypesthesia
  - **Median nerve** most affected by swelling
  - Tx: **forearm fasciotomies**
- **Forearm fasciotomies** – need to open volar and dorsal compartments
- **Dupuytren's contracture** – associated with diabetes, ETOH, Norwegian descent
  - Progressive proliferation of the **palmar fascia of hand** results in contractures that usually affect the **4th** and **5th digits** (cannot extend fingers).
  - Tx: NSAIDs, steroid injections; excision of involved fascia for significant contraction
- **Carpal tunnel syndrome** – median nerve compression by transverse carpal ligament
  - Tx: splint, NSAIDs, and steroid injections; **transverse carpal ligament** release if that fails
- **Trigger finger** – tenosynovitis of the flexor tendon that catches at the MCP joint when trying to extend finger
  - Tx: splint, tendon sheath steroid injections (not the tendon itself); if that fails, can release the pulley system at the MCP joint
- **Suppurative tenosynovitis**
  - Infection that spreads along flexor tendon sheaths of digits (can destroy sheath)
  - **4 classic signs**: tendon sheath tenderness, pain with passive motion, swelling along sheath, and semi-flexed posture of the involved digit
  - Tx: *midaxial longitudinal incision and drainage*
- **Rotator cuff tears** – supraspinatus, infraspinatus, teres minor, and subscapularis
  - Acutely → sling and conservative treatment
  - Surgical repair if the patient needs to retain a high level of activity or if ADL affected
- **Paronychia** – infection under nail bed; painful. Tx: antibiotics; remove nail if purulent.
- **Felon** – fingertip (pad) abscess
  - Tx: incision over the tip of the finger and along the medial and lateral aspects to prevent necrosis of tip of finger

LOWER EXTREMITY

- **Isolated anterior ring with minimal ischial displacement** – Tx: weight-bearing as tolerated
- **Hip dislocation**
  - **Posterior** (90%) – patients have internal rotation and adduction of leg; risk of **sciatic nerve injury**. Tx: closed reduction
  - **Anterior** (10%) – patients have external rotation and abduction of leg; risk of injury to **femoral artery**. Tx: closed reduction
  - Reduce within **24 hours** to prevent avascular necrosis.
- **Hip fracture**
  - **Femoral shaft** – ORIF with intramedullary rod
  - **Intertrochanteric** – ORIF
  - **Femoral neck** – ORIF; risk of avascular necrosis if open reduction delayed

- **Lateral knee trauma** – can result in injury to **anterior cruciate ligament, posterior cruciate ligament,** and **medial meniscus**
- **Anterior cruciate ligament injury** – positive anterior drawer test
  - Present with **knee effusion** and **pain with pivoting action**; MRI confirms diagnosis.
  - Tx: surgery with knee instability (reconstruction with patellar tendon or hamstring tendon); otherwise physical therapy with leg-strengthening exercise
- **Posterior cruciate ligament injury** – positive posterior drawer test
  - Much less common than ACL injury; present with knee pain and joint effusion
  - Tx: conservative therapy initially; surgery for failure of medical management
- **Collateral ligaments**
  - **Medial collateral ligament injury** – lateral blow to knee
  - **Lateral collateral ligament injury** – medial blow to knee
  - Tx: **small tear** – brace; **large tear** – surgery
  - These injuries are associated with injuries to the corresponding **meniscus.**
- **Meniscus tears** – joint line tenderness; can treat with arthroscopic repair or debridement
- **Tibial stress fracture** – young men in forced marches; point tibial tenderness; x-rays initially normal; Tx – cast and repeat x-ray in 2 weeks
- **Posterior knee dislocation** – all patients need angiogram to rule out popliteal artery injury
- **Patellar fracture** – long leg cast unless comminuted, then need internal fixation
- **Tibial plateau fracture** and **tibia–fibula fracture** – ORIF unless open, then need external fixator until tissue heals
- **Plantaris muscle rupture** – pain and mass below popliteal fossa (contracted plantaris) and ankle ecchymosis; Tx: conservative
- **Achilles tendon rupture** – have limited plantar flexion; Tx: open repair for younger patients; casting in older patients
- **Ankle fracture** – most treated with cast and immobilization; bimalleolar or trimalleolar fractures need ORIF
- **Metatarsal fracture** – cast immobilization or brace for 6 weeks
- **Calcaneus fracture** – cast and immobilization if nondisplaced; ORIF for any displacement
- **Talus fracture** – closed reduction for most; ORIF for severe displacement
- **Plantar fasciitis** – older, overweight patients; pain in heel when it strikes ground; Tx: NSAIDs, steroid injections; if conservative measures fail, surgery requires detaching fascia from heel.
- **Morton neuroma** – usually between 3rd and 4th toes; very tender; from pointed shoes; Tx: NSAIDs, can be resected if conservative measures fail
- **Nerve most commonly injured with lower extremity fasciotomy** – superficial peroneal nerve (foot eversion)
- **Footdrop** after **lithotomy position** or after **crossing legs for long periods** or **fibula head fracture** – common peroneal nerve (footdrop)

LEG COMPARTMENTS

- **Anterior** – anterior tibial artery, deep peroneal nerve
  - **Muscles** – anterior tibialis, extensor hallucis longus, extensor digitorum longus, and communis
- **Lateral** – superficial peroneal nerve
  - **Muscles** – peroneal muscles
- **Deep posterior** – posterior tibial artery, peroneal artery, and tibial nerve
  - **Muscles** – flexor hallucis longus, flexor digitorum longus, and posterior tibialis
- **Superficial posterior** – sural nerve
  - **Muscles** – gastrocnemius, soleus, and plantaris

COMPARTMENT SYNDROME

- Most common in the **anterior compartment of leg** (get footdrop) after **vascular compromise, restoration of blood flow**, and subsequent **reperfusion injury** (PMNs) with **swelling of the compartment**
- Can also occur from crush injuries
- Symptoms: swollen and tight extremity: pain with passive motion → paresthesia → anesthesia → paralysis → poikilothermia → pulselessness (late finding)
- **Distal pulses can be present** with compartment syndrome → last thing to go
- Pressure > 20–30 mm Hg abnormal
- Pain under a cast – remove cast and examine limb
- Dx: based on clinical suspicion
- Tx: **fasciotomy**

PEDIATRIC ORTHOPEDICS

- **Hip problems** in children can present with **knee pain** (compensation).
- **Remodeling** and straightening of bone fractures in children occurs even with significant angulation deformities.
- Children heal faster than adults.
- Children do have problems with **supracondylar fractures** and fractures affecting the **growth plate**.
- **Idiopathic adolescent scoliosis** – prepubertal females, right thoracic curve most common, usually asymptomatic
  - Curves 20–45 degrees need bracing to slow progression, which can occur with growth spurt.
  - Curves > 45 degrees or those likely to progress → spinal fusion
- **Acute hematogenous osteomyelitis** – can occur in metaphysis of long bones in children; most commonly staph
  - Symptoms: febrile illness, pain, decreased use of extremity
  - Dx: MRI
  - Tx: antibiotics
- **Septic hip**
  - Toddlers with a febrile illness; refuse to move hip; have elevated ESR
  - Dx: hip aspiration (shows pus)
  - Tx: open drainage
- **Legg–Calvé–Perthes disease** – AVN of the femoral head; children around age 6
  - Can result from a hypercoagulable state; bilateral in 10%
  - Symptoms: painful gait limp; decreased hip motion
  - X-ray: flattening of the femoral head
  - Tx: Maintain range of motion with limited exercise; **femoral head will remodel without sequelae**.
  - Surgery if femoral head is not covered by the acetabulum (casting, crutches)
- **Slipped capital femoral epiphysis**
  - Males aged 10–13; ↑ risk of AVN of the femoral head; painful gait; hip motion limited
  - X-ray: widening and irregularity of the epiphyseal plate
  - Orthopedic emergency
  - Tx: surgical pinning of the femoral head
- **Developmental hip dysplasia** (congenital dislocation of the hip)
  - More common in females; generally diagnosed right after birth
  - Hip can be easily dislocated posteriorly; uneven gluteal folds
  - Dx: sonogram (not XR's as hip is not calcified in newborns)
  - Tx: Pavlik harness for 6 months, which keeps the legs abducted and the femoral head reduced in the acetabulum

- **Osgood–Schlatter disease** – tibial tubercle apophysitis (osteochondrosis); caused by traction injury from the quadriceps in adolescents aged 13–15; have pain over tibial tubercle (there is no knee swelling)
  - X-ray: irregular shape or fragmenting of the tibial tubercle
  - Tx: mild symptoms → activity limitation; severe symptoms → cast 6 weeks followed by activity limitation
- **Genu varum** (bow legs) – normal up to age 3
  - If it persists, likely is **Blount disease** (medial tibial growth plate abnormality) for which surgery can be done
- **Genu valgus** (knock knee) – normal between ages 4 and 8
- **Talipes equinovarus** (clubfoot)
  - Seen at birth
  - Tx: serial casting starts in neonatal period

BONE TUMORS

- Most common is metastatic disease (#1 breast [lytic lesions], #2 prostate [blastic lesions]).
  - Can have localized pain; pathologic fracture may be the initial symptom.
  - Tx: internal fixation with impending fracture (> 50% cortical involvement); followed by XRT
- Bone pain + lesion → very likely malignant
- Primary bone tumors usually present with persistent, low-grade pain for several months.
- **Multiple myeloma** – most common primary malignant tumor of bone
  - Usually in elderly men; fatigue, anemia, and localized bone pain
  - **X-ray** – multiple lytic lesions
  - **Urine** – Bence Jones protein
  - **Blood** – abnormal immunoglobulins
  - Tx: chemotherapy for systemic disease; internal fixation for impending fractures
- **Pathologic fractures** – treat with internal fixation
  - XRT can be used for pain relief in patients with painful bony metastases.
- **Osteogenic sarcoma** – most common primary bone sarcoma, usually around the knee
  - Patients aged 10–25
  - X-ray: **Codman's triangle** → periosteal reaction (sunburst pattern)
  - Tx: limb-sparing resection if possible; XRT and **doxorubicin-based** chemotherapy can be used preoperatively to increase chance of limb-sparing resection.
- **Ewing's sarcoma** – 2nd most common primary bone sarcoma
  - Patients aged 5–15; grows in diaphysis of long bones
  - X-ray – onion skinning pattern
- **Benign bone tumors treated with curettage ± bone graft** – osteochondroma (MC benign bone tumor; resection only if cosmetic defect or causing symptoms), osteoid osteoma, endochondroma (may be able to observe), chondroblastoma, nonossifying fibroma (may be observed), and fibrodysplasia
- **Giant cell** tumor of bone – total resection ± XRT (benign but 30% risk of recurrence; also has malignant degeneration risk)

OTHER ORTHOPEDIC CONDITIONS

- **Spondylolisthesis** – formed by subluxation or slip of one vertebral body over another
  - Most commonly occurs in lumbar region
  - Most common cause of lumbar pain in adolescents (gymnasts)
  - Tx: depends on degree of subluxation and symptoms – ranges from conservative treatment to surgical fusion

- **Cervical stenosis** – surgical decompression if significant myelopathy present
- **Lumbar stenosis** – surgical decompression for cases refractory to medical treatment
- **Torus fracture** – buckling of the metaphyseal cortex seen in children (ie distal radius)
- **Open fractures** – need incision and drainage, antibiotics, fracture stabilization, and soft tissue coverage

43 Pediatric Surgery

INTRODUCTION

- **Foregut** – lungs, esophagus, stomach, pancreas, liver, gallbladder, bile duct, and duodenum proximal to ampulla
- **Midgut** – duodenum distal to ampulla, small bowel, and large bowel to distal ⅓ of transverse colon
- **Hindgut** – distal ⅓ of transverse colon to anal canal
- Midgut rotates 270 degrees counterclockwise normally.
- Low birth weight < 2,500 g; premature < 37 weeks
- **Immunity at birth** – IgA from mother's milk; **IgG** crosses the placenta
- ↑ alkaline phosphatase in children compared with adults → **bone growth**
- **Fetal umbilical contents**
  - **2 umbilical arteries** – become <u>medial</u> umbilical ligaments
  - **1 umbilical vein** – becomes ligamentum teres
  - **Urachus** – becomes <u>median</u> umbilical ligament
  - **Vitelline duct** – can form Meckel's diverticulum
- Unilateral earache, rhinorrhea, or wheezing in a toddler – may be foreign body (Dx/Tx: appropriate endoscopy and removal)

TRAUMA

- **#1 cause of childhood death**
- **Intubation** – use <u>uncuffed</u> tube *only* for neonates/infants (**< 1 year**); cuffed tube if > 1 year
  - **ET tube size** for children aged < 10 = width of patient's pinky nail bed
  - Children can have significant **bradycardia** with intubation (Tx: **atropine**).
- **Trauma bolus** – 20 cc/kg × 2 boluses, then switch to blood 10 cc/kg (if still hypotensive)
  - Usually lactated Ringer's; consider normal saline for younger children (prevents hyponatremia).
- **Tachycardia** – *best indicator of shock in children*; HR indicating tachycardia (apx) →

Neonate/infant (<1)	> 150
Preschool (1–5)	> 120
School age (6–12)	> 110
Teenagers	same as adult

- Blood pressure is the last thing to go → children look well until they crash quickly.
- Appropriate **urine output** (marker of adequate resuscitation):

Age 0–1	> 2–4 cc/kg/hr
Age > 1	> 1 cc/kg/hr

- Children < 6 months only have **25% GFR capacity of adults** (poor concentrating ability).
- Children have increased risk of **hypothermia** (↑ BSA compared to weight) and **head injury**.

MAINTENANCE INTRAVENOUS FLUIDS

- 4 cc/kg/hr for 1st 10 kg
- 2 cc/kg/hr for 2nd 10 kg
- 1 cc/kg/hr for everything after that
- D5 normal saline (0.9% NaCl) preferred

CONGENITAL CYSTIC DISEASE OF THE LUNG

- **Pulmonary sequestration**
  - Lung tissue has **anomalous systemic arterial supply** (thoracic aorta [MC] or abdominal aorta through inferior pulmonary ligament).
  - Have either systemic venous or pulmonary vein drainage
  - **Extra-lobar** – more likely to have <u>systemic</u> venous drainage (azygous system)
  - **Intra-lobar** – more likely to have <u>pulmonary vein</u> drainage
  - Lung tissue does <u>not</u> communicate with the tracheobronchial tree (airway).
  - Most commonly presents with infection; can also have respiratory compromise or an abnormal CXR
  - Tx: Ligate arterial supply first (risk of severe hemorrhage), then **lobectomy**.
- **Congenital lobar emphysema** (overinflation)
  - Cartilage fails to develop in bronchus, leading to air trapping with expiration.
  - Vascular supply and other lobes are normal (except compressed by hyperinflated lobe).
  - Can develop hemodynamic instability (same mechanism as tension PTX) or respiratory compromise
  - LUL most commonly affected
  - Can look like a pneumothorax – do <u>not</u> place a chest tube (will injure lung)
  - Tx: **lobectomy**
- **Congenital cystic adenoid malformation (CCAM)**
  - Communicates with airway
  - Alveolar structure is poorly developed, although lung tissue is present.
  - Symptoms: respiratory compromise or recurrent infection
  - Tx: lobectomy
- **Bronchiogenic cyst**
  - Most common **congenital cysts** of the mediastinum; usually posterior to the carina
  - Are **extra-pulmonary cysts** formed from bronchial tissue and cartilage wall
  - Usually present with a mediastinal mass filled with milky liquid
  - Can compress adjacent structures or become infected; have malignant potential
  - Occasionally are intra-pulmonary
  - Tx: Resect cyst.

MEDIASTINAL MASSES IN CHILDREN

- **Neurogenic tumors** (neurofibroma, neuroganglioma, neuroblastoma) – <u>most common</u> mediastinal tumor in children; usually located posteriorly
- **Respiratory symptoms**, **dysphagia** – common to all mediastinal masses regardless of location
- **Anterior** – T-cell lymphoma, **teratoma** (and other germ cell tumors; most common type of anterior mediastinal mass in children), thyroid CA
- **Middle** – T-cell lymphoma, teratoma, cyst (cardiogenic or bronchiogenic)
- **Posterior** – T-cell lymphoma, neuroblastoma, neurogenic tumor
- *Thymoma is <u>rare</u> in children.*

CHOLEDOCHAL CYST

- **Need to resect** – risk of cholangiocarcinoma, pancreatitis, cholangitis, obstructive jaundice
  - **Type III** have <u>low</u> (2%–3% lifetime) malignant transformation rate and do <u>not</u> always need excision (ie *avoid* doing a Whipple).
- Caused by abnormal **reflux of pancreatic enzymes** into the biliary system **in utero** (from long common biliopancreatic duct)

Choledochal Cyst Surgery

Type	%	Description	Treatment
I	85%	**Fusiform dilation** of entire common bile duct, mildly dilated common hepatic duct, normal intrahepatic ducts	Resection, hepaticojejunostomy
II	3%	A true **diverticulum** that hangs off the common bile duct	Resection off common bile duct; may be able to preserve common bile duct and avoid hepaticojejunostomy
III	1%	**Choledochocele**; dilation of distal intramural common bile duct; involves **sphincter of Oddi**	Transduodenal excision (larger cysts) or endoscopic/transduodenal sphincteroplasty
IV	10%	**Multiple cysts; IVa** – both extrahepatic and intrahepatic; **IVb** – extrahepatic only	**IVa** – hepatic/biliary resection, hepaticojejunostomy **IVb** – biliary resection, hepaticojejunostomy
V	1%	**Intrahepatic cysts** (Caroli's disease); get hepatic fibrosis; may be associated with congenital hepatic fibrosis and medullary sponge kidney	Possible lobectomy if confined to one lobe; liver TXP

LYMPHADENOPATHY

- Usually acute suppurative adenitis associated with URI or pharyngitis
- **If fluctuant** → FNA, culture and sensitivity, and antibiotics; may need incision and drainage if it fails to resolve
  - **Chronic causes** – cat scratch fever, atypical mycoplasma
- **Asymptomatic** – antibiotics for 10 days → excisional biopsy if no improvement
  - This is lymphoma until proved otherwise.
- **Cystic hygroma** (lymphangioma) – usually found in lateral cervical regions in neck; gets infected; is usually **lateral** to the sternocleidomastoid (SCM) muscle
  - Tx: resection

DIAPHRAGMATIC HERNIAS AND CHEST WALL

- Overall survival 50%
- Increased on **left side** (80%; liver protects the right diaphragm)
- Can have severe **pulmonary HTN**
- 80% have associated anomalies (cardiac and neural tube defects mostly; malrotation).
- Diagnosis can be made with prenatal ultrasound.
- Symptoms: respiratory distress
- CXR – bowel in chest
- **Both lungs** are dysfunctional (hernia side is hypoplastic; contralateral side has pulmonary HTN).
- Tx: high-frequency ventilation; inhaled nitric oxide; may need ECMO
  - Stabilize these patients before operating on them.
  - Need to reduce bowel and repair defect ± mesh (abdominal approach)
  - Look for visceral anomalies (run the bowel).
- **Bochdalek's hernia** – most common, usually located left side and posteriorly
- **Morgagni's hernia** – rare, located anteriorly
- **Pectus excavatum** (sinks in) – sternal osteotomy, need strut; performed if causing respiratory symptoms or emotional stress
- **Pectus carinatum** (pigeon chest) – strut not necessary; repair for emotional stress

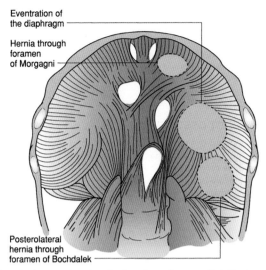

Anatomy of the diaphragm showing the location of congenital diaphragmatic defects.

BRANCHIAL CLEFT CYST

- Leads to cysts, sinuses, and fistulas
- **1st branchial cleft cyst** – angle of mandible; may connect with **external auditory canal**
  - Often associated with **facial nerve**
- **2nd branchial cleft cyst** (<u>most common</u>) – on anterior border of mid-SCM muscle
  - Goes through **carotid bifurcation** into **tonsillar pillar**
- **3rd branchial cleft cyst** – lower neck, **medial** to or through the lower SCM, to the **piriform sinus**
- Tx for all branchial cysts: resection

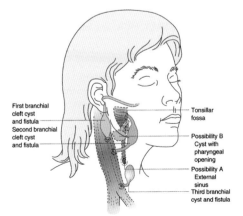

Types of first, second, and third branchial cleft remnants. Sinuses and fistulas are seen most often in infants and young children, whereas cysts usually appear at a later age.

CYSTIC HYGROMA
- Soft, mass-like lesion usually found in the base of the lateral neck (posterior neck triangle)
- Is a multiple, macrocytic lymphatic malformation (nuchal lymphangioma)
- Can get infected, form sinuses
- Dx: CT scan (want to assess depth; can involve mediastinum)
- Tx: **resection**

THYROGLOSSAL DUCT CYST
- From abnormal descent of the thyroid gland from the **foramen cecum**
- May be only thyroid tissue patient has
- Presents as a **midline** cervical mass
- Goes through the **hyoid bone**
- Tx: excision of **cyst**, **tract**, and **hyoid bone** (at least central portion) to the base of the tongue

HEMANGIOMA
- Appears at birth or shortly after
- Most common area – **head** and **neck**
- Rapid growth during first 6-12 months of life, then begins to involute
- Tx: **observation** – most resolve by age 7-8
- If lesion has **uncontrollable growth**, **impairs function** (eyelid or ear canal), or is **persistent after age 8** → can treat with **oral steroids** → laser or resection if steroids are not successful

NEUROBLASTOMA
- **#1 solid abdominal malignancy in children**
- Usually presents as asymptomatic mass
- Can have secretory diarrhea, raccoon eyes (orbital metastases), **HTN**, and opsomyoclonus syndrome (unsteady gait)
- Most often on **adrenals**; can occur anywhere along the sympathetic chain
- Most common in **1st 2 years of life**
  - Children < 1 year have best prognosis (the younger the patient, the better the cure rate).
- Most have ↑ **catecholamines**, **VMA**, **HVA**, and **metanephrines** (HTN).
- Derived from **neural crest cells**
- Encases vasculature rather than invades
- **Rare metastases** – go to lung and bone
- Abdominal x-ray: may show **stippled calcifications** in the tumor
- CT scan – shows **renal displacement** (*not* replacement like Wilms tumor)
- *Worse* prognosis – **NSE, LDH, HVA, diploid tumors**, and **N-myc amplification** (> 3 copies)
- NSE is ↑ in all patients with **metastases**.
- Tx: resection (**adrenal gland** and **kidney** taken; 40% cured)
- Initially unresectable tumors may be resectable after neoadjuvant **doxorubicin**-based chemo.
- One of the few tumors that can involute spontaneously and turn into a benign neuroma

Staging of Neuroblastoma	
Stage	Description
I	Localized, complete excision
II	Incomplete excision but does not cross midline
III	Crosses midline ± regional nodes
IV	Distant metastases (nodes or solid organ)
IV-S	Localized tumor with distant metastases

WILMS TUMOR (NEPHROBLASTOMA)

- Usually presents as asymptomatic mass; can have hematuria or HTN; 10% bilateral
- Mean age at diagnosis – **3 years**
- **WAGR syndrome** – <u>W</u>ilms tumor, <u>A</u>niridia (no iris), <u>G</u>enitourinary malformations, and mental <u>R</u>etardation)
- Prognosis based on **tumor grade** (anaplastic and sarcomatous variations have worse prognosis)
- Frequent metastases to **bone** and **lung**
- Pulmonary metastases – whole lung XRT (same for bone)
- Abdominal CT – replacement of renal parenchyma and <u>not</u> displacement (differentiates it from neuroblastoma)
- Tx: **nephrectomy** (90% cured)
  - If venous extension occurs in the renal vein, the tumor can be extracted from the vein.
  - Need to examine the contralateral kidney and look for peritoneal implants
  - Avoid rupture of tumor with resection, which will ↑ stage.
  - **Actinomycin** and **vincristine** based chemo in all unless stage I and < 500 g tumor
  - Need nephron-sparing surgery for stage V disease

Staging of Wilms Tumor	
Stage	Description
I	Limited to kidney, completely excised
II	Beyond kidney but completely excised
III	Residual nonhematogenous tumor
IV	Hematogenous metastases
V	Bilateral renal involvement

HEPATOBLASTOMA

- Most common malignant liver tumor in children; ↑ **AFP** in 90%
- Fractures, precocious puberty (from beta-HCG release)
- Better prognosis than hepatocellular CA
- Can be pedunculated; vascular invasion common
- Tx: resection optimal; otherwise **doxorubicin**-based chemotherapy → may downstage tumors and make them resectable
- Survival is primarily related to resectability.
- **Fetal histology** has best prognosis.

MOST COMMONS

#1 children's malignancy overall – **leukemia** (ALL)
#1 solid tumor class – **CNS tumors**

#1 general surgery tumor - **neuroblastoma**
  #1 in child < 2 years → **neuroblastoma**
  #1 in child > 2 years → **Wilms tumor**
#1 cause of duodenal obstruction in newborns (< 1 week) - **duodenal atresia**
#1 cause of duodenal obstruction after newborn period (> 1 week) and overall -
malrotation
#1 cause of colon obstruction - **Hirschsprung's disease**
#1 liver tumor in children - **hepatoblastoma**; ⅔ of liver tumors in children are malignant
#1 lung tumor in children - **carcinoid** (#1 benign - hemangioma)
Painful lower GI bleeding - **#1 benign anorectal lesions** (fissures, etc.)
Painless lower GI bleeding - **#1 Meckel's diverticulum**
Upper GI bleeding - 0-1 year → **gastritis, esophagitis**
  1 year to adult → **esophageal varices, esophagitis**

MECKEL'S DIVERTICULUM

- Found on **antimesenteric border** of small bowel
- Embryology - diverticulum represents a **persistent vitelline duct** (omphalomesenteric duct)
- Rule of 2s - 2 feet from ileocecal valve, 2% population, 2:1 male predominance,
  2% symptomatic, 2 tissue types (**pancreatic** - <u>most common</u>; **gastric** - most likely to
  be <u>symptomatic</u>), and 2 presentations (diverticulitis and bleeding)
- **#1 cause of painless lower GI bleeding in children**
- 50% present before **age 5**, 90% before **age 10**.
- Can get Meckel's scan (pertechnetate) if suspicious of Meckel's diverticulum and
  having trouble locating (will only pick up **gastric mucosa**)
- Tx: resection with symptoms, suspicion of gastric mucosa, narrow neck, or
  complication (eg perforation)
  • Diverticulitis involving the base or if the base is > ⅓ the size of the bowel, need to
    perform segmental resection

PYLORIC STENOSIS

- 3-12 weeks, firstborn males
- Sx's - **projectile vomiting** (nonbilious) and **dehydration**
- Can feel **olive mass** in stomach
- Get **hypochloremic, hypokalemic metabolic alkalosis** and **paradoxical aciduria**
- Ultrasound - pylorus ≥ 4-mm thick, ≥ 14-mm long
- For severe dehydration, resuscitate with **normal saline boluses** until making urine,
  then switch to D5 normal saline with 10 mEq K maintenance.
  • *Avoid fluid resuscitation with K-containing fluids (ie lactated Ringer's) in infants with severe
    dehydration as **hyperkalemia** can quickly develop.*
  • *Avoid non–salt-containing solutions in infants as **hyponatremia** can quickly develop.*
  • *Infants should always have a maintenance fluid with **glucose** because of their limited reserves
    for gluconeogenesis and vulnerability for hypoglycemia.*
- Tx: **pyloromyotomy** (RUQ incision; proximal extent should be the circular muscles of
  stomach)

INTUSSUSCEPTION

- Usually 3 months to 3 years
- **Currant jelly stools** (from vascular congestion, <u>not</u> an indication for resection), sausage
  mass, abdominal distention, colicky RUQ pain, and vomiting (**bilious** if obstructed)
- Invagination of one loop of intestine into another (MC - ileum into right colon)
- Lead points in children - enlarged (inflamed) **Peyer's patches** (#1; may have history
  of viral illness), lymphoma, and Meckel's diverticulum
- 15% recurrence after reduction

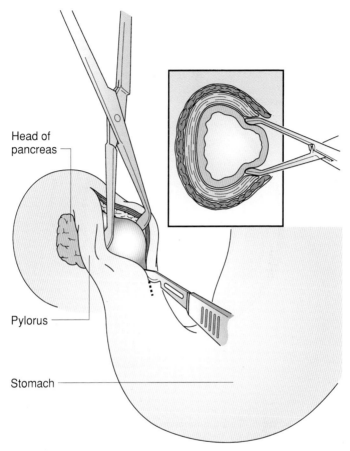

Ramstedt pyloromyotomy for infantile hypertrophic pyloric stenosis. The cross-sectional view shows herniation of the submucosa into the myotomy site, indicative of an adequate myotomy.

- Dx: U/S – shows **Bullseye sign**
- Tx: reduce with **air-contrast enema** → 80% successful; <u>no</u> surgery required if reduced
  - Max pressure with air-contrast enema – **120 mm Hg**
  - Max column height with barium enema – **1 meter (3 feet)**
  - High perforation risk beyond these values → need to proceed to OR if you have reached these values after 1 hour
  - Can try a **2nd time** if it recurs
  - Successful reduction → PO challenge in ED, observe 4 hours, then discharge
  - Need to go to OR with peritonitis, free air (pneumoperitoneum), if unable to reduce, or after 2nd recurrence
    - When reducing in OR, do <u>not</u> place traction on proximal limb of bowel; need to apply pressure to the distal limb and milk intussusception out
    - Usually do <u>not</u> require bowel resection unless associated with complicated Meckel's
- **Adults presenting with intussusception** – patient most likely has **malignant lead point** (ie colon CA in cecum); <u>*no*</u> *air-contrast or barium enema* → go to OR for resection

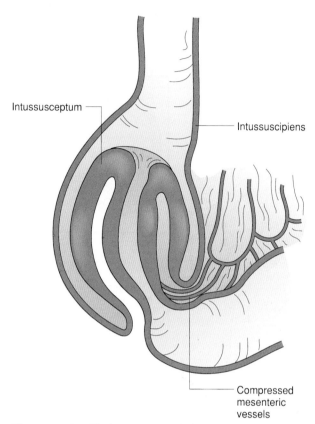

Intussusceptum

Intussuscipiens

Compressed
mesenteric
vessels

Anatomy of intussusception. The intussusceptum is the segment of bowel that invaginates into the intussuscipiens.

DUODENAL ATRESIA

- #1 cause of duodenal obstruction in <u>newborns</u> (< 1 week)
- Usually distal to ampulla of Vater; causes **bilious vomiting** and feeding intolerance immediately after birth
- Associated with **polyhydramnios** in mother (from not swallowing amniotic fluid)
- Associated with cardiac, renal, and other GI anomalies
- 20% of these patients have **Down's syndrome** (check chromosomal studies).
- Caused by failure of **duodenal recanalization**
- Abdominal x-ray – shows **double-bubble sign**
- Tx: resuscitation; duodenoduodenostomy or duodenojejunostomy

OTHER INTESTINAL ATRESIAS

- Develop as a result of **intrauterine vascular accidents**
- Symptoms: bilious emesis, distention; most do not pass meconium
- More common in **jejunum**; can be <u>multiple</u>
- Get rectal biopsy to R/O Hirschsprung's before surgery.
- Tx: resection

TRACHEOESOPHAGEAL FISTULAS (TEF)

- **Type C** – most common type (85%)
  - **Proximal esophageal atresia** (blind pouch) and **distal TE fistula**
  - Symptoms: newborn spits up feeds, has excessive drooling, and respiratory symptoms with feeding; cannot place NG tube in stomach
  - Abdominal x-ray – distended, gas-filled stomach
- **Type A** – second most common type (5%)
  - Esophageal atresia and no fistula
  - Symptoms: similar to type C
  - Abdominal x-ray – patients have gasless abdomen
- **VACTERL syndrome** – **v**ertebral, **a**norectal (imperforate anus), **c**ardiac, **TE** fistula, **r**adius/renal, and **l**imb anomalies
- Before surgery, look at anus for imperforation, x-ray (and sacral U/S) for vertebral/limb anomalies, echocardiogram for congenital heart problems, and renal U/S.
- Tx: **right extrapleural thoracotomy** for most; perform primary repair; and place G-tube
  - Azygous vein often needs to be divided.
- Infants that are **premature**, **< 2,500 g**, or **sick** → Replogle tube (suctions saliva out of the esophagus and prevents aspiration), treat respiratory symptoms; place gastrostomy-tube (for type C; drains stomach and prevents reflux into the lungs); delay repair.
- **Complications of repair** – GERD, leak, stricture, and fistula
- Survival related to birth weight and associated anomalies

MALROTATION

- Sudden onset of **bilious vomiting**
  - Ladd's bands cause duodenal obstruction, coming out from the right retroperitoneum
- Can lead to **midgut volvulus** (bowel twists around mesentery base) – associated with compromise of the **SMA**, leading to **intestinal infarction**
- Due to failure of normal counterclockwise rotation (270 degrees)
- Age at presentation – 75% in the 1st month after birth; 90% present by age 1 year
- *Any child with bilious vomiting needs an emergent UGI to rule out malrotation.*
- Dx: **UGI** – duodenum does not cross midline; duodenal-jejunal junction displaced rightward
- Tx: resect Ladd's bands, counterclockwise rotation (may require multiple turns), place cecum in **LLQ** (cecopexy), place duodenum in **RUQ** (small bowel to the right, large bowel to the left), and appendectomy (avoids future confounding diagnosis)

MECONIUM ILEUS

- Symptoms – no meconium (1st stool) passed in the first 24 hours
- Causes **distal ileal obstruction**, abdominal distention, bilious vomiting, and distended loops of bowel
- Need sweat chloride test or PCR for Cl channel defect
- Occurs in 10% of children with **cystic fibrosis**
- Abdominal x-ray: dilated loops of small bowel without air-fluid levels (because the meconium is too thick to separate from the bowel wall); can have ground glass or soapsuds appearance
- Can cause perforation, leading to meconium pseudocyst or free perforation → requires laparotomy
- Tx: **Gastrografin enema** (effective in 80%); can also make the diagnosis and potentially treat the patient
- Can also use *N*-acetylcysteine enema
  - If surgery required, manual decompression and create an ostomy vent for ***N*-acetylcysteine antegrade enemas**.

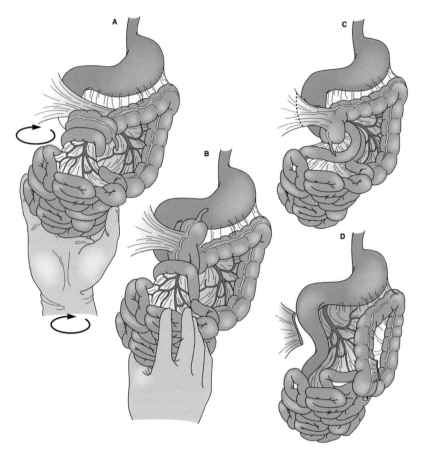

Correction of malrotation. **(A and B)** Detorsion of midgut. **(C and D)** Division of peritoneal attachments (Ladd's bands) of cecum to abdominal cavity.

NECROTIZING ENTEROCOLITIS (NEC)

- Classically presents with **bloody stools after 1st feeding** in **premature neonate**
- Symptoms: lethargy, respiratory decompensation, abdominal distention, vomiting, blood per rectum, thrombocytopenia (sign of sepsis in infants)
- Risk factors: prematurity, hypoxia, sepsis
- Abdominal x-ray: may show pneumatosis intestinalis (_not_ an indication for surgery alone), free air, or portal vein gas
- Need serial lateral decubitus films to look for perforation
- Initial Tx: resuscitation, NPO, antibiotics, TPN, and orogastric tube
- Indications for operation: free air (pneumoperitoneum), peritonitis, clinical deterioration, abdominal wall erythema → resect dead bowel and bring up ostomies
- Need barium contrast enema before taking down ostomies to rule out distal obstruction from stenosis
- Mortality 10%

CONGENITAL VASCULAR MALFORMATION

- Surgery for hemorrhage, ischemia, CHF, nonbleeding ulcers, functional impairment, or limb-length discrepancy
- Tx: **embolization** (may be sufficient on its own) and/or resection

IMPERFORATE ANUS

- More common in males
- Check for associated renal, cardiac, and vertebral (VACTERL) anomalies.
- **High** (above levators) – meconium in **urine** or **vagina** (fistula to bladder/vagina/prostatic urethra)
  - Tx: **colostomy**, later anal reconstruction with **posterior sagittal anoplasty**
- **Low** (below levators) – fistula carries meconium to perineal skin; perform **posterior sagittal anoplasty** (pull anus down into sphincter mechanism); **no colostomy needed**
- Need postop anal dilatation to avoid stricture; these patients are prone to constipation.

GASTROSCHISIS

- Abdominal wall defect
- **Intrauterine rupture of umbilical vein**; does <u>not</u> have a peritoneal sac
- Is usually to the right and inferior to umbilicus
- ↓ congenital anomalies (only 10%) except **intestinal atresia** (MC associated GI finding)
- To the right of midline, no peritoneal sac, stiff bowel from exposure to amniotic fluid
- Tx: initially place saline-soaked gauzes and resuscitate the patient; can lose a lot of fluid from the exposed bowel; TPN, NPO
  - Repair when patient is stable.
  - At operation, try to place bowel back in abdomen, may need silastic mesh silo (abdominal contents are gently squeezed back into the abdomen over a week or so)
  - Primary closure at a later date if silo used

OMPHALOCELE

- **Failure of embryonal development**; <u>has peritoneal sac</u> with cord attached
- Midline defect through the umbilical stalk
- ↑ congenital anomalies (50%)
- Sac can contain intra-abdominal structures other than bowel (liver, spleen, etc.).
- Associated with Down's syndrome
- MC associated GI finding – **malrotation**
- **Cantrell pentalogy**
  - **Cardiac** defects
  - **Pericardium** defects (usually at diaphragmatic pericardium)
  - **Sternal** cleft or absence of lower sternum
  - **Diaphragmatic** septum transversum absence
  - **Omphalocele**
- Tx: initially place saline-soaked gauzes and resuscitate the patient; can lose a lot of fluid from the exposed bowel; TPN, NPO
  - Repair when patient is stable.
  - At operation, try to place bowel back in abdomen; may need silastic mesh silo
  - Primary closure at a later date if mesh used
- Overall <u>worse</u> prognosis for omphalocele compared with gastroschisis secondary to **congenital anomalies**
- **Malrotation** can occur with both gastroschisis and omphalocele.

EXSTROPHY OF URINARY BLADDER

- Abdominal wall defect over the pubis (which is not fused)
- Bladder mucosa comes through defect.
- Tx: surgery to close defect and repair bladder

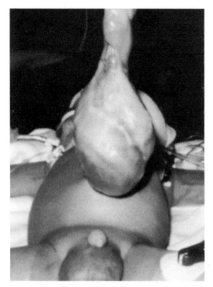

Omphalocele. The herniated intestines and liver are visible inside the sac. The umbilical cord attaches to the sac.

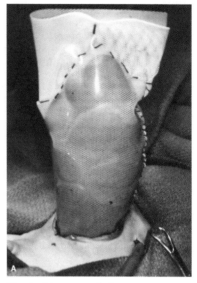

Silastic chimney or silo for temporary coverage of giant omphalocele.

HIRSCHSPRUNG'S DISEASE

- #1 cause of colonic obstruction in infants; more common in males
- **Most common sign** → infants fail to pass meconium in 1st 24 hours
  - Can also present in older age groups as chronic constipation (age 2–3)
- Causes abdominal **distention**; occasionally get colitis
- Can get explosive release of watery stool with anorectal exam
- Suction **rectal biopsy** diagnostic (full thickness; shows **absence of ganglion cells in myenteric plexus**)
- AXR – dilated proximal colon
- Is due to failure of the neural crest cells (ganglion cells) to progress in caudad direction
- Tx: Need to resect rectum and colon until proximal to where ganglion cells appear
  - May need to bring up a colostomy initially
  - Eventually connect the colon to the anus (Soave or Duhamel procedure)
- **Hirschsprung's colitis** – may be rapidly progressive; manifested by abdominal distention and foul-smelling diarrhea; possible sepsis
  - Lethargy and signs of sepsis may be present.
  - Tx: rectal irrigation to try and empty colon; may need emergency colectomy

UMBILICAL HERNIA

- Failure of closure of linea alba; most close by age 3, rare incarceration
- Increased in African Americans and premature infants
- Tx: surgery if not closed by age 5, incarceration, or if patient has a VP shunt

INGUINAL HERNIA

- Nearly all are **indirect** (due to **persistent processus vaginalis**); 3% of infants, M > F
- **Right** in 60%, left in 30%, bilateral in 10%
- Extension of the hernia sac into the internal ring differentiates hernia from hydrocele.
- If not able to reduce (**incarcerated** hernia) – emergent operation
- **Successful reduction** – urgent operation within 24 hours
- **Asymptomatic** – elective repair
- Tx: **high ligation** of the hernia sac (do not necessarily need to remove sac; open sac prior to ligation to avoid bowel/bladder/ovary injury)
- Consider exploring the contralateral side if left sided, female, or child < 1 year.

HYDROCELE

- Similar to inguinal hernia; however, sac does _not_ extend into the internal ring.
- Most disappear by 1 year; noncommunicating will resolve; should transilluminate
- Tx: surgery at 1 year if not resolved or if thought to be communicating (waxing and waning size); **resect hydrocele** and **ligate processus vaginalis**.

CYSTIC DUPLICATION

- Most common in ileum; often on mesenteric border
- Tx: Resect cyst.

BILIARY ATRESIA

- Most common cause of neonatal jaundice requiring surgery
- Most common indication for liver TXP in children
- Progressive jaundice persisting > 2 weeks after birth suggests atresia
- Can involve either the extrahepatic or intrahepatic biliary tree or both

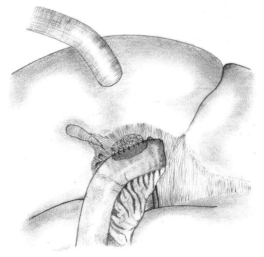

Anastomosis of Roux-en-Y hepatoportoenterostomy to liver.

- Dx: liver biopsy → periportal fibrosis, bile plugging, eventual cirrhosis
  - Ultrasound and HIDA can reveal atretic biliary tree.
- Get continued cirrhosis and eventual hepatic failure.
- Try Kasai procedure (hepaticoportojejunostomy) – ⅓ get better, ⅓ go on to liver transplant, and ⅓ die.
  - Involves resecting the atretic extrahepatic bile duct segment
  - Choleretic agents (eg phenobarbital) and steroids are used to try and increase bile flow.
- Need to perform Kasai procedure **before age 3 months** to avoid irreversible liver damage
- Generally need **liver TXP** if after 3 months

TERATOMA

- ↑ **AFP** and **beta-HCG** (elevated markers suggest transformation to malignancy)
- **Neonates** – sacrococcygeal; **adolescents** – germ cell
- Tx: excision
- **Sacrococcygeal teratomas**
  - 90% benign at birth (almost all have exophytic component)
  - Great potential for malignancy
  - AFP – good marker
  - 2-month mark is a huge transition – **< 2 months** → usually benign; **> 2 months** → usually malignant
  - Tx: **coccygectomy** and long-term follow-up

UNDESCENDED TESTICLES

- Wait **6 months** to treat.
- Higher risk of **testicular CA** in these children
- Cancer risk stays the same even if testicles brought into scrotum.
- Get **seminoma**.
- If undescended bilaterally, get chromosomal studies.
- If you cannot feel the testes in the inguinal canal, you need to get an MRI to confirm their presence.
- If the testicle can be brought into the scrotum, surgery generally not required (is due to overactive cremasteric muscle; 95% will outgrow this and the testicle will remain in the scrotum).
- Tx: **orchiopexy** through inguinal incision; if not able to get testicles down → perform division of spermatic vessels to get length (vas deferens blood supply will collateralize to testicles)

TRACHEOMALACIA

- Elliptical, fragmented tracheal rings instead of C-shaped; collapse with inspiration
- **Inspiratory wheezing**, usually get better after 1–2 years
- Risk factor – TE fistula
- **Surgical indications** – dying spell (MC), failure to wean from ventilator, recurrent infections
- Surgery – **aortopexy** (aorta sutured to the back of the sternum, opens up trachea)

LARYNGOMALACIA

- Most common cause of airway obstruction in infants
- Symptoms: intermittent respiratory distress and stridor exacerbation in the supine position
- Caused by immature epiglottis cartilage with intermittent collapse of the airway
- Most children outgrow this by 12 months.
- Surgical tracheostomy reserved for a very small number of patients

CHOANAL ATRESIA

- Obstruction of choanal opening (nasal passage) by either bone or mucous membrane, usually unilateral
- Symptoms: intermittent respiratory distress, poor suckling
- Tx: surgical correction

LARYNGEAL PAPILLOMATOSIS

- Most common tumor of the pediatric larynx
- Frequently **involutes after puberty**
- Can treat with endoscopic removal or laser but frequently comes back
- Thought to be caused from HPV in the mother during passage through the birth canal

CEREBRAL PALSY

- Many develop **GERD**

Neonatal Intestinal Obstruction			
Diagnosis	**History**	**Physical Examination**	**Diagnostic Studies**
Intestinal atresia or stenosis	Bilious emesis	Abdominal distention	Plain abdominal film
Duodenal atresia or stenosis	Failure to pass meconium	Acholic meconium	Contrast enema
		Gastric distention	Plain abdominal film
	Bilious emesis	Trisomy 21	Upper GI contrast study
Imperforate anus	Failure to pass meconium	Absent anus or visible fistula	Plain chest, abdominal film
	Bilious emesis (late)	Abdominal distention	Ultrasound kidneys, sacrum, rectum
		VACTERL association	Echocardiogram
Necrotizing enterocolitis	High-risk, premature infant	Abdominal distention	Plain abdominal film
	Bilious emesis	Hematochezia, guaiac-positive stool	
Meconium ileus	Cystic fibrosis (10%)	Acholic meconium	Plain abdominal film
	Bilious emesis	Abdominal distention	Contrast enema
Malrotation	Bilious emesis	No abdominal distention	Plain abdominal film
	Term, healthy infant		Upper GI contrast study
Hirschsprung's disease	Delayed passage of meconium	Abdominal distention	Plain abdominal film
	Bilious emesis	Trisomy 21	Contrast enema

GI, gastrointestinal; VACTERL, vertebral, anal, cardiac, tracheal, esophageal, renal, and limb anomalies.

44 Statistics and Patient Safety

INTRODUCTION
- **Null hypothesis** – hypothesis that no difference exists between groups
- **Type I error** (false positive) – rejects null hypothesis incorrectly
  - Falsely assumed there was a difference when no difference exists
  - Represented by the **P value**
  - P value is set at **≤ 0.05** for **statistical significance** ($p \leq 0.05$ rejects null hypothesis).
  - Example: P value = 0.01 indicates 1% chance of type I error.
    - 99% likelihood that the difference between the populations is true
    - 1% likelihood that the difference is not true and occurred by chance alone
- **Type II error** (false negative) – accepts null hypothesis incorrectly due to **small sample size**
  - Falsely assumed there was no difference when a difference actually exists
- **Power of test** = probability of rejecting null hypothesis correctly (likelihood of true positive)
  - Probability a test will find a difference when a difference actually exists
  - Power = 1 – probability of a type II error (power range is 0–1)
  - Power **≥ 0.8** – indicates a sufficiently powered test
  - **Larger sample size** increases the power of a test.
  - Example: power = 0.9 indicates:
    - 90% chance the test will detect the difference when the difference actually exists
    - 10% chance the test will _not_ detect the difference when the difference actually exists
- **Standard deviation** (SD) – indicates amount of variation in a data set compared to the mean
  - **Low SD** – values are close to mean (or expected value)
  - **High SD** – values are more spread out over a wider range
- **Normal distribution** (bell curve) – 1 peak
- **Bimodal distribution** – 2 peaks
- **Parameter** – population
- **Numeric terms** – example: 2, 7, 7, 8, 9, 11, 19
  - **Mode** – most frequently occurring value = 7
  - **Mean** – average = 9 (can be skewed by outliers [extreme values])
  - **Median** – middle value of a set of data (50th percentile) = 8 (used if you have a lot of outliers [resistant to skew]; if even number of values average the middle 2)

TRIALS AND STUDIES
- **Case report** – single patient or event
- **Case series** – accumulation of small number of case reports
- **Retrospective study** – analyzes preexisting data in a selected patient population
  - Has **selection bias** and **information bias**
- **Systematic review** – combining data from multiple different studies
- **Meta-analysis** – combining data from multiple different studies with statistical analysis
- **Prospective study** – data is collected going forward for a patient population and analyzed at a future date
- **Observational studies** – analyzes **risk factors** (or treatments) without changing who or who isn't exposed and **disease** (outcome); all 4 have **nonrandom** patient assignment:
  - **Case-control study** – compares those with **disease** (eg lung cancer) to those **without disease** (eg no lung cancer) and looks at risk factor frequency (eg smoking); _retrospective_
    - Has **selection** and **recall bias**
    - _Can not determine relative risk_; can determine odds ratio

- **Cohort study** – compares those with a **risk factor** (eg smokers) to those **without a risk factor** (eg nonsmokers) and looks at <u>disease</u> rate (eg lung cancer); can be *retrospective or prospective*
  - Has **loss to follow-up bias**
  - Can determine relative risk and odds ratio
- **Cross-sectional study** – looks at population data at **one specific point in time** (now); determines **disease** and **risk factor** <u>prevalence</u> but is <u>*not*</u> used to determine cause and effect (eg smoking and lung cancer)
  - Has **recall bias** and **detection bias**
  - Can determine relative risk and odds ratio
- **Propensity score matched study** – for a population with the **same disease**, a match between a <u>known</u> **treatment group** and an <u>artificially generated</u> **control group** of real patients who have the same risk factors and demographics is generated (finds patients for the control group who have similar covariates as treatment group); *retrospective*
  - Reduces known **confounding variables**
  - Tries to replicate a randomized control trial
  - Does <u>*not*</u> account for **unknown** confounding variables and patient characteristics (RCT does)
- **Randomized controlled trial** (RCT) – prospective study with random assignment to treatment and nontreatment groups
  - *Avoids treatment biases*
- **Cross-over RCT** – randomized and 2 treatments are given (A and B); each group eventually crosses over to the 2nd treatment (A then B <u>*or*</u> B then A)
  - Problem is that one treatment has ***carry-over*** into the 2nd treatment (hard to know influence of each treatment and what actually caused the effect).
- **Single-blinded RCT** – prospective study in which **patient** is blinded to treatment
  - *Avoids placebo effect*
  - Has **observational bias** (physician)
- **Double-blinded RCT** (*best – strongest form of evidence*) – prospective study in which *both* **patient** and **doctor** are blinded to treatment
  - *Avoids observational biases*
  - Avoids previously listed biases as well

QUANTITATIVE VARIABLES

- **Unpaired t test** (student's t test) – 2 independent groups and single variable is **numerical** (quantitative) → compares means (eg mean weight between diabetics and nondiabetics)
- **Paired t tests** – 2 independent groups and variable is **quantitative**; before <u>*and*</u> after studies (eg weight before and after, drug vs placebo)
- **ANOVA** – compares <u>*only*</u> **quantitative** variables (means) for 3 or more groups (eg length of stay for gastric sleeve vs Roux-en-Y vs gastric band)
- **Multiple linear regression** – analyzes influence of 2 or more independent variables (quantitative *or* qualitative) on a <u>**numerical**</u> outcome (eg gastric bypass operating room time)

QUALITATIVE VARIABLES

- **Nonparametric statistics** – compares **categorical** (qualitative) variables (race, sex, medical problems and diseases, medications)
- **Chi-squared test** – compares 2 groups with **qualitative variables** (eg number of obese patients with and without diabetes vs number of nonobese patients with and without diabetes)
- **Multivariate logistic regression** – analyzes influence of 2 or more independent factors (quantitative or qualitative) on a <u>**categorical**</u> outcome (eg factors associated w/ postop DVT)

- **Kaplan-Meyer** – estimates survival (usually small groups)
- **Prevalence** – number of people with disease in a population (eg number of patients in United States with colon CA); *Long-standing disease increases **prevalence***
- **Incidence** – number of **new cases** diagnosed over a certain time frame in a population (eg number of patients in United States newly diagnosed with colon CA in 2021)

Analysis Table

	Positive Test	Negative Test
Have disease	True-positive (TP)	False-negative (FN)
No disease	False-positive (FP)	True-negative (TN)

- **Sensitivity** – likelihood a diseased person will test positive = true-positives / (true-positives + false-negatives)
  - With **high sensitivity**, a negative test result means patient very <u>unlikely</u> to have disease.
- **Specificity** – likelihood a person without disease will test negative = true-negatives / (true-negatives + false-positives)
  - With **high specificity**, a positive test result means patient is <u>very likely</u> to have disease.
- **Positive predictive value** (PPV) = true-positives / (true-positives + false-positives)
  - Likelihood that with a positive result, the patient actually has the disease
- **Negative predictive value** (NPV) = true-negatives / (true-negatives + false-negatives)
  - Likelihood that with a negative result, the patient does not have the disease
- **Accuracy** = (true-positives + true-negatives) / (true-positives + true-negatives + false-positives + false-negatives)
- **Predictive values** (PPV and NPV) – are **dependent** on disease prevalence
- **Sensitivity** and **specificity** – are *independent* of disease prevalence
- **Receiver operating curve** (ROC) – shows trade-off between **sensitivity** and **specificity**; the greater the area under the curve (AUC) the better the test (curve to top left-hand corner quickly indicates a better test)

RISK ASSESSMENT

- **Risk** – probability of adverse outcome
- **Absolute risk** – **probability** of outcome over a stated time period
  - Example: Women with BRCA1 have an <u>absolute risk</u> of 60% (or 60 per 100 women) for developing breast CA in their lifetime.
- **Relative risk** – **probability** of outcome in exposed compared to **probability** of outcome in unexposed
  - Example (same as above): The <u>relative risk</u> of breast CA in women with BRCA1 is 6 (meaning they are 6 times [or 600%] more likely to get breast CA compared to women without BRCA1).
  - Tends to exaggerate risk (better to use absolute risk)
- **Odds ratio** – **odds** of outcome in exposed group compared to **odds** of outcome in unexposed
  - Example (same as above): The <u>odds ratio</u> of breast CA in women with BRCA1 is 5.9 (meaning there is 5.9 times greater likelihood they will get breast CA compared to women without BRCA1).
  - <u>*Not*</u> expressed as a percentage
  - Tends to exaggerate risk for **common diseases** (better to use absolute risk)
- **Confidence interval** – set at **95%**; a range of values where there is a 95% probability the true value exists within it; can be used for both risk (probability) and odds ratio
  - Example (same as above): Women with BRCA1 have an absolute risk of 60% (95% CI 55%–65%) for developing breast CA in their lifetime.
  - A confidence interval crossing 1 means there is <u>*no*</u> difference between the 2 groups.

- **Relative risk reduction** – the _decrease_ in **probability** of outcome in treatment group (or exposed) compared to **probability** of outcome with no (or different) treatment group
  - Example: High-risk women had a 1.5 relative risk reduction (or 50% relative risk reduction) for breast CA with tamoxifen compared to high-risk women with placebo.
  - Tends to exaggerate risk reduction, especially for **rare diseases** (better to use absolute risk reduction)
- **Absolute risk reduction** – the _decrease_ in **probability** of outcome over a stated time period in treatment group (the number of actual percentage points the risk goes down)
  - Example (same trial as above): High-risk women taking tamoxifen had an absolute risk reduction for breast CA of 2.1% (or 2.1 per 100 women) over 5 years.
- **Number need to treat** – number of subjects that must be treated before 1 outcome is avoided (= 1 / absolute risk reduction)
  - Example (same trial as above): The number needed to treat (high-risk women) with tamoxifen for at least 5 years to prevent 1 breast CA is 48 (1/2.1).

BIAS

- **Selection bias** – selecting patients in a **nonrandomized** way (solved with **blinded randomization**)
  - **Allocation bias** – **researcher knows what arm** of the study the next patient will get (treatment or no treatment; this may have been randomized) which influences whether or not they enroll a patient (solved with **concealment** of allocation)
  - **Lead time bias** – **earlier diagnosis** of a disease makes it look like the patient is living longer (ie survival over a time period will be higher compared to those diagnosed later; solved with **lifetime morality rate** [overall mortality] from the disease)
  - **Length time bias** – **screening** is more likely to find slower progressing, asymptomatic cases with longer survival compared to symptomatic, rapidly progressing cases (solved with **pathologic grading** comparisons [_not_ staging comparisons])
- **Information bias** – **misclassification** of exposure or outcomes
  - **Recall bias** – recalled exposure history changes based on **outcome status** (solved with **prospective** studies)
  - **Detection bias** (observer bias) – differences between groups in **how outcomes are determined** due to knowledge of patient's status (ie received therapy or did not receive therapy; solved with **assessor blinding** to patient's status)
  - **Surveillance bias** – differences between groups in **surveillance frequency** (screening or testing) such that the outcome is more likely to be detected in the higher surveyed group (solved with selecting groups with **equal surveillance frequency**)
  - **Hawthorne effect** – subjects **behave differently** when they know they are being observed (solved with either **subject blinding** to the study or **similar observation** between groups)
- **Confounding bias** (confounding variable) – the mixing of effects between exposure and outcome with another variable(s) resulting in a distortion of the true relationship (solved with **prospective randomization** or **propensity matching**)

PATIENT SAFETY

- **National Surgical Quality Improvement Program** (NSQIP) – collects outcome data to measure and improve surgical quality; outcomes are reported as observed/expected ratios.
- **JCAHO prevention of wrong site/procedure/patient protocol:**
  - Preop verification of **patient** and **procedure**
  - **Operative site** and **side** (marking if left or right or multiple levels; must be visible after the patient is prepped)
  - **Time out** before incision made (verifying patient, procedure, position site + side, and availability of implants or special requirements)

- **Promoting culture of safety**
  - Confidential system of reporting errors
  - Emphasis on learning over accountability
  - Flexibility in adapting to new situations or problems
- **RFs for retained object after surgery** (MC sponge) – emergency procedure, unplanned change in procedure, obesity, towel used for closure
- **Sentinel Event** (JCAHO) – unexpected occurrence involving death or serious injury, or the risk thereof; hospital undergoes **root cause analysis** to prevent and minimize future occurrences (eg **wrong site surgery**)
- **GAP protection technique** – gaps in care (eg change in caregiver, divisions of labor, shift changes, transfers) can lead to loss of information and error; **prevention** – **structured handoffs** and **checklists** (face to face best); standardized orders; reading back orders if verbal

↑	increased *or* high
↓	decreased *or* low
2,3-DPG	2,3-diphosphoglycerate
5FU	5-fluorouracil
AAA	abdominal aortic aneurysm
Ab	antibody
Abd	abdominal
ABI	ankle–brachial index
Abx	antibiotic
AC	doxorubicin (Adriamycin) and cyclophosphamide (Cytoxan)
ACE	angiotensin-converting enzyme
Ach	acetylcholine
ACT	activated clotting time
ACTH	adrenocorticotropic hormone
AD	autosomal dominant
ADH	antidiuretic hormone
ADL	activities of daily living
AFP	alpha-fetoprotein
Ag	antigen
AIDS	acquired immunodeficiency syndrome
AKA	above-knee amputation
ALL	acute lymphoblastic leukemia
ALND	axillary lymph node dissection
ALT	alanine aminotransferase
angio	angiography
ANOVA	analysis of variance
AP	aortopulmonary
APACHE	acute physiology and chronic health evaluation
APC	antigen-presenting cells
APR	abdominoperineal resection
APUD	amine precursor uptake and decarboxylation
ARDS	acute respiratory distress syndrome
ARF	acute renal failure
ASA	acetylsalicylic acid
ASD	atrial septal defect
AST	aspartate aminotransferase
ATGAM	anti-thymocyte gamma globulin
AT-III	antithrombin III
ATN	acute tubular necrosis
ATP	adenosine triphosphate
ATPase	adenosine triphosphatase
A-V	arteriovenous
AV	atrioventricular
AVM	arteriovenous malformation
AVN	avascular necrosis
AXR	abdominal radiograph
BCG	bacille Calmette-Guérin
BCT	breast-conserving therapy
BKA	below-knee amputation
BM	bowel movement
BPH	benign prostatic hypertrophy
BSA	body surface area
BT shunt	Blalock-Taussig shunt
BUN	blood urea nitrogen
Bx	biopsy
Ca	calcium
CA	cancer or carcinoma
CABG	coronary artery bypass graft
cAMP	cyclic adenosine monophosphate
CaO_2	arterial oxygen content
CBD	common bile duct
CCAM	congenital cystic adenoid malformation
CCK	cholecystokinin
cCMP	3,5-cyclic monophosphate (cytidine)
CD	cluster of differentiation (eg CD4, CD8)
CEA	carcinoembryonic antigen
CEA	carotid endarterectomy
cGMP	cyclic guanosine-3, 5-monophosphate
chemo	chemotherapy
CHF	chronic heart failure
CI	cardiac index
CLL	chronic lymphocytic leukemia
CMF	cyclophosphamide (Cytoxan), methotrexate, and 5-fluorouracil
CML	chronic myelogenous leukemia
CMV	cytomegalovirus
CN	cranial nerve
CNS	central nervous system
CO	cardiac output
COPD	chronic obstructive pulmonary disease
COX	cyclooxygenase
CPAP	continuous positive airway pressure
CPP	cerebral perfusion pressure
CPR	cardiopulmonary resuscitation
Cr	creatinine

CRH	corticotropin-releasing hormone	ESWL	extracorporeal shock wave lithotripsy
CSA	cyclosporin	ET	endotracheal
CSF	cerebrospinal fluid	ETCO$_2$	end-tidal CO$_2$
CT	computed tomography	ETOH	ethanol or alcohol
CVA	cerebrovascular accident (stroke)	EVAR	endovascular aortic repair
		F/U	follow-up
CvO$_2$	venous oxygen content	FAP	familial adenomatous polyposis
CVP	central venous pressure		
CVVH	continuous venovenous hemodialysis	FAST	focused abdominal sonography for trauma
Cx	complication	Fc	antibody fragment, crystallizable
CXR	chest radiograph		
D/C	discontinue	FEV$_1$	forced expiratory volume in 1 second
DAG	diacylglycerol		
DBP	diastolic blood pressure	FFP	fresh frozen plasma
DCIS	ductal carcinoma in situ	FGF	fibroblastic growth factor
DDAVP	desmopressin acetate, 1-deamino-8-d-arginine-vasopressin	FiO$_2$	fraction of inspired oxygen
		FMD	fibromuscular dysplasia
		FNA	fine needle aspiration
DES	diethylstilbestrol	FRC	functional residual capacity
DIC	disseminated intravascular coagulation	FSH	follicle-stimulating hormone
		FTSG	full-thickness skin graft
DIT	diiodotyrosine	FTT	failure to thrive
DKA	diabetic ketoacidosis	Fx	fracture
DLCO	diffusing capacity of the lung for carbon monoxide	G6PD	glucose-6-phosphate dehydrogenase
		GABA	gamma-aminobutyric acid
DM	diabetes mellitus	GCS	Glasgow Coma Scale
DPL	diagnostic peritoneal lavage	GCSF	granulocyte colony–stimulating factor
DVT	deep venous thrombosis		
Dx	diagnosis	GDA	gastroduodenal artery
DZ	disease	GERD	gastroesophageal reflux disease
EBV	Epstein-Barr virus		
ECA	external carotid artery	GFR	glomerular filtration rate
ECHO	echocardiogram	GH	growth hormone
ECMO	extracorporeal membrane oxygenation	GHRH	growth hormone–releasing hormone
EDRF	endothelium-derived relaxing factor	GI	gastrointestinal
		GIP	gastric inhibitory peptide
EDV	end-diastolic volume	GIST	gastrointestinal stromal tumor
EEG	electroencephalogram	GNR	gram-negative rod
EF	ejection fraction	GnRH	gonadotropin-releasing hormone
EGD	esophagogastroduodenoscopy		
EGF	epidermal growth factor	GPC	gram-positive cocci
EKG	electrocardiogram	GPR	gram-positive rod
ELAM	endothelial leukocyte adhesion molecule	GRP	gastrin-releasing peptide
		GSH	glutathione
EPI	epinephrine	GU	genitourinary
ER	emergency room or endoplasmic reticulum	H and P	history and physical
		HA	headache
ERCP	endoscopic retrograde cholangiopancreatography	HBIG	hepatitis B immunoglobulin
		HBV	hepatitis B virus
ERV	expiratory reserve volume	HCG	human chorionic gonadotropin
ESR	erythrocyte sedimentation rate		

HCl	hydrochloric acid; hydrochloride		LAK	lymphokine-activated killer
Hct	hematocrit		LAR	low anterior resection
HCV	hepatitis C virus		LATS	long-acting thyroid stimulator
HETE	hydroxyeicosatetraenoic acid		LCIS	lobular carcinoma in situ
Hgb	hemoglobin		LD_{50}	dose that will kill 50% of test subjects
HGD	high grade dysplasia			
HIDA	hepatic iminodiacetic acid		LDH	lactate dehydrogenase
HIT	heparin-induced thrombocytopenia		LES	lower esophageal sphincter
			LFT	liver function test
HIV	human immunodeficiency virus		LH	luteotropic hormone
			LHRH	luteinizing hormone–releasing hormone
HLA	human leukocyte antigen			
HMG CoA	_-hydroxy-_-methylglutaryl-CoA		LLQ	left lower quadrant
			LR	lactated Ringer's
HMW	high molecular weight		LS ratio	lecithin:sphingomyelin ratio
HPETE	hydroperoxyeicosatetraenoic acid		LTA_4	leukotriene A_4
			LTB_4	leukotriene B_4
HPF	high-power field		LTC_4	leukotriene C_4
HPV	human papillomavirus		LTD_4	leukotriene D_4
HR	heart rate		LTE_4	leukotriene E_4
HSV	herpes simplex virus		LV	left ventricle or left ventricular
HTLV-1	human T-cell leukemia virus 1		LVEDV	left ventricular end-diastolic volume
HTN	hypertension			
HUS	hemolytic uremic syndrome		LVEF	left ventricular ejection fraction
HVA	homovanillic acid			
IABP	intra-aortic balloon pump		LVESV	left ventricular end-systolic volume
IBW	ideal body weight			
ICA	internal carotid artery		LVOT	left ventricular outflow tract
ICAM	intracellular adhesion molecule		MAC	minimum alveolar concentration
ICP	intracranial pressure		MALT	mucosa-associated lymphoid tissue
ICU	intensive care unit			
Ig	immunoglobulin		MAO	monoamine oxidase
IJ	internal jugular		MAOI	monoamine oxidase inhibitor
IL	interleukin		MAP	mean arterial pressure
IMA	inferior mesenteric artery or internal mammary artery		MEN	multiple endocrine neoplasia
			MHC	major histocompatibility complex
IMF	intramaxillary fixation			
IMV	inferior mesenteric vein		MI	myocardial infarction
INF	interferon		MIBG	radioactive iodine meta-idobenzoguanidine
INH	isoniazid			
INR	international normalized ratio		MIT	monoiodotyrosine
			MRA	magnetic resonance angiogram
IP_3	inositol 1,4,5-triphosphate			
ITP	idiopathic thrombocytopenic purpura		MRCP	magnetic resonance cholangiopancreatography
IV	intravenous		MRI	magnetic resonance imaging
IVC	inferior vena cava		MRM	modified radical mastectomy
IVF	intravenous fluid		MRND	modified radical neck dissection
IVP	intravenous pyelogram			
L	liter		MRSA	methicillin-resistant S. aureus
LA	left atrium		MS	mental status
LAD	left anterior descending (coronary artery)		MSH	melanocyte-stimulating hormone

MSOF	multisystem organ failure		PIP_2	phosphatidylinositol 4,5-bisphosphonate
MTP	metatarsophalangeal		PMHx	past medical history
MTX	methotrexate		PMN	polymorphonuclear leukocytes
N/V	nausea and vomiting		PNA	pneumonia
NADH	nicotinamide adenine dinucleotide		PNMT	phenylethanolamine-*N*-methyl-transferase
NADPH	nicotinamide adenine dinucleotide phosphate		POD	postoperative day
NAPA	*N*-acetylprocainamide		PPI	proton pump inhibitor
NE	norepinephrine		PPN	peripheral line parenteral nutrition
NEC	necrotizing enterocolitis		pRBC	packed red blood cells
NGT	nasogastric tube		PSA	prostate-specific antigen
NHL	non-Hodgkin's lymphoma		PSSS	postsplenectomy sepsis syndrome
NIF	negative inspiratory force		PT	prothrombin time
NO	nitric oxide		PTA	percutaneous transluminal angioplasty
NOMI	nonocclusive mesenteric ischemia		PTC	percutaneous transhepatic cholangiography
NPO	nil per os (nothing by mouth)			
NS	normal saline (solution)		PTCA	percutaneous transluminal coronary angioplasty
NSAID	nonsteroidal anti-inflammatory drug			
			PTFE	polytetrafluoroethylene
NSE	neuron-specific enolase		PTH	parathyroid hormone
NTG	nitroglycerine		PTHrP	parathyroid hormone–related peptide
OCP	oral contraceptive pills			
OKT3	murine monoclonal anti-CD3 antibody therapy		PTLD	posttransplant lymphoproliferative disease
Op-DDD	2,4-dichlorodiphenyl-dichloroethane (mitotane)		PTT	partial thromboplastin time
			PTU	propylthiouracil
OR	operating room		PTX	pneumothorax
ORIF	open reduction and internal fixation		PUD	peptic ulcer disease
			PVC	premature ventricular contraction
PA	pulmonary artery			
PABA	*p*-aminobenzoic acid		PVR	pulmonary vascular resistance
PADP	pulmonary artery diastolic pressure		Qp/Qs	pulmonary-to-systemic flow ratio
PAF	platelet-activating factor		R/O	rule out
PAS	periodic acid–Schiff stain		RA	right atrium
PCN	penicillin		RBC	red blood cell
PCR	polymerase chain		RLL	right lower lobe
PDA	patent ductus arteriosus		RLN	recurrent laryngeal nerve
PDGF	platelet-derived growth factor		RND	radical neck dissection
PE	pulmonary embolism		ROM	range of motion
PECAM	platelet/endothelial cell adhesion molecule		RPR	rapid plasma reagin
			RQ	respiratory quotient
PEEP	positive end-expiratory pressure		RR	respiratory rate
			RUG	retrograde urethrogram
PEG	percutaneous endoscopic gastrostomy		RUL	right upper lobe
			RUQ	right upper quadrant
PGD_2	prostaglandin D_2		RV	residual volume *or* right ventricle
PGE_1	prostaglandin E_1			
PGE_2	prostaglandin E_2		S/E	side effect
PGF_2	prostaglandin F_2		SBFT	small bowel follow-through
PGG_2	prostaglandin G_2		SBO	small bowel obstruction
PGH_2	prostaglandin H_2			
PGI_2	prostaglandin I_2 (prostacyclin)			

SBP	spontaneous bacterial peritonitis		TRALI	transfusion-related acute lung injury
SBP	systolic blood pressure		TRAM	transverse rectus abdominis myocutaneous
SCC	squamous cell carcinoma		TRH	thyrotropin-releasing hormone
SCD	sequential compression device			
SCM	sternocleidomastoid		TRUS	transrectal ultrasound
SCV	subclavian		TSH	thyroid-stimulating hormone
SFA	superficial femoral artery		TSI	thyroid-stimulating immunoglobulin
SIADH	syndrome of inappropriate antidiuretic hormone			
			TTP	thrombotic thrombocytopenic purpura
SIRS	systemic inflammatory response syndrome		TURP	transurethral prostatectomy
SLE	systemic lupus erythematosus		TV	tidal volume
SLNBx	sentinel lymph node biopsy		Tx	treatment
SMA	superior mesenteric artery		TXA_2	thromboxane A_2
SMV	superior mesenteric vein		TXP	transplant
SOB	shortness of breath		U/S	ultrasound
STEMI	ST-segment elevation myocardial infarction		UC	ulcerative colitis
			UDCA	ursodeoxycholic acid
STSG	split-thickness skin graft		UES	upper esophageal sphincter
SVC	superior vena cava		UGI	upper gastrointestinal
SvO_2	mixed venous oxygen saturation		URI	upper respiratory tract infection
SVR	systemic vascular resistance		UTI	urinary tract infection
SVRI	systemic vascular resistance index		UV	ultraviolet
			V/Q	ventilation/perfusion
SVT	supraventricular tachycardia		VC	vital capacity
Sx	symptom		VCAM	vascular cell adhesion molecule
T bili	total bilirubin		V-fib	ventricular fibrillation
TAG	triacylglyceride		VIP	vasoactive intestinal peptide
TAH	total abdominal hysterectomy		VIPoma	vasoactive intestinal peptide–producing tumor
TB	tuberculosis			
TBG	thyroid-binding globulin		VLDL	very-low-density lipids
TCOM	transcutaneous oxygen measurement		VMA	vanillylmandelic acid
			VO_2	oxygen consumption
TCR	T-cell receptor		VP-16	etoposide
TE	tracheoesophageal		VRE	vancomycin-resistant *Enterococcus*
TEN	toxic epidermal necrolysis			
TFT	thyroid function test		VSD	ventricular septal defect
TGF-β	transforming growth factor-beta		V-tach	ventricular tachycardia
			vWD	von Willebrand's disease
TIA	transient ischemic attack		vWF	von Willebrand factor
TIPS	transjugular intrahepatic portosystemic shunt		W/U	workup
			WBC	white blood cell
TLC	total lung capacity		WDHA	watery diarrhea, hypokalemia, achlorhydria
TLSO	thoracolumbosacral orthosis			
TMJ	temporomandibular joint		wedge	pulmonary artery wedge pressure
TNF	tumor necrosis factor			
TOS	thoracic outlet syndrome		WLE	wide local excision
tPA	tissue plasminogen activator		XRT	radiation therapy
TPN	total parenteral nutrition		Z–E/ZES	Zollinger–Ellison syndrome

INDEX

Note: Page numbers in *italics* denote figures; those followed by t denote tables.